Primary Care in a Public Health Emergency

Anthony Cheng • Jennifer E. DeVoe
Lauren S. Hughes
Editors

Primary Care in a Public Health Emergency

Lessons from the Frontlines of the COVID-19 Pandemic

Springer

Editors
Anthony Cheng
Family Medicine
Oregon Health & Science University
Portland, OR, USA

Lauren S. Hughes
Farley Health Policy Center
University of Colorado
Aurora, CO, USA

Jennifer E. DeVoe
OHSU Center for Primary Care Research and Innovation and OHSU-PSU School of Public Health
Portland, OR, USA

ISBN 978-3-032-12486-9 ISBN 978-3-032-12487-6 (eBook)
https://doi.org/10.1007/978-3-032-12487-6

This Springer imprint is published by the registered company Springer Nature Switzerland AG
The registered company address is: Gewerbestrasse 11, 6330 Cham, Switzerland

Contents

Chapter 1
Introduction

Lauren S. Hughes, Anthony Cheng, and Jennifer E. DeVoe

Primary care teams across the globe were among many unsung heroes during the early years of the COVID-19 pandemic. Despite immense challenges, primary care clinicians and practices everywhere innovated in the face of significant resource constraints and in rapidly evolving policy, public health, educational, and clinical environments to be on the frontlines caring for patients, families, and communities. This book dives deep into the experiences of primary care teams, educators, researchers, learners, and patients to examine the heroics of primary care during the pandemic, from accelerating new ways of delivering care (e.g., telehealth) to discovering and treating novel clinical diagnoses (e.g., Long COVID) while continuing the day-to-day work of delivering primary care and partnering with communities to improve population health. We focus on examples from the United States (U.S.), but we believe this book still offers valuable insights for a much broader, international audience. In addition to the rich history included here, it is our hope that primary care practices, community organizations, and health systems leaders can use the wisdom of the past to respond to the future. We hope that lessons learned and detailed in this book can be leveraged to care for patients and communities before, during, and after the next inevitable crises, including infectious disease outbreaks.

Both primary care and public health entered the pandemic with fragile infrastructure, in large part due to years of chronic underinvestment. Poor cross-sector risk communication and workforce development; nascent electronic health record

L. S. Hughes (✉)
Farley Health Policy Center, University of Colorado, Aurora, CO, USA
e-mail: lauren.hughes@cuanschutz.edu

A. Cheng
Department of Family Medicine, Oregon Health & Science University, Portland, OR, USA

J. E. DeVoe
OHSU Center for Primary Care Research and Innovation and OHSU-PSU School of Public Health, Portland, OR, USA

A. Cheng et al. (eds.), *Primary Care in a Public Health Emergency*,
https://doi.org/10.1007/978-3-032-12487-6_1

(EHR) and communicable disease surveillance interoperability between primary care and public health, and highly variable local and regional public health laboratory capacity were examples of failing infrastructure and serious cracks in a shaky foundation that existed at the start of the pandemic. These cracks impeded optimal coordination and often led to a difficult dance of roles, responsibilities, and functions as leaders in both fields worked hard to respond and coordinate.

Chapter 4 discusses one of the key challenges for both primary care and public health: how to effectively communicate to patients and communities about transmission, risk factors, and SARS-CoV-2 variants, as well as mask types and their effectiveness, how to interpret diagnostic tests, and the basics and effectiveness of different COVID-19 vaccine types. Public health often struggled to convey new terms and concepts to the public, including isolation, quarantine, and contact tracing, and had a difficult time keeping up with changing public health orders, especially early in the pandemic. The lack of a coordinated communications campaign across primary care and public health led to primary care clinicians and practices being inundated with individual patient questions and care coordination needs. Outdated technology platforms and lack of interoperability between clinical EHRs, public health surveillance systems, and vaccine registries negatively impacted availability of accurate, real-time data to inform messaging to the public. Exacerbating these difficulties, turmoil in the public discourse included misinformation that inhibited public health education. The authors of Chap. 4 reflected, "The evolving nature of the COVID-19 pandemic, ever-changing scientific evidence, and misinformation complicated effective, trustworthy communication."

In addition to the fragile state of the primary care and public health infrastructure at the start of the pandemic, U.S. health policy leaders were grappling with the continued high costs of health care, inequities in access to care, and poor health outcomes. While some progress had been made in providing health insurance coverage to more people, access to and affordability of health insurance coverage remained a huge problem in 2020. In Chap. 13, the authors reflect on the U.S. health policy landscape in the decade leading up to the start of the pandemic and discuss changes in policy that occurred between the start of the pandemic through the end of the federally declared "public health emergency" (PHE) on May 11, 2023.

In the 10 years before the arrival of the COVID-19 pandemic in the U.S. in early 2020, the state of health policy in the U.S. was dynamic: health care coverage and access expanded with passage of the Patient Protection and Affordable Care Act (ACA) in March 2010 and then contracted with changing federal priorities. For primary care clinics, these changes created a whipsaw effect. Medicaid expansion provided insurance coverage to low-income, childless adults in most states and greater sustainability for safety net clinics, while also increasing demand for health care services. Subsequent real and threatened contractions created great uncertainty and operational challenges.

The ACA enhanced access by requiring all health insurance plans to cover certain benefits, including preventive services and mental health and substance use disorder treatment. Individuals could not be denied health insurance coverage because of pre-existing conditions, and caps on annual and lifetime benefits were prohibited. However, seemingly immediately after its passage, the ACA has been subject to numerous legal challenges. In June 2012, the Supreme Court of the United States (SCOTUS) rendered Medicaid expansion optional without risking loss of funding. While the SCOTUS ruled that the individual mandate within the ACA was constitutional, the Tax Cuts and Jobs Act of 2017 eliminated the tax penalty related to the individual mandate in 2019, effectively repealing this policy designed to ensure access to health insurance and to control insurance premium costs by including healthy people in the risk pool. In the years that followed this landmark SCOTUS decision, individual states made decisions about whether and how to expand Medicaid, and Congress continued to pass laws to facilitate expansion for certain populations in all states, even among those who chose not to expand Medicaid more broadly, e.g., an expansion of Medicaid postpartum coverage to 12 months.

On the heels of a decade of seesawing health policy changes at the federal and state levels, the COVID-19 pandemic prompted substantial loss of employment due to businesses slowing or suspending operations and record numbers of temporary layoffs. With job loss came the loss of employer-sponsored health insurance. As a result—and due to the countercyclical nature of Medicaid during economic downturns—enrollment and spending increased across the country, especially in expansion states. Several federal pandemic-related relief packages ensued, providing continuous Medicaid enrollment, reimbursement for virtual visits and telehealth for a range of conditions, and early refill and waiver of fill limit provisions for prescriptions. Barriers to COVID-19 testing and treatment were eliminated. Changes in workforce scope were also implemented, such as permitting community pharmacists to administer vaccines. After the PHE ended on May 11, 2023, over 25 million children and adults lost Medicaid coverage when continuous enrollment was lifted.

In Chap. 13, the authors share several policy lessons learned: (a) regarding continued access to health insurance, "We recommend that federal and state policies facilitate continuous enrollment such as developing systems to streamline enrollment and eligibility determination. We recommend that all states expand Medicaid coverage to support low-income adults, without imposing burdensome provisions such as work requirement reporting. Further, several states have expanded eligibility regardless of citizenship status to promote health care for all. Lessons from the ACA Medicaid expansion suggest that such eligibility expansion will benefit the overall population health of the state. We recommend that states broaden their eligibility criteria to encompass all individuals and reduce disparities in access." (b) regarding the adoption of telehealth, "We recommend that federal policies be established to (1) standardize telemedicine regulations across states; (2) include a comprehensive set of services; and (3) ensure parity of reimbursement for all services to all providers or organizations, including audio-only services." (c) regarding ensuring an adequate health care workforce, "We recommend the following: (1) a comprehensive review of the scope of practice be completed to expand service delivery, which could assist with workforce shortages; (2) efforts be accelerated to promote and facilitate an expansion of the health care workforce in specialties and areas of greatest need by providing financial incentives and increased availability of community-based residencies and curriculum; (3) alignment of federal and state funding (and ongoing accountability) with training benchmarks targeting the nation's needs (e.g., primary care, mental health care) and (4) narrow the salary gaps between providers in different specialties to not dissuade future graduates from entering specialties with the greatest needs (e.g., primary care, mental health care)."

A necessary innovation rapidly implemented by nearly all health systems and primary care practices nationwide was telehealth, which is described in Chap. 9. Before the pandemic, the use of telephone and video visits in primary care was highly variable and sporadic at best. In the span of a 6-week period beginning in March 2020, the use of such visits exploded by >600% out of necessity to provide some semblance of continuity and access to clinical care at a time when primary care clinics were concerned about the safety of their patients and the need for continued access to care. In addition to delivering all the essential primary care services, demand for primary care skyrocketed to "keep people out of the hospital" with mild cases of COVID-19 or other respiratory illnesses to limit the spread of the disease to hospital workers and inpatients. Seminal policy changes in The Coronavirus Preparedness and Response Supplemental Appropriations Act (2020) and The Coronavirus Aid, Relief, and Economic Security Act (2020) led to the U.S. Centers for Medicare and Medicaid Services (CMS) and private insurers instituting waivers to change telehealth reimbursement policies, allowing parity in payment for telehealth consultations akin to in-person visits across a range of technology platforms. At first, data systems had a hard time keeping up, and privacy regulations were concurrently being developed. Primary care clinicians and practices launched natural experiments in real-time and made several critical discoveries ranging from *how* to deliver effective clinical care via telehealth (> e.g., synchronous versus asynchronous) to *which types* of conditions could be addressed in this way (e.g., preventive care, chronic disease management, mental and behavioral health, medication review, education about lab results).

As detailed in Chap. 9, health systems and practices rapidly gained experience with telehealth, while also discovering a range of strengths, weaknesses, opportunities, and threats for its continued implementation. A hallmark strength of telehealth is that it supports flexible scheduling and increases access to care, especially for patients who do not have a designated primary care provider or for those who cannot physically travel to a clinic for an in-person visit. Telehealth's convenience and expansion in access helped to mitigate challenges related to sick leave, childcare, and/or transportation. It also helped to limit spread of infection by providing an alternative to being close together in an enclosed space where the virus could easily spread. During this time of rapid deployment and experimentation, teams also discovered several weaknesses. For example, delivering high-quality and equitable telehealth requires substantial infrastructure and investment, especially for the broadband needed to deliver high-speed internet and the purchase of necessary equipment, e.g., cameras, tablets, new scheduling software. Some technology platforms can be challenging for non-native English speakers and less tech-naive patients to navigate, as well as some rural and/or elderly patients. Depending on where the patient is located, confidentiality can be difficult or impossible to preserve. Telehealth does present many new opportunities. For example, these modalities provide insight into a patient's lived environment, are effective for managing chronic diseases, and reduce costs. However, numerous threats also exist. Telehealth may diminish relationship-centered care and reinforce or widen health inequities related to accessing these platforms and some patients perceiving the interactions to feel impersonal or stilted. Regulations also are constantly evolving. After the end of the PHE, several states changed reimbursement policies for Medicaid, while CMS did the same for Medicare. At the time of this writing, reimbursement policies vary widely, including allowed visit types, reimbursement (or not) of phone-only visits, where telehealth visits can be conducted, and which types of patients, e.g., established patients only, are eligible for reimbursement.

While the use of telehealth has declined since the height of the pandemic and its early popularity, telehealth remains a permanent fixture of primary care delivery that was accelerated and shaped by a necessity for virtual care that was unique to this time in history. In general, many patients and clinicians express a strong preference for in-person visits for establishing care, when a physical exam is required, and for the purpose of building relationships. Lowest rates of telehealth use are seen among uninsured individuals and young adults, while higher rates are seen among Medicaid and Medicare beneficiaries. As with many care delivery innovations, visionary leadership is essential to advancing telehealth to help secure financing, technology, and staff resources.

Implementing telehealth was not the only innovative care delivery change that required flexibility and resourcefulness to design and execute within days. Chapter 8 highlights two case studies, one that describes an urban federally qualified health center (FQHC) outdoor COVID-19 testing site and the other that explores a vaccination clinic in a rural health clinic (RHC), both of which were conceived and set up within a week. In the urban example, the team moved fast given rapidly evolving protocols and adopted a "beg for forgiveness later" approach. They leveraged trust with community partners, made do with what they had, and stayed in close contact with infection control experts at their local academic teaching hospital. This urban FQHC faced several decisions, including who should or should not be tested; how to acquire and distribute available personal protective equipment (PPE); which testing options could be acquired and the characteristics (e.g., sensitivity and specificity of each), and what information (e.g., how long to isolate or quarantine) and treatment recommendations (e.g., effective medications for symptom relief) patients needed to receive if they were to test positive. As a group, the FQHC team at this urban clinic navigated changing testing guidelines, the need to deliver other, non-COVID-19 related care, evolving telehealth capabilities, emotionally charged social media messages, and inevitable challenges staff faced at home (e.g., sick family members, no childcare, virtual-only schools).

The RHC weekend and evening vaccination clinic was offered in partnership with the local county public health department. Together, they approached this project in four phases: (1) developed and piloted vaccine clinic workflows; (2) recruited volunteers and increased vaccine clinic capacity to meet community demand; (3) expanded access further and addressed vaccine hesitancy, and (4) closed the vaccine clinic and moved vaccination into the regular clinic setting and workflows. The

RHC and public health leaders jointly created a plan that addressed several factors, including how to procure needed vaccines, obtain a special refrigerator to store them, schedule patients for initial and return vaccine appointments, get and train additional staff, and bill for services, among other considerations. Phase 4 was complicated by significant staff burnout after a wave of resignations due to state vaccine mandates, leading to a substantial loss of long-time colleagues and a blow to clinic morale. Reflecting on their experience, leaders of this effort recognized the great value in partnering with local public health and the state's Medicaid program and the challenge of managing shifts in vaccine supply from scarcity and rationing to surplus, as well as dealing with gamification and equity issues when urban and/or more tech-savvy residents signed up online for vaccine slots at the RHC. The clinic's pre-existing quality improvement culture and team-based care approach were essential to balancing the chaos and designing and deploying effective vaccination processes.

Beyond near-constant policy and systems changes and new ways of delivering primary care services, another challenge began to take shape early on the pandemic: the emergence of what we now know as Long COVID and how to address it in the primary care setting. Chapter 12 shares a comprehensive overview of what we understand about this condition, such as risk factors (e.g., obesity, pulmonary disease), protective or perpetuating factors, clinical presentation, and management. Presentation is highly variable, with over 200+ clinical signs and symptoms that have been attributed to this condition, including chronic fatigue, post-exertional malaise, cognitive impairment or "brain fog," sleep and orthostatic changes, gastrointestinal disturbances, and altered sensory perception. No biomarker or diagnostic test yet exists to rule Long COVID in or out. Clinical symptoms can vary in severity, and prognosis can fluctuate. It is important for clinicians to consider other conditions that may mimic or co-exist with Long COVID, including fibromyalgia or myalgic encephalomyelitis/chronic fatigue syndrome, in addition to assessing how symptoms impact patients' function and quality of life. Management often entails a multi-modal approach, leveraging trauma-informed care principles. Patients may need chronic pain and orthostatic symptom management, mental, emotional, and/or behavioral health support, physical, occupational, and/or speech therapy, environmental modifications to reduce triggers, peer support, and in some cases, access to therapeutic trials.

Chapters 10 and 11 address two issues that were foundational to all aspects of the primary care COVID-19 response, including clinical care, care delivery innovation, medical student and resident education, and more: how to care for employees' well-being and how to manage teams in a stressful, rapidly evolving environment. For example, Oregon Health & Science University (OHSU) quickly identified several policies they needed to create to protect their employees, including quarantine, symptom self-check and self-report, prioritized access to PPE and related medical and religious exemptions to PPE use, vaccine mandates, and more. The authors of Chap. 10 conveyed, "Employee health is a critical aspect of any organization, encompassing various functions and principles aimed at ensuring the physical, emotional, and psychological well-being of workers. Basic principles of employee health include promoting a safe work environment, providing access to health care services, and implementing preventive measures."

The COVID-19 pandemic presented numerous management challenges, such as handling temporary or permanent reductions in force (RIFs), re-deployment of staff to other areas, vaccine hesitancy, and state and/or health system vaccine mandates, among others. The authors of Chap. 11 offer the SCARF (Status, Certainty, Autonomy, Relatedness, Fairness) framework as a management approach that helped leaders at Northwest Permanente tee up and address issues as they arose by centering the social needs of individuals within an organization. Status signifies how important someone feels relative to someone else. Certainty signals the ability to predict the future, while autonomy indicates a sense of control over events in one's life or place of work. Relatedness symbolizes a sense of safety or friendship with others, and fairness represents a sense of justice and/or impartiality. This chapter pays special attention to guiding an organization through a voluntary or involuntary RIF. If considering reductions that impact women, minorities, workers older than 40, or LGBTQ+ individuals, consulting human resources experts and employment lawyers is essential. Separation packages and agreements should be crafted in such a way to protect the practice or system from future potential legal disputes. Caring for the individuals who survive RIFs is paramount to help move the organization forward. This may mean allowing them to process the stages of grief for colleagues who have left the organization, reconnecting team members to the mission, recognizing staff for a job well done, creating individual development plans, and more. Departures impact both the individuals who were let go and those who were chosen to stay.

The pandemic upended so many facets of primary care and the broader health care system, including undergraduate and graduate medical education. Chapters 5 and 6 dive into the experiences of medical students and residents, respectively, and how 2020 especially impacted their training in both positive and negative ways. On March 17, 2020, the Association of American Medical Colleges (AAMC) issued guidance calling for a 2-week suspension of educational activities where students interact with patients, thus effectively suspending clinical rotations. While medical students made a staggered return to in-person studies between April and August 2020, the plans for return and the impacts of these disruptions varied widely across the country. For students in the pre-clinical years, their transition to virtual learning happened almost overnight, and for those newly starting their medical careers, they didn't get to participate in typical "white coat" or other welcoming ceremonies, given fears of spreading the virus. Students also faced scattered access to mentorship. Students in the clinical years navigated exposure to a potentially deadly virus with limited PPE, uncertain roles on care teams, and the challenge of learning clinical medicine during virtual rotations. Preceptors had to balance caring for patients, worrying about their own families, and what the loss of in-person teaching time would mean for the next generation of physicians.

Despite these setbacks, novel and high-quality educational innovation emerged. An unprecedented pandemic provided opportunities for students to learn how to respond to a public health crisis. They helped design and implement COVID-19 testing and vaccination centers, provided childcare for health care workers, and staffed call centers, answering a wide array of clinical questions from patients and families. In some schools, students formed 12-week "social bubbles" combining an apprenticeship model, face-to-face clinical exposure, educational seminars, and research and quality improvement projects that groups of students did together as a unit to minimize risk of viral transmission.

The transition from medical school to residency was also unusual. Fewer opportunities to travel for interviews or to be a visiting student at another school were available, and the application process moved fully virtual. While this move reduced the environmental footprint and saved students money, it was challenging for them to get a full sense of residency programs and to be well-informed about the place(s) where they were signing up to spend the next several years of their lives as resident physicians.

Several changes in the national medical student education realm ensued. In January 2021, the United States Medical Licensing Examination (USMLE) changed Step 1, the first of three USMLE exams that tests medical students' knowledge of basic science principles and how they apply to medicine, to pass/fail while increasing the passing threshold. For a variety of reasons, students felt greater pressure to perform on USMLE Step 2 CK—or Clinical Knowledge—a 1-day, computer-based exam that assesses a student's ability to apply medical facts and understanding of clinical science to patient care. Depending on local viral transmission, testing centers for Step 2 CK had erratic opening and closing hours, which made scheduling more difficult. The USMLE Step 2 CS—or Clinical Skills—a 1-day, in-person exam where students' ability to interact with standardized patients and demonstrate clinical skills was evaluated, was suspended because of the pandemic. In January 2021, Step 2 CS was permanently cancelled.

The authors of Chap. 6 offer the following lessons learned for future pandemics: (1) advocate for specific and meaningful roles for learners; (2) implement flexible learning models; (3) adjust accreditation standards if needed; (4) enhance simulation-based learning and encourage interprofessional training; (5) refine assessments for virtual learning; and (6) promote public health and epidemiological literacy.

Residency education suffered similarly. Chapter 5 cites examples of educational impacts from programs in Oregon, Texas, New York, and California. In March 2020, there were 144,988 residents and fellows in the US in 12,092 programs nationwide. Of those, just over 20% represented trainees in internal medicine programs, nearly 10% in family medicine programs, and just over 6% in pediatric programs. The Accreditation Council for Graduate Medical Education (ACGME) issued guidance on how to balance the needs of hospital systems with resident learning and safety.

Many primary care physicians are trained in family medicine residencies, located in all 50 U.S. states, Puerto Rico, and the District of Columbia. Family medicine residents faced numerous educational disruptions. Elective cases were cancelled, all in-person didactics were moved to virtual platforms, and stress mounted about how trainees would meet their required outpatient clinical numbers to graduate. Residents were exposed to several unexpected clinical and operational challenges in both the inpatient and outpatient settings, e.g., diagnosing and treating greater acuity cases related to delays in care, facilitating end-of-life conversations virtually with family members who weren't allowed to visit, navigating fluctuating supply levels of medications, blood products, ventilators, and PPE, and quickly being forced to work outside of their training level under attendings who may not have been as knowledgeable in this unpredictable and unfamiliar environment. Residents—like students and attendings—were also impacted by childcare center closures and worried about infecting their own families.

The author team for Chap. 5 recommends the following changes to prepare for subsequent pandemics: (1) establish longer-term jeopardy or extended leave coverage policies involving senior residents; (2) invest consistently in computer-based simulation programs, standardized patients, and virtual reality simulators to aid learning in the event of in-person training disruptions; (3) develop support systems to help residents attend to basic needs, e.g., grocery shopping, childcare; (4) incorporate pandemic-related training into residency curricula, including contact tracing, outbreak response, communications skills, combating misinformation, telehealth, and ethical decision-making in resource-limited settings; and (5) expand access to wellness resources such as tele-mental health, physician coaching, and resiliency and adaptability training.

Looking back on the early years of the COVID-19 pandemic, primary care weathered extraordinary challenges and rose to the occasion multiple times and in multiple ways. Despite entering 2020 with fragile infrastructure and facing numerous health policy changes, primary care clinicians and practices launched telehealth practically overnight, quickly deployed testing sites and vaccination clinics, monitored and supported patients navigating Long COVID, cared as best they could for themselves and their employees, and strived to meet the educational needs of medical students and residents. All these heroics were accomplished with threats to their livelihood as many practices faced a precipitous drop in patient volume, a subsequent seismic drop in reimbursement, and/or significant delays in payment due to cancelled appointments, bureaucratic red tape, and rapidly changing billing policies. Chapter 2 examines the impact of these challenges on ten features of high-performing primary care. The Ten Building Blocks of High-Performing Primary Care, developed by the Center for Excellence in Primary Care (CEPC) at the University of California—San Francisco in 2014, has served as a valuable framework for practice improvement since its release. Created based on detailed site visits of 23 exemplar primary care practices, the Building Blocks include four foundational elements—engaged leadership, data-driven improvement, empanelment, and team-based care—that are essential to assist the implementation of the other six: patient-team partnership, population management, continuity of care, prompt access to care, comprehensiveness and care coordination, and a template of the future.

Chapter 2 authors crosswalk the Ten Building Blocks framework elements against what happened to primary care during the pandemic. Chapter authors describe how leadership within primary care practices had to be flexible, nimble, and creative to deal with so much uncertainty, especially in the face of ever-changing clinical and regulatory guidelines. From a data-driven improvement standpoint, practices witnessed a rapid shift in their ability to meet quality metrics with an abrupt drop in in-person visits during the early months of the pandemic. Chapter 2 authors reflect on empanelment, "… the shrinking of the primary care workforce through illness and attrition and having fewer patients engaged with primary care practices, has made it harder to empanel patients and to foster these important relationships." In the early months of the pandemic, primary care teams scrambled to make abrupt shifts to telehealth, and medical assistants were frequently re-deployed or furloughed after demand for in-person visits rapidly declined, and patients sought virtual visits or asynchronous care. As co-location was not possible or limited for many months, the institutional memory for team-based care eroded. Disruptions to the patient-team partnership also occurred. In many instances, patients experienced care with only one individual, rather than the broader team, and frequently remotely, both of which impact the building and maintenance of relationships with all members of the team. Most population health management efforts had to be paused or abandoned altogether during this time. In terms of continuity of care, the authors in Chap. 2 share the following, "At present, continuity of care is not achievable for large proportions of the population, and the COVID-19 pandemic accelerated this trend. Given that continuity of care is associated with better health outcomes, this workforce shortage is problematic." While telehealth has led to improvement in access to care for some patients, the broader trend of workforce shortages and increasing difficulty in finding a primary care provider or team has negatively impacted access overall. Comprehensiveness and care coordination also suffered. So much attention—understandably so—was directed at the COVID-19 response. In its wake, non-COVID-19 conditions worsened or remained undetected for months, delaying timely diagnosis and management. The pandemic also underscored the urgency of screening for and adequately addressing the social drivers of health, e.g., housing, transportation, food. The final Building Block—a template of the future—highlights the importance of moving primary care away from the constraints of fee-for-service, visit-based payment to value-based care. This future orientation, focused on improving health outcomes, includes opportunities for care to be delivered by extended members of the interprofessional primary care team, asynchronous care, and telehealth, all of which grew significantly during the COVID-19 pandemic.

Chapter 7 details key lessons learned from a multi-site community health center in Cleveland, OH, learnings that hold great potential for primary care practices that wish to implement best practices and prepare for the next pandemic or major disruption to clinical care. The authors of this chapter encourage practices to put down roots and build authentic relationships within the community <u>before</u> the next crisis hits. Making a commitment to transparency and keeping patients and staff safe, as well as leading with humility and data-driven quality improvement will engender trust that is essential to weathering clinical and operational crises. Leveraging creative problem-solving skills to tackle challenges as they arise is a foundational skill set for any organization. In this community health center, a senior clinician went door-to-door to ensure immigrant families felt safe with pandemic protocols, and to minimize overhead, voluntary and temporary furlough arrangements were offered to employees. The authors of Chap. 7 suggest ensuring that pandemic-era learnings are sustained. For example, the virus had long-lasting impacts on student and resident education. In this clinic, learners gained leadership skills and hands-on insights into decision-making regarding clinical and operational issues. This approach can be incorporated moving forward.

Chapter 3 explores patient experiences during the pandemic, highlighting the value patients place on strong primary care relationships and informing how we can design high-quality, relational primary care moving forward. Between May 2020 and December 2022, the Larry A. Green Center fielded 14 patient surveys. The research team qualitatively analyzed a total of 162 free-text responses to the question, "Is there anything else you would like us to know about your experience with primary care during the COVID-19 pandemic?" Four themes emerged from this analysis related to patient expectations and needs, both met and unmet: (1) personal relationship and connection with a clinician, (2) clinician as someone a patient could turn to, (3) mutual care/reciprocity, and (4) appreciation/adaptability/flexibility. Of all the responses, a total of 102 addressed the core functions of primary care: access, continuity, comprehensiveness, and coordination. The authors of Chap. 3 note about theme one, "This was apparent in the data when patients noted their clinician was kind, compassionate, reassuring, or supportive and paid attention to patient's issues/interests as the patient described them." They go on to comment on theme two, "Evidence of patient interest and value in having a 'clinician as someone to turn to' was seen in comments that expressed desire or gratitude for reliance, comfort, confidence in the clinician expertise, professionalism, or knowledge." Related to theme three, the research team identified examples such as patients expressing concerns for their clinician and the pressures the pandemic had placed on them, sometimes delaying care because of this. And, regarding theme four, survey responses also indicated the expectation that primary care clinicians should be adaptable or flexible. This translated into gratitude for clinicians who offered multiple ways of connecting or providing clinic visits that were not routine before the pandemic began.

The authors of Chap. 3 suggest four ways we can return to the heart of high-quality primary care: "(1) Fully and explicitly embrace the core of primary care as relationship-based, (2) Utilize the well-developed theories and concepts of relationship science to improve the effectiveness and efficiency of relationship building in primary care through education, training, and research, (3) Enable creative, positive, disruptive innovations to establish more functional primary care models that in turn promote relational care, and (4) Embrace social movements to empower patients and communities to get the primary care that they want and need, which is fundamentally about relationships."

In conclusion, the devastation during and since the COVID-19 pandemic has been real, painful, and extensive, the human and economic toll of which we are only just now beginning to fully understand. The pandemic's immediate and profound shock waves that upended established norms and traditions of providing and receiving primary care continue to reverberate. As primary care teams, patients, and communities attempt to recover, we are all forever changed. We have learned we are tougher, smarter, braver, more resilient, and more flexible than we ever imagined. We have also collectively experienced fragility, fear, hopelessness, and uncertainty. Walls between our professional and personal lives were shattered. These experiences deepened our knowledge and belief in the power of social connection, compassionate human touch, and reminded us that no one is invincible. We learned how important it is that primary care keep striving to serve all people at all times, and especially in their times of need. To realize this bold vision, primary care must not only survive but rather thrive.

We hope you enjoy and learn from this book. Our hope is that lessons shared in this text can be leveraged to help primary care enter the next pandemic stronger and more prepared and emerge even more resilient and grounded.

Chapter 2
COVID-19's Impact on the Building Blocks of High-Performing Primary Care

Thomas Bodenheimer and Rachel Willard-Grace

> *The COVID-19 pandemic has changed the face of healthcare and has also called into question long-standing structures, beliefs, and habits that have now proven inadequate. [1]*

For the past 30 years, primary care has rapidly evolved. Paper charts have given way to electronic medical records and patient registries. Standards for evidence-based care have proliferated, with the onus falling on primary care to ensure that a host of guidelines are met. The focus has shifted from treating the concerns of people during their clinic appointments to taking responsibility for populations, whether or not they seek care. Primary care now must ensure that people are up to date on vaccines, cancer screenings, and preventive and chronic care. A recognition of the impact of social determinants and trauma on health has sparked greater attention to screening for and addressing larger societal factors within the clinical setting. Primary care has been involved in multiple improvement initiatives such as building teams with combinations of skills to meet patients' needs and designing information systems to facilitate population health and information exchange across the medical neighborhood and within local communities. The COVID-19 pandemic had a major impact on these initiatives, on the one hand relegating primary care improvement to the back burner, and on the other hand accelerating some areas of progress.

One primary care improvement model is the Ten Building Blocks of High-Performing Primary Care, initially published in 2014 by members of the Center for Excellence in Primary Care at the University of California, San Francisco (Fig. 2.1). The Building Blocks framework was developed from detailed site visits to 23 highly regarded primary care practices around the United States: 8 hospital-based clinics, 7 integrated delivery system sites, 6 federally qualified health centers, and 2 independent private practices. Our team discerned a set of elements—building blocks—that occurred with regularity among well-functioning practices [2]. We

T. Bodenheimer (✉) · R. Willard-Grace
Center for Excellence in Primary Care, University of California, San Francisco, San Francisco, CA, USA

A. Cheng et al. (eds.), *Primary Care in a Public Health Emergency*,
https://doi.org/10.1007/978-3-032-12487-6_2

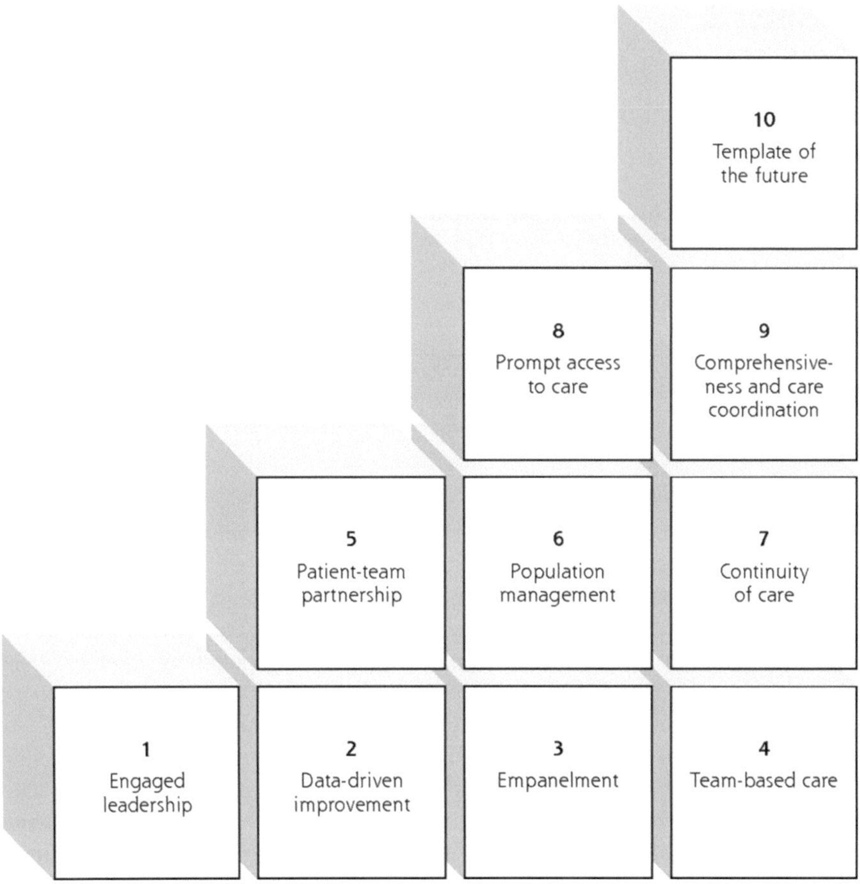

Fig. 2.1 The ten building blocks of high-performing primary care. This model outlines key elements that support high-quality, patient-centered care, organized from foundational structures to advanced functions. (Reprinted with permission from Bodenheimer et al. [2]. © 2014 Annals of Family Medicine, Inc. All rights Reserved)

cross-referenced these elements with themes articulated by other improvement initiatives such as Patient Centered Medical Home, Change Concepts for Practice Transformation [3, 4], and published research on practice improvement.

We observed ten key areas for practice improvement: leadership, data-driven improvement, empanelment, teams, patient-team partnership, population health, continuity, access, coordination, and a template for the future. These elements were meant not simply as descriptions of high-performing practices, but as areas to prioritize in improvement efforts. Over a 10-year period, our team has utilized the Building Blocks framework in coaching many practices to improve their functioning.

Writ large, COVID-19 has had major impacts on (1) the abrupt movement to telehealth and asynchronous communication, (2) health worker shortages due to redeployment and burnout resulting in personnel leaving the workforce, and (3) the recognition of glaring health care inequities as evidenced by COVID-19 mortality data. This chapter briefly summarizes the pandemic's effects on each of the ten Building Blocks.

Primary Care Building Block #1: Leadership COVID-19 presented unique challenges to primary care leaders. An article early in the pandemic laid out the vital role of primary care in ensuring the sustainability of the health care system during a pandemic, including reinforcing public health messaging, helping ensure that many patients could manage infections at home, and checking on vulnerable populations [5]. Good leaders followed the ever-changing public health guidelines, adapting them to their particular circumstances. They guided development of new protocols to minimize transmission in the clinic setting, such as separating people with possible COVID-19, masking, and limiting the number of people on site. They helped establish new workflows for telehealth. Some leaders drew upon methods such as human-centered design to engage their teams in rapid adaptation [6]. They also drew upon their networks to develop regional and statewide strategies to garner resources to support primary care, for example with nursing triage [7]. They set up testing and immunization sites in their parking lots. They supported community partners, bringing knowledge, testing, vaccines, and treatment to shelters, retirement communities, churches, and community centers. Leaders stepped up to serve as spokespeople delivering messages to diverse audiences. For example, as the first waves of vaccines rolled out, physicians at San Francisco General Hospital formed a speakers bureau to share reliable information about vaccines at community events [8].

Overall, strong leaders developed a mindset of flexibility, recognizing the necessity to shift priorities as the world around them evolved. They faced uncertainty, terrified teams, and patients in need of answers to countless unanswerable questions. Their day-to-day efforts to be nimble, creative, and responsive were usually met with appreciation and gratefulness; but sometimes, they encountered mistrust or outward hostility.

Primary Care Building Block #2: Data-Driven Improvement Many standardized pre-COVID-19 primary care quality metrics were defined based on in-person visits and preventive care activities, which were dramatically reduced during the pandemic [9]. Health care personnel experienced strain from continued demands to meet quality metrics despite reduced capacity and patients' justified reluctance to seek in-person care where care gaps could be closed [10]. The absence of in-person staff meetings meant fewer opportunities for discussion of practice data, and even remote meetings took second place to COVID-19 prevention and treatment. On the positive side, momentum grew to strengthen approaches being developed by primary care teams to stratify and assess quality measures by patient and population demographics (e.g., race and ethnicity), which helped in identifying and addressing COVID-19 inequities. This work guided prioritization and targeting of public health efforts. For example, when COVID-19 vaccines were first released, the San Francisco Health Network used data about neighborhoods hardest hit by COVID-19 to plan vaccine drop-in sites in those neighborhoods, with resulting vaccine rates higher among Black and Latino communities than across the city as a whole [11]. The improved data systems and methods for increased work in this area show promise for the future. However, primary care's post-pandemic workforce shortages and financial challenges are certain to constrict data-driven improvement opportunities.

Primary Care Building Block #3: Empanelment This Building Block refers to the process of linking patients with a personal primary care clinician and team, providing the structure for the therapeutic relationships at the heart of primary care. During the early months of the pandemic, many primary care teams were pulled in multiple directions, were overwhelmed by meeting patients' acute needs, and suffered exhaustion from the additional burden COVID-19 placed on their already busy workload. Now, a few years later, the shrinking of the primary care workforce through illness and attrition and having fewer patients engaged with primary care practices, has made it harder to empanel patients and to foster these important relationships. At a time when patient-clinician trust was particularly important, the chaos of COVID-19 eroded that trust. Rebuilding the long-term personal relationship between patients and clinicians will be another post-COVID-19 challenge for primary care, especially with the worsening workforce shortages faced by primary care in the coming years.

Primary Care Building Block #4: Teams The abrupt shift to remote work and telehealth, coupled with redeployment of health care staff for testing and vaccination efforts, destabilized team-based workflows [12]. Within clinics, rooming workflows that allowed medical assistants and nurses to bring patients up to date on cancer screenings, immunizations, and other preventive care were difficult to integrate into new virtual workflows. With few patients making in person visits to their clinics and practices, the need for medical assistants—often the glue holding teams together—dropped. Some organizations were able to redeploy medical assistants for new COVID-related tasks such as patient education, COVID-19 testing and immunizing, and contact tracing; others simply furloughed their medical assistants. The COVID-19 pandemic rolled back the evolution from clinician-only care to team-based care. Even after in-person visits resumed and the need for these visits increased beyond pre-pandemic levels, primary care workforce shortages and turnover meant that the institutional memory for robust team-based care was lost, and clinicians were left managing population health responsibilities that had previously been shared across the team [13]. With many clinicians and staff working off site, most practices were unable to recreate virtual spaces to retain the great value of minute-to-minute conversations. Virtual meetings and email updates rarely provided opportunities to seamlessly share information relevant to patient care.

In many places, team-based care has moved away from the traditional model with team members working together in person each day in a co-located pod, caring for a stable panel of patients who receive all their care from their personal team.

Hybrid care models are becoming more prevalent with team members spending more time delivering asynchronous and virtual care in isolated work settings. High turnover among team members has also made it more difficult to build long-term relationships among patients and teams.

Primary Care Building Block #5: Patient-Team Partnership Partnership between patients and their health care teams means creating a space in which the lived expertise of patients and their agency in decision making is recognized alongside the medical expertise of the clinical team. Patient-team partnership may occur at the level of the clinical relationship or in organizational improvement, as patients and community members are invited to contribute their expertise to improving organizational policies. Longitudinal relationships of trust facilitate partnership at both levels. The disruptions to team-based care meant that patients experienced care with only their clinician rather than their team, and often remotely, posing a challenge for patient-team partnerships. Established relationships helped to weather the pandemic, but new relationships were more difficult to build. Patient and community involvement as advisors for quality improvement efforts often fell by the wayside due to other urgencies during the pandemic. In many places, the continuous relationships among patients, clinicians, and teams will need extra time and resources to rebuild and sustain.

Primary Care Building Block #6: Population Management Pre-COVID-19, many primary care practices were achieving high marks in their chronic and preventive care metrics. Workflows designed to excel at population management aided practices in their COVID-19 response efforts. For example, one large medical system in Massachusetts developed an algorithm to flag their most vulnerable patients who had tested positive for COVID-19, so that primary care teams could reach out to support them as they convalesced at home [14]. Others reached out to patients with chronic conditions or social vulnerability in the early days of the pandemic in order to check on them and link them to resources as needed [15]. While some practices refocused their population health infrastructure to serve COVID-19 needs, most of the broader population management efforts had to be paused or completely abandoned. This was due to a loss (or redeployment) of medical assistants who were doing the population-oriented work as part of their in-person visits and a sharp decline in patients seeking in-person care.

With the disruptions to team-based care, the reluctance of patients to seek preventive care [16], and the challenge of performing routine chronic and preventive care during virtual visits, population management took a back seat during the early years of the pandemic and has not recovered. In many practices, patients fell behind in receiving preventive care, such as childhood immunizations, cancer screening, blood pressure monitoring, and diabetes management. Population management does not work well if there is a breakdown in empanelment, meaning that clinicians and teams cannot easily identify who is in their population. An inability to do empanelment well is a direct threat to primary care's ability to recover pre-COVID-19 population health capabilities.

Primary Care Building Block #7: Continuity of Care The emergence of telehealth on the scene has improved continuity of care, at least in the short-term. Phone- and video-visit options have made it easier to arrange a visit with a patient's personal clinician when an in-person visit is not convenient for the patient or the clinician. However, an increase in early retirements among some primary care physicians and mid-career departures from primary care among many others has disrupted longer-term continuity. There are currently not enough primary care clinicians to allow every person in the country to have a personal clinician who can provide continuity. At present, continuity of care is not achievable for large proportions of the population, and the COVID-19 pandemic accelerated this trend. Given that continuity of care is associated with better health outcomes, this workforce shortage is problematic. For some patients, continuity with a clinic location or a system of care might work well. New models of primary care are emerging, but it is too soon to know if they will be sufficient replacements for traditional patient-clinician continuity.

Primary Care Building Block #8: Access As the work of prevention and care of COVID-19 consumed a great deal of primary care's capacity, in-person access for patients with non-COVID needs fell. As a result, timely diagnoses of new conditions as well as routine care services were delayed [17]. Telehealth has long held the promised potential to overcome geographic and transportation barriers to access. Indeed, rates of patients failing to show up for telehealth visits were lower than no-show rates for in-person visits. But studies show that lower-income and marginalized populations were encountering high barriers to telehealth, which exacerbated existing inequities in access. For example, large scale telephone triage systems did not reduce health disparities in access to testing [18]. Amid the challenges of COVID-19, primary care practices sought out ways to improve access. Recognizing that they were trusted sources of care and information, some opened testing or vaccination sites, often utilizing pop-up tents in parking lots. A detailed case study is presented in Chap. 8 of this book. When hospital systems in Connecticut realized that web-based sign-up systems were excluding older residents and those without computers, they partnered with churches to arrange pop-up vaccine sites [19]. To facilitate access to preventive care, some practices set up drive-through systems to collect laboratory specimens [15]. In general, COVID-19 inspired telehealth has led to sustained improvement in access for some patients; however, the larger trend of workforce shortages and declining opportunities for patients to find and establish continuity relationships with primary care clinicians has thwarted prompt access for many others.

Primary Care Building Block #9: Comprehensiveness and Care Coordination With the primary focus on COVID-19 response, non-COVID illnesses went undetected, and timely diagnosis and referral patterns were often upended. At the same time, the pandemic underscored the urgency of assessing and addressing social determinants of health, such as access to housing, food, transportation, and jobs. Some health care organizations developed stronger relationships with community-based organizations, while others connected people with resources. For example, primary care physicians in Santa Rosa, California, founded a not-for-profit called IsoCare to support their most at-risk patients during quarantine and isolation. IsoCare created intervention teams for people awaiting test results, providing food, laundry, and financial support services to ensure they could remain in isolation during their most infectious period [20]. But as we have seen with so many of the Building Blocks, the overall trend has been disruption.

Primary Care Building Block #10: Template of the Future This tenth Building Block refers to freeing primary care from the constraints of visit-based payment. Templates of the future are envisioned to include group visits, care delivered by other members of the care team, asynchronous care (e.g., messaging via a portal), and telehealth. Primary care has long sought to find new modalities to meet the needs of patients, but payment models have thwarted many efforts. The pandemic-era necessity of moving to telehealth and asynchronous care broke inertia and resistance to change among practices and payers. For example, the Centers for Medicare and Medicaid Services instituted waivers allowing payment for telehealth visits irrespective of the location of the clinician, and many commercial insurance companies adopted similar measures [21]. Thanks to the exigencies of the pandemic and removal of payment barriers, the use of telehealth exploded in a very short timeline: telehealth claims in the U.S. increased by more than 4000% between March 2019 and March 2020 [22]. Some of the facilitators to telehealth and other innovations have dissipated with a return to in-person care; for example, payers have dramatically scaled back on payments for telephonic visits [23]. Consumers, on the other hand, have embraced new modalities, with some unexpected consequences. For example, asynchronous messaging by patients to their health care providers has increased by more than 150% of pre-pandemic levels [24] and has not abated [25].

Most payers have not adapted their payment to match these new trends, resulting in an explosion of unpaid work for clinicians, for example in-basket messaging. Atrius Health, an ambulatory care health system in Massachusetts, embarked on a multi-year process to streamline in-basket messaging, with a goal to reduce the volume of in-basket messages by eliminating or automating unnecessary messages. The result was a 25% reduction of in-basket messaging, with a substantial reduction in unreimbursed work [26]. However, the focus on virtual care risks creating new inequities for patients. People with limited digital literacy or English proficiency are often unable to use electronic portals to make appointments, send messages to their clinicians, or order prescription refills. One key learning of the pandemic was that equitable primary care access requires supporting patients and families that may struggle to use these new platforms [27]. Within the first months of the pandemic, the Center for Care Innovations developed and produced a Telemedicine for Health Equity Toolkit. The toolkit assesses a patient's digital access and provides support when needed [28]. These emerging practices offer a path forward toward a more equitable template of the future. But payer resistance and workforce shortage trends place that future in jeopardy.

Conclusion In summary, the pandemic stalled improvement in some Building Blocks, but accelerated change in other Building Blocks. Many primary care practices rose to the challenge of the COVID-19 pandemic, applying tools and principles of population health and equity-focused data-driven improvement to the challenges of protecting vulnerable patients, addressing critical social needs, and ensuring equitable vaccine outreach. Other practices sought innovative ways to promote access, ranging from drive-through labs to telehealth supports. Realistically, these positive examples are more than balanced by pandemic challenges to access, continuity, population health, and team-based care.

With the end of the emergency period of the pandemic, practices have options on how to move forward in the future:

- Revisit which data-driven improvement metrics are priorities to monitor and utilize;
- Rely on the population management Building Block and re-engage patients in preventive care;
- Revitalize team-based processes of care; and
- Pay close attention to patient access and continuity of care in the new telehealth and workforce-constrained environment.

Prior to the pandemic, a number of primary care practices self-assessed their performance for each of the ten Building Blocks and used that assessment to guide their improvement activities. Considering their learnings from the pandemic, practices may find it worthwhile to re-visit the Building Blocks of Primary Care Assessment [29] and use that assessment to re-imagine their short- and long-term goals for the future.

References

1. Berwick DM. How has the pandemic changed improvement? Presented at: International Forum on Quality and Safety in Healthcare. 2021. Virtual.
2. Bodenheimer T, Ghorob A, Willard-Grace R, Grumbach K. The 10 building blocks of high-performing primary care. Ann Fam Med. 2014;12(2):166–71. https://doi.org/10.1370/afm.1616.
3. Jackson GL, Powers BJ, Chatterjee R, et al. The patient centered medical home. A systematic review. Ann Intern Med. 2013;158(3):169–78. https://doi.org/10.7326/0003-4819-158-3-201302050-00579.
4. The Commonwealth Fund. The Safety Net Medical Home Initiative. https://www.commonwealthfund.org/publications/other-publication/2014/oct/safety-net-medical-home-initiative?redirect_source=/publications/resources/2010/the-safety-net-medical-home-initiative.
5. Krist A, DeVoe J, Cheng A, Ehrlich T, Jones S. Redesigning primary care to address the COVID-19 pandemic in the midst of the pandemic. Ann Fam Med. 2020;18:349–54. https://doi.org/10.1370/afm.2557.
6. Levander XA, VanDerSchaaf H, Barragán VG, et al. The role of human-centered design in healthcare innovation: a digital health equity case study. J Gen Intern Med. 2024;39(4):690–5.

7. DeVoe JE, Cheng A, Krist A. Regional strategies for academic health centers to support primary care during the COVID-19 pandemic: a plea from the front lines. JAMA Health Forum. 2020;1(4):e200423.
8. Sanchez T, Ho C, Moench M. California says equity is vital for vaccine distribution, but the data is almost non-existent. San Francisco Chronicle.
9. Alexander GC, Tajanlangit M, Heyward J, Mansour O, Qato DM, Stafford RS. Use and content of primary care office-based vs telemedicine care visits during the COVID-19 pandemic in the US. JAMA Netw Open. 2020;3(10):e2021476. https://doi.org/10.1001/jamanetworkopen.2020.21476.
10. Cunningham AT, Felter J, Smith KR, et al. Burnout and commitment after 18 months of the COVID-19 pandemic: a follow-up qualitative study with primary care teams. J Am Board Fam Med. 2023:jabfm.2022.220226R1. https://doi.org/10.3122/jabfm.2022.220226R1.
11. Stern RJ, Rafferty HF, Robert AC, et al. Concentrating vaccines in neighborhoods with high COVID-19 burden. NEJM Catalyst. 2021;2(2). https://doi.org/10.1056/CAT.21.0056.
12. DePuccio MJ, Sullivan EE, Breton M, McKinstry D, Gaughan AA, McAlearney AS. The impact of COVID-19 on primary care teamwork: a qualitative study in two states. J Gen Intern Med. 2022;37(8):2003–8. https://doi.org/10.1007/s11606-022-07559-5.
13. Rheuban K, Jin J. Telehealth integration and optimization. American Medical Association. Updated 22 Jan 2025. https://edhub.ama-assn.org/steps-forward/module/2813038.
14. Blazey-Martin D, Barnhart E, Gillis J Jr, Vazquez GA. Primary care population management for COVID-19 patients. J Gen Intern Med. 2020;35(10):3077–80. https://doi.org/10.1007/s11606-020-05981-1.
15. Albert SL, Paul MM, Nguyen AM, Shelley DR, Berry CA. A qualitative study of high-performing primary care practices during the COVID-19 pandemic. BMC Fam Pract. 2021;22(1):237. https://doi.org/10.1186/s12875-021-01589-4.
16. Cutler D. How will COVID-19 affect the health care economy? JAMA Health Forum. 2020;1(4):e200419. https://doi.org/10.1001/jamahealthforum.2020.0419.
17. Williams R, Jenkins DA, Ashcroft DM, et al. Diagnosis of physical and mental health conditions in primary care during the COVID-19 pandemic: a retrospective cohort study. Lancet Public Health. 2020;5(10):e543–50. https://doi.org/10.1016/s2468-2667(20)30201-2.
18. Cheng A, Hart K, Baron A, et al. Unbiased care, unequal outcomes: a nursing telehealth intervention reveals systematic inequities in COVID-19 care delivery. BMC Nurs. 2024;23(1):622. https://doi.org/10.1186/s12912-024-02270-8.
19. Altimari D. Data show mass vaccination sites are reaching the general population — not the vulnerable areas they are supposed to target. 2021. https://ctmirror.org/2021/03/08/data-show-mass-vaccination-sites-are-reaching-the-general-population-not-the-vulnerable-areas-they-are-supposed-to-target/.
20. Beck J. Doctor launches IsoCare to help residents isolating during pandemic. The Press Democrat. https://www.pressdemocrat.com/article/specialsections/sonoma-gives-doctors-aha-moment-drives-effort-to-build-safety-net-with/.
21. Sinsky CA, Jerzak JT, Hopkins KD. Telemedicine and team-based care: the perils and the promise. Mayo Clin Proc. 2021;96(2):429–37. https://doi.org/10.1016/j.mayocp.2020.11.020.
22. Gelburd R. Examining the state of telehealth during the COVID-19 pandemic. New York, NY: United Hospital Fund; 2020.
23. Henry TA. Commercial payer patchwork is holding back telehealth's promise. American Medical Association. https://www.ama-assn.org/practice-management/digital/commercial-payer-patchwork-holding-back-telehealth-s-promise.
24. Holmgren AJ, Downing NL, Tang M, Sharp C, Longhurst C, Huckman RS. Assessing the impact of the COVID-19 pandemic on clinician ambulatory electronic health record use. J Am Med Inform Assoc. 2022;29(3):453–60. https://doi.org/10.1093/jamia/ocab268.
25. Arndt BG, Micek MA, Rule A, Shafer CM, Baltus JJ, Sinsky CA. More tethered to the EHR: EHR workload trends among academic primary care physicians, 2019–2023. Ann Fam Med. 2024;22(1):12–8.

26. Fogg JF, Sinsky CA. In-basket reduction: a multiyear pragmatic approach to lessen the work burden of primary care physicians. NEJM Catal Innov Care Deliv. 2023;4(5):CAT. 22.0438.
27. Lyles CR, Sharma AE, Fields JD, Getachew Y, Sarkar U, Zephyrin L. Centering health equity in telemedicine. Ann Fam Med. 2022;20(4):362–7.
28. Center for Care Innovations. Telemedicine for health equity toolkit. https://www.careinnovations.org/resources/telemedicine-for-health-equity-toolkit/.
29. Willard-Grace R, Dube K, Grubach K, Bodenheimer T. The 10 building blocks of primary care. Building blocks of primary care assessment https://cepc.ucsf.edu/sites/cepc.ucsf.edu/files/Building%20Blocks%20Assessment.pdf.

Chapter 3
Patient Experiences During the Pandemic Highlight the Value of Established Relationships with Primary Care and Identify a Focus for the Future of Primary Care

Ashley P. Duggan, Rebecca S. Etz, Martha M. Gonzalez, Sarah R. Reves, and Bernard Ewigman

> *Knowing our doctor for over 10–15 years and having a great relationship with her, helped get through covid. Having that relationship with her helped with many of our decisions we took, like should we get a shot or not. We felt we were able to trust her judgment and her honesty.* —A patient

The COVID-19 pandemic disrupted health care systems, bringing into sharp focus what matters most in health care. The pandemic also offered a unique opportunity to take the pulse of primary care, from many different perspectives, including the patient perspective. Patient expectations of primary care are often multifaceted: expecting their primary care provider (PCP) to provide expert care and be someone they can count on to be there whenever needed. These expectations were greatly

A. P. Duggan (✉)
Communication Department, Boston College, Chestnut Hill, MA, USA
e-mail: ashley.duggan@bc.edu

R. S. Etz · S. R. Reves
The Larry A. Green Center, Richmond, VA, USA

Department of Family Medicine and Population Health, Virginia Commonwealth University, Richmond, VA, USA

M. M. Gonzalez
Department of Family Medicine and Population Health, Virginia Commonwealth University, Richmond, VA, USA

B. Ewigman
Tufts University School of Medicine, Department of Family Medicine, Boston, MA, USA

A. Cheng et al. (eds.), *Primary Care in a Public Health Emergency*,
https://doi.org/10.1007/978-3-032-12487-6_3

amplified during the early years of the pandemic and collectively became much more frequent and acutely pressing at a population scale.

This chapter is devoted to patients and their experiences with primary care during the COVID-19 pandemic. In this chapter, we capture patient voices generated through a series of surveys relevant to primary care that were fielded by the Larry A. Green Center during the pandemic to learn what really mattered from the patient perspective. We analyze free-text responses to an open-ended question about what patients want to share, with the goal of capturing patients' experiences and expectations of primary care. We frame the significance of patients' words through the lens of relationship science in analyzing and interpreting these findings. We conclude by outlining key strategies for assuring a positive future for primary care including: research, training, and policy designed to restore meaning and purpose driven by the science of relational processes; systems-based positive disruptive innovations that facilitate better relational care; disengaging from our dysfunctional health care system; and counter-cultural social movements powered by patients and clinicians seeking to restore purpose and meaning in primary care through systems-level policy changes [1–3].

Methods

Survey Creation and Data The patient perspectives used in our analyses were collected as part of a larger set of Larry A. Green Center [4] surveys of primary care clinicians and patients. The surveys focused on the experiences, responses, and capacity of primary care clinicians and practices during the pandemic. The Green Center also collected 14 waves of patient surveys between May 2020 and December 2022.

Patient surveys included a combination of structured questions and open-ended questions. For this chapter, we focus on patient open-text comments received from a single question included in every patient survey: "Is there anything else you would like us to know about your experience with primary care during the COVID-19 pandemic?" We focused on this "anything else" text data because such responses offer breadth, reflective opportunities, and sense-making, and are not directed toward a specific aspect of patient experience. Respondents choosing to write answers to this question were likely speaking to the matters of great importance to them at the time.

Survey Procedures Each patient survey started with a screener question. Potential survey participants were first presented with the following definition of primary care:

Primary care is:

1. a place and/or team that recognizes what's important to you,
2. makes sense of your health concerns in ways meaningful to you, and
3. is available to you when you need it and in the way(s) you need it.

Following this definition, potential participants were asked if they had had any experience with primary care in the preceding 12 months. Only those who were 18 years of age or older and who said yes to the screener question were eligible to take the survey.

Surveys were made available to the general population through the online survey tool SurveyMonkey (www.surveymonkey.com) and a service they provide called SurveyMonkey Audience which allows for the user to request a specified number of respondents fitting study criteria. This SurveyMonkey service has been used effectively in previous health service research [5–7]. The Green Center team specified that demographic criteria for recruitment be consistent with the US Census in terms of balancing gender, age, race, ethnicity, income, and education. The first four patient surveys included a minimum sample of 1000 participants screening yes to an experience with primary care in the past 12 months, over the age of 18, and with overall representation matching requested demographics. For the remaining ten surveys, the team requested a general minimum sample of 1000 plus an additional sample of 400 participants, focused primarily in rural and/or low-income participants. The result is a convenience sample with enrollment discontinued as specific demographic categories were filled.

All patient surveys collected were anonymous, voluntary, and took approximately 5–10 minutes to complete. Survey questions were informed by a multistakeholder national advisory committee and focused on these topical areas: access, continuity, coordination, telehealth, cost of care, experience with COVID-19, opinions on vaccination, and perceptions of primary care experience. Surveys largely consisted of structured questions, with some open-ended questions, and all surveys ended with an open space for final comment. This research protocol was reviewed and approved as exempt by the Virginia Commonwealth University Institutional Review Board. Funding was provided by the Agency for Health care Research and Quality (R01 HS028253-01), the Samueli Foundation, and the Andrew and Corey Morris-Singer Foundation.

Sample Demographics The demographics of all patient respondents are summarized in Table 3.1.

Analysis The research team developed a template-based approach to analysis using an *a priori* codebook based on concepts from relationship science [8, 9]. Relationship science provides theoretical and methodological tools to explain the processes of relationship development; the nature and functions of personal relationships across the life span; individual differences and their influence on relationships; relationship processes such as cognition, emotion, and communication; relational qualities such as satisfaction and commitment; environmental and contextual influences on personal relationships; and maintenance and repair of relationships [9]. Relationship science emerged as a defined interdisciplinary field of study in the late twentieth century, drawing upon theory, methods and empirical findings from sociology, psychology, communication and other disciplines.

Table 3.1 Patient participant demographics

Patient participant demographics	# of responses	% of responses
Total number of responses[a]	23,238	100%
Highest formal education		
High school	7275	33.2
4-year college degree	5311	24.2
Graduate or professional degree	3282	15.0
Household income		
Less than $50,000	9364	42.7
Greater than $150,000	2236	10.2
Participants who identify as living in a rural area		
Yes, rural area	5811	25.0
Participants who identify as Hispanic or Latinx?		
Yes, Hispanic or Latinx	1332	9.8
Race/ethnicity?		
American Indian/ Indigenous or Alaska Native	330	4.7
Asian	640	4.7
Black or African American	2089	15.3
Native Hawaiian or Pacific Islander	101	0.7
White	9281	68.1
Prefer not to say	198	1.5
Other (please specify)	149	1.1
Age		
18–35	6996	30.1
Over 65	4021	17.3
Gender		
Male	9452	40.7
Female	12,613	54.3
Other	310	1.3
Unemployment status		
Unemployed	6789	29.2

[a]We note "responses" here, instead of "respondents" because each survey was a unique fielding, and respondents were anonymous. It is possible that the same person could have answered more than one survey; however, this possibility is unlikely.

First, three team members (RE, MG, and AD) read through all open-text responses to the "anything else" question independently, identifying themes and content areas that emerged from the open-text responses, focusing on relational aspects of care as discussed by patient respondents. Next, each of these team members worked independently to identify examples of relational or social aspects of care in the text and shared these independent findings with the group. Those initial conversations led to the creation of the *a priori* thematic codebook which was then used by the lead author and a research assistant (AS) to identify and code responses that included relational aspects of primary care, such topics as trust, rapport, and feeling known or social aspects such as support or connection in social life (both subsequently referred to as relational). In addition to relational thematic coding, the general functions of primary care, including access to care, continuity of care, comprehensiveness and coordination of care, and whether those functions were met or unmet expectations, were coded by the last author (BE) and the research assistant (AS) when a description or reference to these functions was present in the responses previously identified as social or relational aspects of primary care.

Viewed through a lens of relationship science, medical care is about more than diagnosis and treatment; effective care is also about the development of relationships that engender trust, compassion and understanding. Scholars in this field focus on the core elements of relationships such as trust, interdependence, communication, empathy, and emotional intimacy using measures such as self-report scales, observational coding systems, behavioral experiments, and physiological measurements. Relationship science provides theoretical and conceptual models and has great potential to inform impactful applications for understanding and improving the processes, skills, and outcomes of patient-clinician relationships [8, 10].

Data were imported into Atlas.ti 9 to assist with team-based coding and analysis. Code frequencies and team discussion allowed for the systematic development of themes, consistent with the observational epidemiology approach described by Miller and Crabtree [11] and informed by grounded theory, as discussed by Kennedy and Lingard [12]. During discussion of themes as they were developed, research team members collectively agreed through consensus on naming "expectations/ implicit assumptions" as well as explicit expectations within the relational data identified in the "anything else" comments. In cases of disagreement, or questions, the team shifted and reorganized instances of relational issues until consensus was reached.

Results

Within the 23,238 total responses, we identified 678 "anything else" open text comments related to social or relational aspects of care. We further found that 309 of these comments (48% of the total relational or social comments) were focused on patient (explicit or tacit) expectations for relationships with clinicians. Within those comments, we then narrowed to indications of relationships with *primary care* clinicians, focusing on 162 comments. These 162 comments were then coded and organized into four main themes as they fit the *a priori* codebook about patient expectations. Patient expectations and needs, both met and unmet, coalesced around the following: (1) personal relationship, connection with clinician, (2) clinician as someone to turn to, (3) mutual care/reciprocity, and (4) being appreciative of adaptability and flexibility. Below we present representative participant responses that are both positive (sharing a fulfilled expectation or need met) and negative (sharing an unfulfilled expectation or need unmet). Of these relational responses, 102 of the statements alluded to core functions of primary care: access, continuity, comprehensiveness, and coordination.

Relational Themes

Relational Theme 1: Personal Relationship/Connection with a Clinician

Patient responses indicative of an expectation for a personal relationship (n = 71) expressed desire or gratitude for feeling known and understood by their clinician or gratitude towards their clinician for caring for them as a person. This was apparent in the data when patients noted their clinician was kind, compassionate, reassuring, or supportive and paid attention to patients' issues/interests as the patient described them.

Positive patient responses (n = 69), indicative of "personal relationship" as a met need, included:

I go to a clinic that specializes in people over 65 years old. I was very touched when my health coach called me just to see how I was doing during the pandemic.
It would be hard if you did not know your doctors.
I have the absolute best doctor. She has helped me and my friends through many situations. I wish everyone had a doctor like her. She really makes a difference.
She knows I am very concerned about my health and very inquisitive, so she always takes time with me to talk about my health and what I can do to live my best life. I love my primary care doctor!

We found only two negative patient responses (n = 2), indicative of personal relationship as an *unmet* need, both of which might apply to the broader primary care team rather than a specific clinician. The two comments were:

I have a primary care provider that I wouldn't call that personal or close. So while I trust the care, I don't have a super close relationship with them.
I feel that my appointments with my new provider have been professional but not personal, but maybe that's the nature of managed health care.

Relational Theme 2: Clinician as Someone to Turn to

Evidence of patient interest and value in having a "clinician as someone to turn to" (n = 41) was seen in comments that expressed desire or gratitude for reliance, comfort, confidence in the clinician expertise, professionalism, or knowledge.

Examples of positive patient responses (n = 39) include:

I rely heavily on my primary care doctor; she is a comfort to me.
My doctor/nurse practitioner is the best and more than understanding, and always helps to ease my mind when I'm worried about the pandemic.
My doctor has been very informative about vaccines. My doctor doesn't try to force a vaccine on me though.
She spoke to me at eye level. That made me feel more comfortable. Also didn't sugar coat possible symptoms. I really trusted her.

Again within this theme, only two negative patient responses were found. In each case, they included a specific mention by the patient of not getting what they wanted—an unmet need—as they perceived regarding their COVID-19 symptoms. For instance, said one, "I would say he really didn't know much about COVID-19 and minimized my symptoms until he got it himself. I no longer see him."

Relational Theme 3: Mutual Care/Reciprocity

In addition to wanting to be known and cared for, patients' responses also showed their reciprocal concern for their primary care clinician. Examples of this theme were seen in the data when patients shared an expectation for mutual care or reciprocity (n = 18) with their clinician, expressed their concerns for their clinician, support for clinicians' future beyond the pandemic, or their choice to put off care due to pandemic pressure on the clinician.

Positive examples (n = 10) of mutual care and reciprocity as met needs included:

I am concerned that my primary care physician may be losing income due to the virus and that is unfortunate. I want him to stay in business.
My doctor has been amazing; never making me feel rushed during appointments and making sure we address all my concerns even though I know he has been busier than normal.
I do not want to burden the health care system, specifically my primary care provider, with anything less than serious. They have enough to worry about and I'm doing my part.
I just feel like the people that work in the medical field, bless their souls, are so worn out from this pandemic that they just basically don't care anymore. They are exhausted, overworked, and I'm sure underpaid.

For this theme, "negative" responses (n = 8) were found when patients made comments clinicians were under strain but with a focus on how this resulted in an unmet need for patients, rather than a concern for the clinician's wellbeing. This was most often expressed as patient frustration, and included such examples as:

Doctors were overworked and rushed appointments and couldn't give patients the time they needed.
It's been horrible; doctors are all exhausted and don't have the time nor energy for chronic or otherwise non-acute patients.

Relational Theme 4: Appreciative of Adaptability & Flexibility in Meeting Patient Needs

Patient survey responses also included an expectation that their primary care clinician be adaptive or flexible (n = 32). This expectation was expressed as desire or gratitude for clinicians who offered multiple modalities for connecting to patients or for providing clinical visits that were not part of routine care before the pandemic. While the use of telehealth was adaptive during the pandemic, it was also required for a practice to function. Comments coded in this theme did not simply recognize use of telemedicine as a flexibility or adaptation. They also included evidence of positive patient sense-making or affect, such as appreciation of the clinician as adaptive to this new requirement and flexible in how it was employed with their patients.

Patient expressions of gratitude and recognition of clinician adaptability (n = 21) included:

Had my first zoom visit and it went very well. It was reassuring to be able to speak with my doctor to have my prescriptions renewed without endangering my welfare.
If it wasn't for the concessions my doctor made to have zoom meetings, I wouldn't have received the care I needed.
Telehealth makes [care] more accessible when your doctors are far.

Negative responses (n = 11) included lack of flexibility as perceived by patients and could be examples of patient's inability to adapt or feeling that recognition of their preference in modality of care was being ignored. Examples include:

Although I didn't object when my doctor asked if I'd participate in a remote, zoom-type appointment, I also didn't care for it, and would never voluntarily engage in such meetings unless my doctor felt it would be important. This sort of appointment is impersonal with too many glitches.
Telehealth is severely limited by the number of observations that are not available through a screen. My doctor can't tell my blood pressure, skin texture, pulse or blood oxygen level through a zoom call. She can't hear if my lungs have fluid in them. These are all items that affect her ability to diagnose and my quality of care. Also, using a walk-in clinic means that the person seeing me has no idea of my medical history or what is "normal" for my body. Since that varies a great deal from patient to patient, health care for anything other than Covid-19 at that time was not very helpful.

Functional Elements of Primary Care Within Relational Themes

Within the 162 comments focused on relationships with primary care clinicians, 102 comments also indicated one or more of four functional elements of primary care that was either directly stated or implied. The four functional elements included: access to care, continuity of care, comprehensive care, and coordinated care. These patient comments indicated these functional elements as present or absent. Key examples below illustrate the relevance of building personal relationships as interconnected to functional elements of primary care. The following are examples of patient responses that are indicative of functional categories.

Category 1: Access to Care

I have been able to see my doctor whenever I wanted to.
When I was tested positive and my doctor called me immediately and assure me of her assistance, day or night and shared her personal mobile number for any emergency and gave me advice on home quarantine method.
When I had covid I called my doctors office/they told me what to take/do... is as if they were in my home.
I wish people had more access and that wait times weren't ridiculous. I also wish people would answer the phone more, but I also hate to be a bother.

Category 2: Continuity of Care

Knowing our doctor for over 10–15 years and having a great relationship with her, helped get through covid. Having that relationship with her helped with many of our decisions we took, like should we get a shot or not. We felt we were able to trust her judgment and her honesty.
They have taken care of me and my family especially when we all were infected with covid and that's all I could have asked for.
My primary care {doctor} checked with me weekly, just checking in by email/message to see how I was, even when no appointment. She was there for my admissions and all the tests and follow up. She was amazing.
Primary care was with me the whole time and together we got thru the pandemic.

Category 3: Comprehensive Care

I had a stroke in October 2019. Received my referral for my primary care physician in December 2019 and she took the time to phone me as the pandemic began and then we scheduled my first appointment in August of 2020. She knows I am very concerned about my health and very inquisitive so she always takes time with me to talk about my health and what I can do to live my best life. I love my primary care doctor!
I would say he really didn't know much about it and minimized my symptoms until he got it himself. I no longer see him. That brought me Long Covid afterwards. That's when he helped me with the asthma.
My doctor has been amazing, never making me feel rushed during appointments and making sure we address all my concerns even though I know he has been busier than normal.

Category 4: Coordinated Care

I had a great experience with my primary care provider, who quickly answered my request for her referral to get the vaccine. She immediately drew up the referral and had it ready for me to use the very next day!!!
Had a visit via web and was prescribed Paxlovid and my Dr. worked with the pharmacy until 8 o'clock at night to make sure I got it.
I wish my primary care doctor would look at other doctor's care and put it all together and see me as a total person. It is too easy to just refer all the things out that they don't want to mess with.

Discussion

The COVID-19 pandemic shined a light on patient expectations and experiences of primary care, which reflect many of the core values of primary care. Patients' responses to the surveys we analyzed bear witness to what they valued most from primary care clinicians, gratitude for what was working, as well as frustration with unmet expectations about relationships. Notably, the pandemic experience prompted unanticipated vulnerability both individually and collectively. The patient comments reviewed in this chapter speak to the essence of primary care—the importance of having a relationship with a doctor/clinician—especially in times of vulnerability.

What we see in this data is that relationship matters to patients, and attending to relationship processes may be an everyday salve and positive disruptor to the depersonalized and fragmented US health care delivery system [13, 14]. Patient expectations of their primary care clinician were boldly declared either through expression of deep gratitude or great disappointment when reflecting on their pandemic experiences of primary care. Their expressions of gratitude or disappointment indicated just how much patients assumed that they should be able to count on feeling understood and supported by their primary care clinician. Expressions of gratitude included feeling seen as the person they are, feeling grounded during a chaotic time, and feeling a sense of being known and belonging. Disappointment was expressed as unmet desires for access to care or coordination of resources or feeling alone and vulnerable.

When offered the opportunity to answer an open-ended question about "anything else," patients wanted to communicate about primary care. Several patients (unprompted) highlighted foundational features of primary care—being known and understood as a person and having relationships with clinicians who are accessible, provide continuous and comprehensive care, and coordinate the care of their patients. Of note, 82% (84/102) of responses mentioned at least one primary care core function in addition to social and relational expectations. In addition to identifying met and unmet expectations regarding the core functions of access, continuity, comprehensiveness and coordination, this data also reveals that interpersonal closeness, trust, appreciation and reciprocity are foundational to meeting patient expectations and needs.

When clinicians care for patients in the ways patients most want to be seen and understood, they get back to what matters to clinicians; and, it restores their meaning and purpose, which in turn energizes, builds resilience and reduces the risk of burnout. The core principles of Family Medicine are grounded in person-centered care, and in the lived experience of health/illness [15–18]. In many ways, the mindset, focus, and values of Family Medicine were counter-cultural when the specialty was founded and continue to be at odds with the priorities of the technology-heavy, subspecialty-oriented, business driven US health care system. This divergent status of Family Medicine has always existed and historically has energized advocates and practitioners of the discipline. Today, Family Medicine faces a crisis of role and relevance within a deeply flawed system [1–3]. A renewed emphasis on the importance of the patient-clinician relationship and adequate funding to strengthen it will benefit patients and clinicians as well as help to reinvigorate Family Medicine, and primary care in general, and improve functional delivery of health care.

Hopeful Pathways to Get Back to the Heart of Primary Care

We see four hopeful pathways for restoring access to what patients truly need, as was illustrated so graphically by the patient voices captured in these surveys during the pandemic; (1) Fully and explicitly embrace the core of primary care as relationship-based, (2) Utilize the well-developed theories and concepts of relationship science to improve the effectiveness and efficiency of relationship building in primary care through education, training, and research, (3) Enable creative, positive, disruptive innovations to establish more functional primary care models that in turn promote relational care, and (4) Embrace social movements to empower patients and communities to get the primary care that they want and need, which is fundamentally about relationships.

In this chapter, we use our findings to re-orient and re-center health care around the central role of relationships to recognize not just what matters, but also how to get there. Relationships make a difference individually and collectively, but meaningful relationships don't just happen by saying they are important. We need tools to move to the future, to address how primary care and relationships complement each other for the common good. Author and columnist David Brooks argues in his 2023 bestseller ("How to Know a Person") that the act of seeing another person is profoundly creative and that seeing something large in another person, in turn, allows us to see something larger in ourselves. Brooks identifies the one skill that lies at the heart of any healthy person, family, school, community, or society: the ability to see someone deeply and make them feel deeply seen, to accurately know another person, to have them feel valued, heard, and understood [19]. And yet, Brooks says, we humans do not do this well; thus, people all around us feel invisible and misunderstood. Brooks describes tools from the humanities, tools that we appreciate and that give us broad frameworks. Relationships are foundational, not an add on, and yet our discussion of their importance is not yet an explicit part of primary care as known among health systems and business planners. The result is an unnecessary increase in unmet patient needs and a damaging lack of support for those tools and strategies clinicians use when relationship needs are met. Integrating relationship science as a lens for drawing out the significance of our findings and providing a vocabulary that might make the role of patient-clinicians more tangible to those most able to support it through structures and systems of care delivery.

I Matter. You Matter. And We're in This Together: Relationship as Central in Primary Care

Our findings underscore the importance of each person feeling individually seen and understood in an interaction or conversation in primary care, as well as the mutual interplay or dyadic understanding of how one person influences and is influenced by the other.

Individually Seen and Understood In health care, the yearning to be seen and experience trust as an individual is particularly poignant because the relationship between clinician and patient is in many ways so intimate—and often at the most vulnerable moments of an individual's life—and, at the same time, the learning and practice of relationships in clinical care can commonly feel so distant [20]. Clinicians bring individual traits to the health care interaction, starting points for both positive and negative aspects of what we do, who we are, and what we expect. Relationship-centered care focuses on relationship with self, relationship with patients, team relationships and community relationships. Truly seeing and understanding another person is an indispensable aspect of all relationships [21].

Dyadic Understanding The reciprocal interplay that happens in clinical interactions makes a profound difference in clinical outcomes [22]. People affect each other, and behavior in specific interactions influences the general course of a relationship. As an example, interdependence theory explains *interactions* among people in relationships [23, 24]. Interdependence theory was developed and tested in applications such as altruism, attribution, coordination, conflict, cooperation, trust, sacrifice, self-presentation, stereotyping, and hostility and aggression in the context of dyads, as well as a myriad of group applications, environmental issues, organizational issues, and political issues [25, 26].

Using a relationship science framework reveals a way forward to conceptualize and measure the pathways that get us where we want to go [27]. For example, each of the themes from this study could be considered in terms of relational trust, and relationship science gives us a way to disentangle the dimensions of trust and to measure how specific patient and clinician behaviors co-create trusting interactions over time. Trust occurs when individuals feel they can be vulnerable to others because of the sincerity, benevolence, truthfulness and sometimes the competence they perceive [28]. People may extend trust to individuals, organizations, or societal structures that could act to further our interests or protect what we see as vulnerable [20]. Future research using tools from relationship science to articulate how patient experiences build a scientific foundation for the relational aspects of trust, and how that trust also requires considering the broader social context will inform how to more effectively meet patients' relational needs.

What Can Be Done? How Can a Focus on Relationship Help Primary Care?

Given that the core of primary care is relational, we need to become more proficient at this essential element [20, 29], including explicit clinician and patient attentiveness to relational elements as well as building systems to facilitate, support, and strengthen relationships. While it will also be necessary to advocate, innovate and change the structure of health care to better enable relationship development, learning to be a better listener, a more effective communicator, and to have greater capacity for empathy and compassion will serve to greatly strengthen relationships with patients even in the currently dysfunctional system.

The crucial role of primary care in all health care systems includes the fundamental need for trusting relationships as powerfully voiced by these patients as well as serving as the foundation for achieving longevity and quality of life at a societal level. Despite the overwhelming evidence documenting the essential need for robust primary care systems to achieve these aims, the US health care system has pushed primary care to a precarious state characterized by declining capacity, burnout, and the threat of demise [1, 3, 14, 30, 31]. Key leaders and scholars in primary care and family medicine argue that past efforts to change the trajectory of the decline of US primary care have failed and that the hope lies in a social movement empowered by patients and a refusal by primary care clinicians to continue enabling a broken system. The comprehensive review of this problem and the recommendations of the National Academies of Sciences, Engineering, and Medicine (NASEM) [2] Committee on Implementing High-Quality Primary Care, if put into action, would be transformative and likely greatly enhance the capacity to offer strong relationship-centered primary care. Unfortunately, past NASEM reports have largely been ignored. While a flurry of activity occupied the first 2 years after the *Implementing High-Quality Primary Care* report was published, the current political environment has shifted and does not seem conducive to such radical change.

Such a social movement must have as its driving motivation the enhancement of trusting relationships in primary care and that "planting the seeds for the rebirth of health care that starts with the whole person and then focuses on the parts only in the context of knowing and connectedness" [3]. Just as clinical research on diagnosis, prognosis, prevention, and treatment has elevated medical care to be informed by more rigorous evidence through the evidence-based medicine movement, so too the empowerment and reform of health care will be better informed through the science of relationships, the essence of primary care.

Implications

During the pandemic, new information was generated at lightning pace creating mass confusion for patients regarding what information to follow, what information to trust, and how best to care for routine, chronic, and preventive health care needs. In the usual course of patients' lives, they need support, information, advice, trust and empathy from PCPs, even more so when patients are experiencing vulnerability due to illness, injury or loss. The pandemic further heightened these needs. Unfortunately, the capacity to meet even usual needs in primary care in the US has been severely compromised over the past several decades. The forces driving our health care system emphasize efficiency, standardization, and profit with inadequate funding for primary care and little to no attention on clinician-patient relationships, to the great detriment of primary care [1–3].

Patient voices captured in this analysis speak to where we need to focus our attention on what really matters. Primary care in general, and the relational nature of primary care specifically, is essential to meeting the health care needs of patients in all health care systems. In the context of declining interest in primary care disciplines among medical students, reductions in capacity and fragmentation in scope of practice in primary care, and commercial pressures to improve efficiency and profit, the relational essence foundational to this model of care delivery is being lost. The heart of primary care is failing.

Efforts to reinvigorate primary care are emerging. One example is Etz et al.'s [32] Person-Centered Primary Care Measure (PCPCM), which captures the patient experience of person-centered care as a more relevant measure of the performance of excellent primary care than the well-intended but fragmenting quality measures that dominate value-based care (VBC) and the reimbursement tied to VBC models. Ultimately, major structural changes in the US health care system will be necessary if we are to achieve an equitable health care system with outcomes comparable to other developed countries at a cost that is not several-fold greater, as is currently the case. Until that happens, a focus on the essential nature of primary care as relational through positive disruptive innovations and a social movement provides a hopeful pathway.

In summary, patient voices described in this chapter highlight their experiences with the value of relationships with clinicians during the pandemic. As Gayle Stephens wrote in his (1982) book mapping out the intellectual basis of Family Practice, "medicine is always the child of its time and cannot escape being influenced and shaped by contemporary ideas and social trends." He said that "history does not just explain the past but also, by providing the framework for understanding the present, helps us move forward." When patients were asked if there was "anything else" that they wanted to communicate about their experiences with primary care, they overwhelmingly focused on relationships, and this was the focus whether their expectations had been met or unmet. This important and historical tenet of the relational focus of primary care is longstanding and still critically important today. Moreover, the relational element becomes even more important in crisis such as during the pandemic. Although the transactional elements of primary care are also crucial, the relational focus is eroding. The pandemic was a critical warning signal to change course and get back on track to move toward building and sustaining relationships as the heart of primary care. Primary care risks losing a lot if the system continues to veer off this path. If primary care further erodes, the system risks losing a lot, too. Some would argue a loss of heart and soul.

Acknowledgements Audrey Sparano, Asher Cohen, Christine Bechtel, and 3rd Conversation were central to the development and implementation of surveys and data analysis.

Funding Support AHRQ (R01 HS028253-01), Andrew and Corey Morris-Singer Foundation, Samueli Foundation.

References

1. Grumbach K. Forging a social movement to dismantle entrenched power and liberate primary care as a common good. Ann Fam Med. 2023;21(2):180–4.
2. National Academies of Sciences Engineering Medicine. Implementing high-quality primary care: rebuilding the foundation of health care. Washington, DC: National Academies Press; 2021.
3. Stange KC. Time for family medicine to stop enabling a dysfunctional health care system. Ann Fam Med. 2023;21:202–4.
4. Larry Green Center. COVID-19 survey [survey data]. www.green-center.org/covid-survey. Accessed 10/30/2024.
5. O'Callaghan E, Belanger H, Lucero S, Boston S, Winsberg M. Consumer expectations and attitudes about psychotherapy: survey study. JMIR Form Res. 2023;7(1):e38696.
6. Patel SJ, Truong S, DeAndrade S, et al. Respectful maternity care in the United States—characterizing inequities experienced by birthing people. Matern Child Health J. 2024;28(7):1133–47.
7. Youn B-Y, Moon S, Mok K, et al. Use of traditional, complementary and alternative medicine in nine countries: a cross-sectional multinational survey. Complement Ther Med. 2022;71:102889.
8. Simpson JA, Campbell L. The Oxford handbook of close relationships. Oxford University Press; 2013.
9. Vangelisti AL, Perlman D. The Cambridge handbook of personal relationships. Cambridge University Press; 2018.
10. Beach MC, Inui T, Network R-CCR. Relationship-centered care: a constructive reframing. J Gen Intern Med. 2006;21:3–8.
11. Crabtree BF, Miller WL. Doing qualitative research. Sage Publications; 2023.
12. Kennedy TJ, Lingard LA. Making sense of grounded theory in medical education. Med Educ. 2006;40(2):101–8.

13. Hoff T. Next in line: lowered care expectations in the age of retail-and value-based health. Oxford University Press; 2018.
14. Hoff TJ. Searching for the family doctor: primary care on the brink. JHU Press; 2022.
15. Freeman TR. McWhinney's textbook of family medicine. Oxford University Press; 2016.
16. Green LA, Puffer JC. Reimagining our relationships with patients: a perspective from the Keystone IV Conference. J Am Board Fam Med. 2016;29(Supplement 1):S1–S11.
17. Hashim MJ. Principles of family medicine and general practice–defining the five core values of the specialty. J Prim Health Care. 2016;8(4):283–7.
18. Stephens GG. The intellectual basis of family practice. Tucson: Winter Publishing Co; 1982.
19. Brooks D, Benedetti G. How to know a person: the art of seeing others deeply and being deeply seen. Natl Forum Phi Kappa Phi J. 2024:15–5.
20. Shaughnessy AF, Vicini S, Andrea, Zgurzynski M, O'Reilly-Jacob M, Duggan AP. Indicators of the dimensions of trust (and mistrust) in early primary care practice: a qualitative study. BMC Prim Care. 2023;24(1):150.
21. Gaines SO. The self in relationships: social-personality theory, research, and new directions. Oxford University Press; 2023.
22. Jonas W. How healing works: get well and stay well using your hidden power to heal. Lorena Jones Books; 2018.
23. Reis HT, Arriaga XB. Interdependence theory and related theories. In: Gawronski B, Bodenhausen GV, editors. Theory and explanation in social psychology. The Guilford Press; 2015. p. 305–27.
24. Holmes JG. Interpersonal expectations as the building blocks of social cognition: an interdependence theory perspective. Pers Relat. 2002;91(1):1–26. https://doi.org/10.1111/1475-6811.00001.
25. Irani E, Buck HG, Lyons KS, et al. Examining how congruence in and satisfaction with dyadic care type appraisal contribute to quality of life in heart failure care dyads. Eur J Cardiovasc Nurs. 2023;22(2):158–65.
26. Lyons KS, Lee CS. The theory of dyadic illness management. J Fam Nurs. 2018;24(1):8–28.
27. Duggan AP. Health and illness in close relationships. Cambridge University Press; 2019.
28. O'Reilly-Jacob M, Vicini A, Duggan AP. Ethical considerations of telehealth: access, inequity, trust, and overuse. J Health Ethics. 2022;18(1):3.
29. Scott JG, Cohen D, DiCicco-Bloom B, Miller WL, Stange KC, Crabtree BF. Understanding healing relationships in primary care. Ann Fam Med. 2008;6(4):315–22.
30. The plight of primary care, part 1. Intention to treat. N Engl J Med. 2023. https://www.nejm.org/doi/full/10.1056/NEJMp2303852.
31. The plight of primary care, part 2. Intention to treat. N Engl J Med. 2023. https://www.nejm.org/doi/full/10.1056/NEJMp2305758.
32. Etz RS, Zyzanski SJ, Gonzalez MM, Reves SR, O'Neal JP, Stange KC. A new comprehensive measure of high-value aspects of primary care. Ann Fam Med. 2019;17(3):221–30.

Chapter 4
Into the Storm: Primary Care, Public Health, and the COVID-19 Pandemic

William D. Nettleton and Sarah D. Present

We made the best decisions we could with the information we had at the time during a constantly evolving situation, period of rapidly changing scientific evidence, and amidst circumstances outside our control. —William Nettleton, MD, MPH

In the first year and a half of the pandemic, I was incredibly proud of myself as a Health Officer, my public health department and emergency operations centers, and my region for our response. We had relatively low death rates, many successes in finding equitable vaccine distribution processes, and many successes in connecting with the community through unprecedented partnerships to understand and address needs of our most vulnerable residents. But I still struggled to explain everything that was going on even to my own family. Trying to be the trusted source of information when I didn't have access to all the information myself was exhausting. I lost faith in myself and then let the onslaught of hatred towards public health affect me. I would wake up in the morning and try not to look at the county's Facebook page but inevitably would. I would feel awful, but get up, drink my coffee, and just try to do better each day. Even today, I find myself not telling strangers when they ask that I'm a Public Health Officer. I tell them I'm a Family Physician, which is half of my job, but I don't tell them I'm also a public health official until I feel I can trust them not to automatically judge me for my role. It's as if I feel responsible for the pandemic itself. —Sarah Present, MD, MPH

W. D. Nettleton
Department of Family and Community Medicine, Western Michigan University Homer Stryker M.D. School of Medicine, Kalamazoo, MI, USA
e-mail: william.nettleton@wmed.edu

S. D. Present (✉)
Clackamas County Public Health Division, Oregon City, OR, USA
e-mail: spresent@clackamas.us

A. Cheng et al. (eds.), *Primary Care in a Public Health Emergency*,
https://doi.org/10.1007/978-3-032-12487-6_4

Introduction

Both primary care and public health are difficult to characterize because of their wide scope and breadth of practice. Primary care is a model of health care that supports first-contact, accessible, continuous, comprehensive, and coordinated person-focused care of individuals [1]. Public health is a discipline and perspective that aims to protect and improve the health of communities and populations [2]. There is overlap between primary care and public health as both emphasize optimizing health, preventing disease, and mitigating health risks to individuals and populations. Further, historical models of public health included primary care services and shared population health improvement efforts.

The opportunities and challenges of the close relationship between primary care and public health became clear in many communities during the COVID-19 pandemic. In some cases, public health and primary care teams worked collaboratively to mount an effective response. However, potential synergies were not always realized because public health and primary care had been undergoing significant transformation and modernization in the decades leading up to the pandemic. Primary care was moving closer to public health with efforts to do population health management. Public health was transitioning away from providing primary care and other direct clinical care provision while increasing emphasis on promotion of policies, systems, and overall community conditions to achieve optimal health for all in their local communities. These shifts had not yet been coordinated or synchronized leaving uncertainty around core functions, roles, and responsibilities. Theoretical collaborative models had been proposed but remained untested. Additionally, both disciplines had experienced long histories of being undervalued and under-resourced, so there were significant gaps in capacity, infrastructure, and preparedness. In some regions, there was competition for limited resources. Still, shared goals of community safety and optimizing health led to many creative and innovative partnerships and coordination of systems that built a foundation for future collaborative efforts toward disease prevention and response.

This chapter is intended to focus on the interface between primary care and public health during the early years of the COVID-19 pandemic. This story has a long history; for example, public health efforts and improved clinical quality of care from 1900–1999 led to a 30-year increase in US life expectancy, 25 years of which were attributable to public health advances [2]. However, we focus on the decades immediately leading up to the COVID-19 pandemic and the period between 2020 and 2023. We write from our experiences as primary care physicians who also serve as local public health officials in three different jurisdictions, collectively responsible for more than 800,000 lives prior to and throughout the COVID-19 pandemic (Clackamas County, Oregon [approx. 425,000 population] and Calhoun and Kalamazoo Counties in Michigan [approx. 400,000 combined population]). As physicians with combined training in family medicine as well as public health and general preventive medicine, we have a unique set of perspectives regarding the primary care and public health responses to the COVID-19 pandemic from 2020 to

2023. In this chapter, we draw on historical and contemporary elements of primary care and public health practice while sharing pragmatic and sobering illustrations from the field, success stories, and partnership achievements. The chapter culminates in recommendations about how primary care and public health partnerships can more effectively serve communities in future pandemics.

COVID-19: Before the Storm

Primary Care Transformation and Public Health Modernization Moving Forward on Parallel Tracks

In the decades leading up to the COVID-19 pandemic, there were efforts to redefine primary care. In 2008, Berwick et al. and the Institute for Health care Improvement published the Triple Aim, a concept stating for overall health care systems to improve, they must aim to improve population health, improve the patient experience, and reduce the cost of health care per capita [3]. This work fueled innovation in primary care, and along with groundbreaking Medicaid expansion in the same timeframe, helped facilitate the establishment of patient-centered medical homes (PCMH), population-based metrics to drive population health work in primary care, quality incentives for Federally Qualified Health Centers (FQHC), and many other initiatives at the federal, state, and local levels to bolster primary care and transform the system. Through primary care transformation, many communities worked to build a more robust primary care network that has the ability and tools to serve patients' health needs in a supportive and holistic framework addressing multiple determinants of health.

During the early twenty-first century, the number of FQHCs increased, Medicaid expansions were implemented, and primary care embraced population health management, which reduced the need for uninsured and underinsured patients to rely upon local public health departments (LHD) for clinical care services. Technological advancements with electronic health records and registries further increased primary care's capabilities. While the transfer of preventive care and population management functions into primary care for many patients was successful, public health continued to serve as a backup to the safety net that FQHCs and other primary care clinics provide, depending on the needs and systemic gaps in each community. For example, LHDs continue to provide communicable disease investigations and many offer wrap-around services for pregnant people, infants, and children including nutritional services like the Women, Infants, and Children (WIC) program [4]. Many LHDs have closed clinical sites and instead assure clinical services in partnerships with FQHCs or other community-based settings. Still other LHDs directly maintain immunization, sexually transmitted infection, tuberculosis, HIV testing and prevention, and Title X family planning clinics. Some provide HIV and hepatitis C treatment, oversee school nursing programs, and direct school-based health centers for primary care services. Where clinical services are maintained by LHDs, the clinical volume is often dwarfed by health care systems but focuses on access for low-resource patients with conditions of public health significance (Table 4.1) [5].

As these shifts were taking place, public health was being redefined. In 1988, the Institute of Medicine (IOM) published *The Future of Public Health* to begin to address the concern that "this nation has lost sight of its public health goals and has allowed the system of public health activities to fall into disarray" [10]. A federal working group presented the 10 Essential Public Health Services (EPHS) in 1994, which were then revised and finally updated in September 2020 during the first year of the COVID-19 pandemic (Fig. 4.1).

After several assessments of the status and risk to the public health system, its ability to address emerging threats, and how public health best fit into health care changes with the Affordable Care Act and its required National Prevention Strategy, the process of public health modernization began in earnest in the early 2010s. The US Department of Health and Human Services and national public health partners characterized this transformation as Public Health 3.0—an effort to enhance public health practice beyond public health department functions and programs [11]. A key component of Public Health 3.0 includes local public health leaders embracing chief health strategist roles for their communities in an effort to address social determinants of health [11]. Development of structured, cross-sector partnerships to drive change is thus inherent to such Public Health 3.0 initiatives. Under guidance from the DeBeaumont Foundation and the Public Health National Center for Innovations (PHNCI), the EPHS framework evolved into defining Foundational Public Health Services to provide a minimum package of public health capabilities and programs and to establish a Public Health Accreditation Board (PHAB) to assess and accredit public health agencies at different levels and sizes to

Table 4.1 Selected foci of primary care transformation and public health modernization efforts in the decades leading up to 2020. [6–9]

Primary care transformation	Public health modernization
Patient-centered medical home	Communicable disease control
Multidisciplinary team-based care	Chronic disease and injury prevention
Increased access to care	Environmental public health
Active chronic disease management	Maternal and child health
Population health management	Access and linkage to clinical care
Value-based care	Assessment and disease surveillance
Continuous, comprehensive, coordinated care	Community partnership development
Engaged leadership	Policy development
Patient empanelment	Emergency preparedness and response
Data-driven improvement	Communications

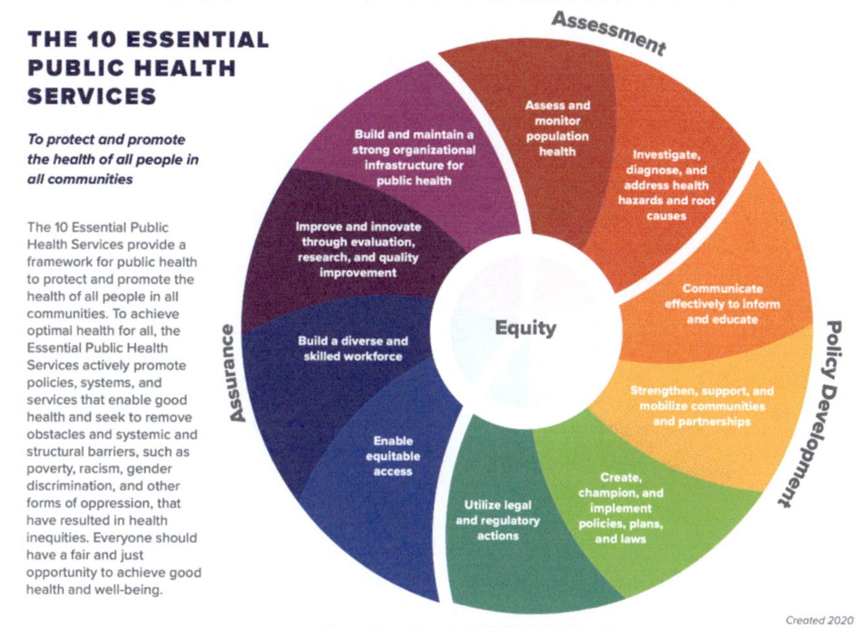

Fig. 4.1 10 Essential Public Health Services Futures Initiative Task Force. 10 Essential Public Health Services. September 9, 2020. https://phaboard.org/wp-content/uploads/EPHS-Graphic-Image.png [2]. This framework is an open-access public health resource and is freely available from the Public Health National Center for Innovations

demonstrate they were meeting these goals [12]. Public Health 3.0 initiatives would require actionable, sub-county level data with clear metrics linked between public and private sectors in addition to enhanced and innovative funding mechanisms.

Oregon was one of the few states leading the process of public health modernization and passed House Bill 2348 in 2013 establishing the Task Force on the Future of Public Health Services to develop a set of foundational capabilities and programs that define core public health services across the state. The first "Public Health Modernization Manual" in Oregon was published in 2017 with this framework described in detail [13]. Figure 4.2 shows a summary of the framework. In essence, as public health decreased its focus on direct clinical care, the responsibilities became increasingly strategic. Public health modernization goals included modernizing data collection, evaluation, and visualization. The envisioned strategic role relies on public health officials maintaining ties with health care leaders. A decrease in reportable diseases such as tuberculosis or varicella due to successful disease control or vaccination may have ironically weakened ties between public health and health care leaders given less frequent interaction for response.

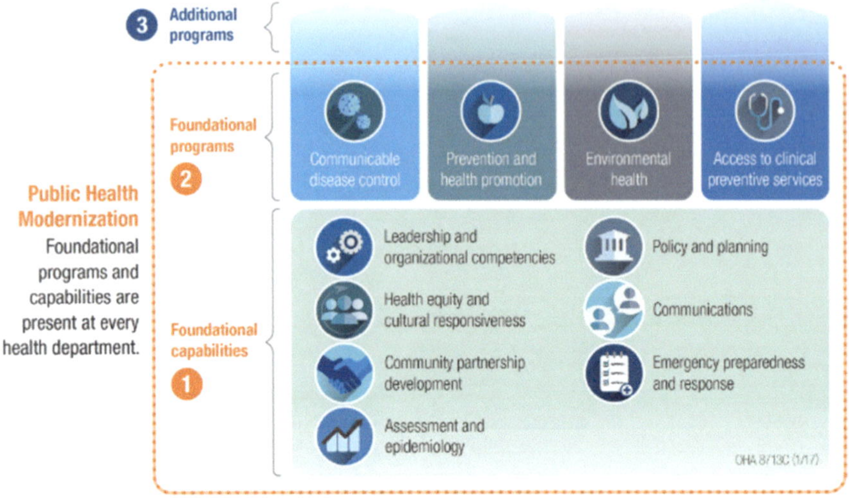

Fig. 4.2 Oregon's modernized framework for governmental public health services. (*Figure reprinted from "Modernized Framework for Governmental Public Health Services," in* Statewide Public Health Modernization Plan, *Oregon Health Authority, December 2016. Used with permission.*)

Despite Individual Progress, Theoretical New Roles for Primary Care and Public Health Were Not Empirically Tested

Similar to Oregon's framework, structures were developed in Washington and Ohio, and as of early 2024, approximately 20 states were using the Foundational Public Health Services framework [12, 14]. It is important to note that nowhere in these capabilities or programs is direct care a requirement. Although noting the need to tailor individual community needs, the framework encourages public health departments to move more into the capabilities of data and epidemiology, policy, and partnership development to drive the programs, while leaving clinical services to covered entities. The intent was that public health could inform and convene health care partners to be effectively coordinated and ready to prevent disease and respond to emerging threats [15].

It is important to note that FQHCs, major health systems, and payers were often neither involved in nor adequately informed of this public health transformation. The experience of this role expectation uncertainty was variable across the different state and public health jurisdictions across the country, but a general divergence of knowledge and coordination between public health and primary care was a common experience. Thus, at the beginning of the pandemic, 3 years after public health modernization was adopted in the state of Oregon, health care partners may not have been ready for how heavily public health would need to lean on them for providing care.

Despite Modernization Efforts, Public Health Continued to Struggle

Public Health Was Chronically Underfunded

One aspect that certainly impacted public health modernization and that routinely directs the role of public health in any community was (and continues to be) a lack of adequate funding. The health system of the US continues to be complex, as noted by The Commonwealth Fund in 2020:

> *The U.S. health system is a mix of public and private, for-profit and nonprofit insurers and health care providers. The federal government provides funding for the national Medicare program for adults age 65 and older and some people with disabilities as well as for various programs for veterans and low-income people, including Medicaid and the Children's Health Insurance Program. States manage and pay for aspects of local coverage and the safety net. Private insurance, the dominant form of coverage, is provided primarily by employers. The uninsured rate, 8.5 percent of the population, is down from 16 percent in 2010, the year that the landmark Affordable Care Act became law. Public and private insurers set their own benefit packages and cost-sharing structures, within federal and state regulations* [16].

While the US spends over four trillion dollars each year on health care, it has historically spent less than 3% of that on public health [17]. Further, national health care expenditures increased by about 50% from 2008 to 2018, but state public health expenditures saw no growth except in injury prevention [18]. This lack of investment translated to challenges in local public health response during the pandemic despite the influx of pandemic relief dollars. Table 4.2 lists some of the ongoing public health infrastructure gaps.

This systemic underfunding can be illustrated by a few events in recent history, when public health emergencies have called for a rapid response that the public health system has struggled to mount. One was the anthrax attacks that occurred in

Table 4.2 Ongoing public health infrastructure gaps

Workforce development
Cross-sector skills in risk and crisis communications
Communicable disease surveillance system interoperability within states and between states
Electronic health record interoperability between public health and health care
Reliance on aged communication technologies like fax machines and voice mail
Local and regional public health laboratory capacity
Existing scheduling system for mass vaccination

fall 2001. Responding to bioterrorism as an unlikely but very severe threat was not something frontline physicians in primary care or emergency departments had the tools to cohesively address. As Marmagas et al. noted in 2003, the attacks:

> ...strained the abilities and resources of the Centers for Disease Control and Prevention (CDC) and state and local health departments to react effectively... as a nation, we were unable to prepare an effective risk communication strategy after the anthrax events that could alleviate nationwide panic, and we were unprepared for the volume of laboratory samples that had to be processed [19].

Marmagas et al.'s strong recommendation at that time was for policymakers and the public health community to invest in overall public health capacity to effectively address modern threats, "...whether they be emerging infectious diseases, terrorist attacks, or chronic illnesses." The bioterrorism threat of the early 2000s did lead initially to funding emergency preparedness efforts focused on medical countermeasure distribution planning. For example, the CDC's Cities Readiness Initiative (CRI) [20] was established in 2004 to enhance preparedness in large cities and still informs public health emergency preparedness today. CRI-funded regions have continued to plan for and exercise mass distribution of medical countermeasures, and many of these plans were dusted off from the shelves in preparation for a COVID-19 vaccine. However, since funding had slowly declined over time as the threat seemed less imminent, the plans were often only known to the emergency response teams within public health who all assumed coordination would occur with partners across the health care system.

Aside from bioterrorism, the threat often considered by public health emergency preparedness practitioners was pandemic influenza. Pandemic influenza preparedness was tested in 2009 with the threat of the H1N1 influenza virus. While there were many local successes that led to increased visibility of public health and to local partnership building, some lessons from the response included increasing communication and vaccine distribution infrastructure, as well as coordination between emergency response and frontline health care workers. While over $1.4 billion was distributed for response efforts in 2009–2010, ongoing planning funding decreased year over year, and when COVID-19 appeared, the infrastructure to maintain the cooperation with communities and primary care had lapsed for many public health departments [21].

Some states were studying their readiness and the resources needed to implement new frameworks that had been developed. For example, the state of Oregon put significant effort into identifying the foundational programs and capabilities for each LHD as well as how much funding would be needed to achieve this level of function for every LHD across the state. In a 2016 baseline assessment, the state found that with increased investments from the legislature in response to nascent modernization legislation, in 2016, "Governmental public health authorities are already significantly executing the public health modernization framework, with

$209 million in 2016 dollars being spent annually on the foundational capabilities and programs. This is approximately two-thirds of the cost of full implementation of the framework, with the current service delivery model. The preliminary estimated additional spending needed for full implementation is approximately $105 million annually in 2016 dollars" [13]. Oregon was at the national forefront of modernizing public health and just learning what investments would really be needed to fully support public health when COVID-19 began testing the system.

Public Health Data Systems Did Not Receive Adequate Investment

In 2009, the Health Information Technology for Economic and Clinical Health (HITECH) Act was passed into federal law and provided billions of dollars for adoption of health information technology, mostly to clinicians and hospitals. There were initial requirements in this Act meant to enhance two-way communication between health care delivery providers and public health systems, starting with transmission of data to local, state, and federal public health departments on notifiable conditions, syndromic surveillance by hospitals, and immunizations. While some funding was to go into public health data infrastructure, the majority went into incentives for "meaningful use" of the electronic health records, including direct patient care functions such as e-prescribing and into reporting of certain quality indicators to the Centers for Medicare and Medicaid Services (CMS) [22]. While this helped in population health management, there was not meaningful development on data system integration between health care and public health which would have allowed for a streamlined response to a new health threat. Although little progress was made to integrate systems, new electronic reporting systems for public health were emerging. For example, public health in Oregon gained access to the Electronic Surveillance System for the Early Notification of Community-based Epidemics (ESSENCE) [23] data with syndromic surveillance of emergency room diagnoses, and an Immunization Information System [24] which houses immunization records, and an All Payer All Claims (APAC) database for diagnosis-based billing data, which is necessarily delayed from the date of service. Vital records are housed within public health but with significant delays in aggregating data that does not give real-time information. The reportable conditions database was still lacking a bidirectional ability to send information to providers, and it was difficult to produce real-time monitoring reports.

There was growing recognition that achieving bidirectional exchange between public health information and clinical health records would require a significant investment into data modernization for public health. As one clinician shared, "I get notified when my patient has a stroke in Pennsylvania, but not if my pregnant patient is diagnosed with syphilis in Maine." These efforts were still in their infancy when the COVID-19 pandemic hit.

COVID-19: The Storm Hits

No one was prepared for what was to come: the scientific uncertainty surrounding a novel virus, the difficulties of communication, and the lack of coordination that challenged every community in the US. The infrastructure risks had been identified, but not to a point of stress testing the readiness necessary to address the threats COVID-19 posed in the twenty-first century. As described above, primary care and public health responses were not set up well in most parts of the country to provide a coordinated, prolonged pandemic response. Despite some public health and primary care teams having run through emergency response scenarios in their individual siloes, they had been practicing separately and not across sectors and systems. This hampered the ability to coordinate action, know what each other was doing, and exchange accurate, timely information between public health agencies and primary care providers, and thus to patients during the pandemic.

Public health and primary care systems were undergoing dynamic changes on parallel tracks with limited resources, making it difficult for them to be quickly scaled up, coordinated, or sustained for pandemic response. Despite these challenges, partnerships created and sustained between local public health and health systems, including primary care, strengthened and ultimately saved lives. This section describes some examples drawn from our own experiences.

Public Health Decision Making

Public health emergencies or threats present unique challenges to decision making. During a public health threat, public health professionals often make decisions in context of significant uncertainty and unequal distribution of risk across a population. Public health officials must first assess the facts, nature of the threat, consequences, probability of occurrence, and potential action steps; second, they must deliberate when to act and the consequences of acting too soon or too late; and third, they must decide what and when to communicate to the public [25]. Public health officials might also take executive action that requires assessment of legal authority and duty to act and ultimately reasonable discretion on whether to act [26]. Historically, the National Incident Management System (NIMS) [27] guided governmental and non-governmental organization incident prevention, mitigation, response, and recovery efforts. However, the novelty, scope, and duration of the COVID-19 pandemic complicated every level of public health decision making and challenged the functionality of NIMS. The federalist structure of the US, differing state public health governance, and politicization of the pandemic created varied incident responses across the nation that left many health care entities looking to their LHDs for guidance. In this context, local public health physicians drew upon their clinical and public health expertise to synthesize information garnered from scientific literature, professional colleagues, clinical experience with COVID-19 patients, and state, federal, and international health authorities to then make decisions, recommendations, and policies that impacted entire populations.

Educating Different Audiences

The evolving nature of the COVID-19 pandemic, ever-changing scientific evidence, and misinformation complicated effective, trustworthy communication. Local public health physicians participated in public education, risk communication, and crisis communication throughout the pandemic. Public education included media interviews, press conferences, town halls, teleconferences, social media videos and posts, and virtual meetings on the basics of COVID-19, masking efforts, vaccine information, SARS-CoV-2 variants, and interpretation of public health orders, among other topics. In some cases, this work was rapidly published and disseminated. For example, in April 2021, Dr. Nettleton published a summary on interpreting COVID-19 diagnostic tests to assist practicing family physicians across the country at a time of evolving test understanding and availability [28]. Risk communication included efforts to communicate how COVID-19 posed hazards to communities and efforts to reduce risk. LHDs also were often caught in the middle of ever-changing state and federal policy and communications. For example,

> National and state agencies did not include LHDs in decisions that affected their communities, which made LHDs appear to be ill-prepared and/or incompetent. Moreover, due to the lack of a unified approach...LHDs were not often notified of top-down decisions of local, state, and national leaders or were given minimal time to prepare to implement those decisions [29].

Local crisis communications included emergency updates, public health orders, and responses when situations changed. For example, Dr. Nettleton noted,

> *In the summer of 2021, we in local public health were trying to catch our breath after seven months of mass vaccination clinics and tailored community vaccination events. But the Delta variant was now spreading and causing increased hospitalizations. Michigan's state public health masking order had expired months ago. Like other local health departments, we had worked closely with local school districts on infection control plans for the approaching school year and had recommended a mask optional approach based on pre-Delta variant status and current state epidemic orders. Then, on July 27, 2021, the CDC recommended universal masking in K-12 schools. Immediately, school districts and communities were asking what we and other local health departments were recommending or ordering in our respective jurisdictions. The local health officer planned to issue a masking order for schools. I reached out to our local hospitals and medical school and garnered public support from our children's hospital and medical school. I also supplied the most current information and evidence that supported the indication for a masking order.*

Dr. Nettleton recalls also updating local school superintendents while logged into a virtual meeting on his phone, as he stepped away from rounding in a hospital unit dedicated to COVID-19 patients. Local public health physicians with backgrounds in family medicine also highlighted their roles as family doctors to augment credibility and increase trust. In November 2021 when the COVID-19 vaccine became available for children 5 years or older, Dr. Nettleton publicly stated,

> *As a family doctor, I recommend the COVID-19 vaccine for children and adolescents aged five years or older. As a parent, I will be vaccinating my five-year old. I encourage parents with questions to talk with their family doctor, pediatrician, or nurse about getting the COVID-19 vaccine for their child.*

Both authors also created social media videos on Facebook and participated in dozens of television, radio, and print news interviews. Table 4.3 gives examples of the many topics local public health physicians were being asked to present to different audiences during the COVID-19 pandemic.

Although located in communities, primary care and local public health had variable staffing for community health workers to effectively assist in community engagement. One strategy during the pandemic was to partner with trusted messengers, particularly for vaccination outreach. These trusted messengers included religious leaders, community leaders, local physicians, and community members dedicated to outreach. In Calhoun County, Michigan, local "vaccine ambassadors" [30] supported by a local non-profit and hospital grant engaged community groups and households in vaccine hesitancy, and Dr. Nettleton provided a training session on vaccine basics. In February 2021, Dr. Nettleton participated in a Battle Creek NAACP community information meeting about the COVID-19 vaccine in which a local pastor stated, "When I took the shot I made sure our congregation knew…It's

Table 4.3 Examples of topics public health officials were being asked to present to different audiences during the pandemic

Asymptomatic transmission of SARS-CoV-2
Isolation, quarantine, and contact tracing
Mask types and effectiveness
Interpretation of COVID-19 diagnostic tests
SARS-CoV-2 variant threat differences (e.g., Delta and Omicron)
COVID-19 vaccine basics
Vaccine prioritization categories during initial roll out
Vaccine effectiveness in reduction of disease severity vs. transmission
Correcting misinformation
Correcting disinformation
Keeping local audiences aware of federal or state pronouncements or orders
Helping local audiences interpret state public health orders
Explaining local public health orders
Navigating the local public health communication infrastructure

important as an African American church leader that I do everything I can to get information to our churches and make sure people we trust get that information to people." During the meeting, Dr. Nettleton noted, "The messenger and partnership are really what matters…I look forward to partnerships that come out of this conversation today. This is what community is all about, the importance of partnership and highlighting that this is an issue of justice" [31]. Dr. Nettleton also organized a press conference in December 2021 with physician leaders from three hospital systems to share information and plead with the community for help in reducing the burden on health care systems and the COVID-19 spread during the Omicron variant surge. He and other public health and primary physicians around the country also participated in television and social media advertisements with fellow physicians to encourage vaccination.

Technology and Communication

Data System Challenges and Opportunities

When COVID-19 hit Oregon and Michigan, the reportable condition databases—the Oregon Public Health Epidemiologists' User System (ORPHEUS) and the Michigan Disease Surveillance System (MDSS)—were set up to receive only positive lab results. The HITECH requirements of EHRs were met by a system of electronic case reports in which EHRs could transmit diagnoses to ORPHEUS and MDSS. But the systems also were not set up to track negative tests or point-of-care tests. Michigan's state immunization registry also did not have a field to track race or ethnicity in December 2020 when COVID-19 vaccination began [32]. Therefore, to track potential racial disparities in vaccination access and uptake, the system had to be modified; public health workers and National Guardsmen then had to retrospectively fill in data on tens of thousands of patients.

Few in health care were prepared for the lack of nimbleness in knowing real-time information, such as percent positivity of test results or which health system was seeing more cases of COVID-19. Lack of data portability added to lack of coordinated care for individuals with COVID-19 well into the pandemic. And most importantly, lack of data portability, combined with lack of systemic communication systems contributed to both primary care and public health losing credibility. Table 4.4 outlines opportunities for health information technology integration between primary care and public health.

Communication Challenges and Opportunities

The mantra "be first, be right, be credible" of Crisis and Emergency Response Communication (CERC) [33] was established in a time in which news outlets were often the main source of information around emergency response. It was

Table 4.4 Health information technology integration opportunities

	Public health	Primary care	Opportunities
Reportable conditions	Disease surveillance databases • Some electronic submissions possible with human processing or manual input • Rarely includes negative tests • Public health case management may be documented • Differences between states; no overall federal standard Data outputs: incidence reports and trends	Electronic health records • May or may not have automatic or manual electronic reporting to public health–rarely reports any clinical information • Do not routinely have inputs from public health • Differences between EHRs as well as system-specific usage of each Data outputs: clinical care and progress for individuals	Investments in interoperability • Negative test result reporting can improve percent positivity • Two-way communications about individual patient care and response • Improve EHR access to public health to decrease manual reporting and outdated communication styles (e.g., fax)
Disease surveillance	Multiple databases looking at entire population of a jurisdiction. Birth and death records not real time, data delay typically in months. Some LHDs have real-time access to medical examiner data. Able to evaluate and respond to social determinants of health needs at a population level with publicly funded services directed to areas of need.	EHR ability to pull reports on patients with specific diseases or on provider/clinic-based performance metrics Able to track and respond to social determinants of health needs for patients in a system of care with specific coverages	• Work together on developing surveillance programs such as AI that can improve disease prediction and risk factor identification across a population using EHR details • Invest in shared epidemiology/data management to provide covered services and publicly funded services efficiently • Invest in shared solutions to data privacy in rapidly evolving HIT fields

(continued)

Table 4.4 (continued)

	Public health	Primary care	Opportunities
Incident response	National Incident Management System (NIMS) is practiced regularly News and social media are ways to share information LHDs have varying ways to communicate with primary care providers.	Incident management is often focused on clinical response needs. Systemic response information often comes from larger health systems, payers, and public health partners, leaving local leaders needing to translate many information sources to make patient information in EHRs as well as clinic workflows around providing clinical information to patients.	The NIMS guides all levels of government, non-governmental organizations, and the private sector to work together to prevent, protect against, mitigate, respond to, and recover from incidents. Invest in LHDs practicing together with primary care and community-based organizations in addition to hospitals and large health care systems. Invest in disaster communication planning with current technologies being used.
Immunizations	State-level databases, with no standard for communication with other states	Ability to enter patient historical immunizations Many EHRs can communicate with and update state databases or be updated by state databases	Invest in interstate immunization record sharing. Continue to develop apps and other electronic resources for patients to easily access their full immunization records.
Billing/ payment for services	Funded by tax dollars and grants Billing systems set up for fee-for-service payments for clinical services are difficult to apply to public health practice. Investment needed to build billing infrastructure can be a barrier to LHDs to bill insurance payer for services that would otherwise be covered if performed in a primary care setting.	Robust billing infrastructure Variety of structures including fee-for-service, per-member-per-month and incentives for meeting metrics set out by CMS and other payers.	Continue to find creative ways locally and at the state/federal levels for health care dollars to support coordinated prevention efforts and clinical services provided by public health to the populations that include covered and non-covered individuals.

challenging to experience the communication infrastructure of the public health system not keeping up with the communication infrastructure of social media platforms. Thus, determining who was first, who was right, and who was credible was confusing and frustrating for many.

Public health leaders realized despite years of work in response plans, a modern communication framework that could adapt to a dynamic situation and reach partners, governments, health care, and the public was missing. The last pandemic of this magnitude had occurred 100 years prior. The Spanish Flu in 1918 was a novel influenza A virus that ravaged the world, infecting roughly one third of the population at the time, with a mortality rate somewhere around 10% (approximately 50 million deaths). As opposed to 1918 when orders were placed in prominent locations in towns and cities across the country [34], public health could not simply post orders or information in a town square or local newspapers. Communication is a pillar of the developing modern public health system that was needed during the early days of the COVID-19 pandemic prior to being fully ready.

It is well known that misinformation and disinformation flooded media markets, but even without that, credible and timely information came from disparate sources throughout the world and public health and primary care faced many challenges in determining what was the most up-to-date and applicable information for their communities and patients. Governmental public health agencies at both federal and state levels lacked infrastructure to accept, analyze, and distribute helpful health information during the rapidly evolving pandemic. Furthermore, public health lacked infrastructure and workforce to effectively counter misinformation or disinformation. Supply chain disruptions led to recommendations of safety precautions that were not feasible. Additionally, the range of organizations and entities in emergency response mode was unprecedented–all with a need to disseminate information.

The information flow, and ways to communicate to the public, were severely taxed. Information exchange with primary care had several hurdles. First, public health engaged all sectors during the pandemic. With this level of engagement, interaction was often with leaders of institutions, including health care institutions, or liaisons to public health updates. The employed nature of many physicians meant they depended upon their leadership or health systems to communicate information. Before getting to primary care or other disciplines within a health care system, the recipient of information had to then forward or adapt the information for its own communication process. Successful LHDs like Kalamazoo County Health & Community Services (HCS) established structures to hold conference calls with community organizations, schools, health care systems, skilled nursing, and elder care facilities prior to and during the early days of the COVID-19 pandemic response. Computerized virtual meetings then became widespread and made it possible for emergency operations centers to work remotely and effectively, an approach to emergency response that was truly unprecedented. For example, on March 27, 2020, Calhoun County opened a unified command with the City of Battle Creek that served as a cross-sector, in-person, and virtual emergency operations center throughout the pandemic. An interim After Action Report (AAR) from the Regional Disaster Preparedness Organization (RDPO) [35], which serves the Portland Metro region in

Oregon, also identified one of the successes for this region to be developing creative ways to address the chaos:

> Despite an overload of information and fast moving, ever-changing incidents, the strong internal communication and professionalism of the Region's EOC/ECC logistics teams enabled them to design and implement local communication systems that worked well given the circumstances [35].

At the same time, the challenge was not overlooked as an area of improvement:

> There was both an overload of and an over-reliance on electronic communication. Many AAR participants reported that initially the information flow was "like drinking through a fire hose." This overuse resulted in some historically effective emergency communication tools….being lost and/or forgotten [35].

Another area where communication was strained and more proactive collaboration was needed between public health and primary care was in providing information directly to patients. Early in the COVID-19 pandemic, what clearly emerged from national public health messaging was instruction for patients to reach out to their primary care providers (PCPs) for personalized guidance. Without a system that empowered PCPs with information, clinics were inundated with phone calls. The public was under an immense amount of psychological distress and needed answers to questions about their health [36, 37]. Simultaneously, clinics were overwhelmed by the volume of calls and the rapidly changing information landscape. They were also being forced to rapidly change their clinical operations to include telehealth [38–40] to mitigate the spread of illness during initial quarantine efforts. The next sections describe more about the primary care experiences with these challenges.

Primary Care: On the Frontline of COVID-19 Clinical Information

While public health reached out directly to community-based organizations with education, personal protective equipment, and access to care, a demand for wider COVID-19 clinical information fell to primary care. In the broader public eye, health care and public health were losing credibility. Whether this was based on the communication infrastructure challenges, politicization, resistance to mandates, social media disinformation, or other reasons, by May 2022, only about half of Americans rated public health officials and elected state and local officials as having done an excellent or good job of responding to the pandemic. In a survey across sociodemographic groups of 443,455 US adults, trust in "physicians and hospitals" decreased from 71.5% in April 2020 to 40.1% in January 2024 [41]. However, 95% of 2007 individuals from various demographics and across political parties polled in 2023 still considered their *personal* physician as a trusted source of health information [42].

To meet a demand for incoming calls to primary care for information, some health systems developed telephone-based COVID-19 hotlines. Previous studies had shown that telephone triage services can positively affect behaviors [43, 44].

These hotlines were typically started very quickly using redeployed nurses and doctors [44] and health professions students [45, 46]. Others used existing infrastructure such as poison control centers [47] or units started during prior pandemics [48]. Some successful ones involved local and state public health professionals as well. The efforts were sometimes led by a single individual [49]. The hotlines provided clinical guidance to patients and other health care professionals. Of note, they sometimes also provided psychological support [50, 51]. Data suggests that the hotlines were able to answer a large volume of clinical questions and reduce unnecessary emergency room utilization [52, 53].

In the Portland Metro area, Dr. Sarah Present worked with family medicine colleagues at the Oregon Health & Sciences University to ensure coordination between primary care communications and local public health response while setting up what became a highly utilized hotline service for the whole state of Oregon. The COVID Connected Care Center (C4) "was developed with the idea that providing a low-barrier telephone nurse hotline would increase access to health care information and services for systematically harmed groups who face significant obstacles to necessary information and care" [54].

Vaccine Equity Planning and Response

Despite communication challenges and siloed work prior to 2020, vaccine planning and response led to innovation in primary care and public health coordination of mass vaccination and tailored vaccination outreach for specific communities. In the Portland Metro Region, public health leaders knew early that equitable vaccine distribution was going to be a monumental challenge. The five major health systems in the area set up an unprecedented partnership to staff and coordinate mass vaccine distribution sites. This was a huge success reflecting a modern coordinated public health and health care system coming together to meet the needs of the community in appropriate ways. Most of the direct care, including vaccine distribution, was spearheaded by health care systems, and public health was able to focus on more specific communities with individual needs. Public health and primary care practitioners knew that not everyone, particularly the nation's most medically vulnerable populations, would be able to access vaccines at the mass vaccination sites. A vaccine coordination meeting naturally formed, soon warmly termed the "Breakfast Club" due to meeting routinely at 7:30 am. This group consisted of representatives from public health from each of the three major counties in the region, emergency management, and representatives from the coordinated Medicaid providers in the region. The group met 3–5 times per week to review vaccine plans for the day and other tasks that needed to be completed to work towards equitable distribution of vaccines across the region. Data from multiple organizations helped identify vaccine rates among age, race/ethnicity, and zip codes, as well as work to identify medically fragile individuals, and even homebound individuals covered by

Medicaid services. From this, partnerships with clinical practices, health systems, community-based organizations, and more could be formed in a focused manner to get vaccines to those people and places with identified needs [55].

Vaccine Distribution

LHDs were successful in not only the equity of vaccine distribution but also in the logistics of mass vaccination and tailored vaccination clinics at churches, schools, homeless shelters, drop-in centers, and senior centers. Throughout 2020, Kalamazoo County partnered with local health systems and the local medical school on communications, personal protective equipment distribution, and community education. Between December 2020 and May 2021, Kalamazoo County Health & Community Services administered 81,403 COVID-19 vaccine doses with the help of 324 unique community volunteers, including 8000+ volunteer hours to staff 68 vaccine clinics. Kalamazoo County partnered with Kalamazoo Valley Community College, Western Michigan University School of Nursing, Western Michigan University Physician Assistant program, and Western Michigan University School of Medicine which provided 223 medical students and faculty to assist in vaccination clinics and a COVID-19 call center.

Several logistical factors limited primary care distribution of COVID-19 vaccines during the initial vaccine roll out of 2020–2021. mRNA vaccines required ultra-cold storage with freezers and dry ice that most primary care offices did not possess. Initial mRNA vaccines were also packaged in multi-dose vials and given limited allocation; distribution prioritized health care and public health entities that could vaccinate higher volumes of patients. To receive federal allocation of COVID-19 vaccine, entities had to enroll as a COVID-19 vaccine provider and attest they could meet all requirements of storage, handling, administration, and safety reporting. Smaller or less experienced primary care practices which did not previously store and administer vaccines on site, particularly those not enrolled or proficient with the Vaccines for Children program, were not readily equipped for emergency distribution of a medical countermeasure during a pandemic. LHDs brought expertise in vaccine education, storage and handling, administration, and logistics and then leveraged community and health care partnerships to vaccinate large populations that they could not do alone.

Another innovation that could only occur with partnerships across the health care and public health systems was the in-home vaccination program in Clackamas County, Oregon. This program received national attention for its innovation [56]. Homebound individuals were identified through data sharing from health systems, payers, county Department of Human Services (DHS) programs working with individuals with disabilities, and primary care providers. However, once the county offered a nursing program to do this, the requests were overwhelming. The New York Times reported, *"In Clackamas County in Oregon, G.I.S. data has become the backbone of efforts to vaccinate people who are homebound. 'Because we are a large county with somewhat rural areas, we do have some transportation issues and access is a challenge for many of our residents,' said Kim La Croix, a public health program manager for the county. 'Those mass vaccination sites were just not accessible to homebound seniors and homebound people with mental, developmental or physical disabilities'"* [57]. The In-Home Vax team was able to set up a dataset with all requests from any individual or organization, then worked with a GIS specialist to develop an interactive map and a phone app for the nurse to streamline her route throughout the county each day [56]. This innovative tool could schedule appointments, keep track of first and second doses of vaccines, and plot appointments on a map for maximum travel efficiency. The tool also allowed the nurse to do "safety checks" throughout the day and had a dashboard for easy reporting. Nurses could also keep track of other providers from health systems who were giving in-home services and potentially refer covered individuals to their primary care system for this service.

The In-Home Vax team consisted of many people organizing efforts but only two nurses in the field vaccinating. Nurses administered over 1000 vaccines to homebound residents over the course of a year. In Michigan, both Calhoun and Kalamazoo Counties utilized their Area Agencies on Aging to identify homebound individuals, garner nursing staff, leverage GIS mapping, and publicly promote at-home vaccination programs. Moving forward, public health may not be able to continue to provide such services, but covered entities could work with other partners to deliver similar health care services.

Moral Injury to Family Physicians and Public Health Professionals

Physicians, including public health physicians, were witness to preventable suffering and death during the COVID-19 pandemic. The key word above is *preventable*. While suffering and death were tragic and expected during the pandemic, the scope of preventable suffering and death was unexpected. An analysis from Brown School of Public Health found that 100% uptake of the COVID-19 vaccine for Americans eligible between January 2021 and April 2022 could have prevented at least 318,000 COVID-19 deaths; in other words, half of Americans who died of COVID-19 during that period might not have died if they had received the COVID-19 vaccine [58]. The knowledge that further death and suffering could have been prevented directly conflicted with the values of many health care and public health professionals and contributed to moral injury. Moral injury can occur when, "in traumatic or unusually stressful circumstances, people may perpetrate, fail to prevent, or witness events that contradict deeply held moral beliefs and expectations" [59]. Although historically characterized among veterans, moral injury has been increasingly recognized in health care workers and public health professionals and worsened during the COVID-19 pandemic [60].

Furthermore, harassment of public health officials contributed to the demoralization of the public health workforce and led to negative health impacts such as depression, post-traumatic stress disorder, and suicidal ideation [29]. The recovery phase of the pandemic response required and continues to require supporting the well-being and strengthening of the public health workforce. Recovery also includes planning, so the future workforce and the work is tailored to the needs of the local community. Identifying the trusted sources of information and incorporating them into the public health system will increase job satisfaction if the community is better served. Finding the technology, the people, the primary care clinicians or community health workers that can deliver messages that are first, right, credible, and culturally acceptable to our incredibly diverse public is key to the success of future public health responses.

After the COVID-19 Storm: Lessons for the Future

The authors of this chapter represent only two family physicians who were uniquely equipped to navigate and bridge the worlds of primary care and public health during the pandemic. Family physicians, in particular, view an individual's health in the greater context of family, environment, culture, and the interplay between community and individual health. The American Academy of Family Physicians describes some features of family medicine as:

- *Caring for patients regardless of age or health condition, sustaining an enduring and trusting relationship*
- *Understanding community-level factors and social determinants of health*
- *Serving as a patient's first contact for health concerns*
- *Navigating the health care system with patients, including specialist and hospital care coordination and follow-up*
- *Using data and technology to coordinate services and enhance care*
- *Considering the impact of health on a patient's family*

These traits translate well into providing medical consultation for a public health department and providing care to whole populations. While there is no official training for being a local public health physician, the attributes outlined in Table 4.5 that family medicine brings to public health practice are further augmented by training in a preventive medicine residency program.

Overall, greater focus is needed to augment and support the shared missions of primary care and public health in the US. Local public health physicians practicing family medicine and preventive medicine/public health offer a tangible example of how the shared missions can be bridged on an individual level. On a systems level, deep investment in public health infrastructure and workforce is sorely needed, and health care needs to be involved in informing public health systems that meet clinical care needs of local communities. Data integration and interoperability across clinical and public health systems are essential, but connections and clearer roles

Table 4.5 Contribution of family medicine attributes to practicing local public health physicians during the COVID-19 pandemic

Family medicine attributes	Application to local public health practice during the COVID-19 pandemic
Scope of practice	Pediatric and adult vaccination familiarity Maternity care and vaccination familiarity Ability to converse with a variety of medical specialties Familiarity of providing direct preventive and acute patient care
Health systems knowledge	Relationships with hospitals and medical center structures, medical staff, and leadership Coordination of mass vaccination clinics with health system partners
Family and community perspective	Engagement beyond the individual and outside a health care setting Community and demographic specific COVID-19 testing and vaccination outreach
Personal relationship with patients	Ability to relate with people of diverse backgrounds
Trustworthiness	Increased credibility as a local, practicing family doctor
Work in underserved communities	Understanding need and who to engage Outreach pitfalls Cultural humility
Rural and urban practice	Understanding of different perspectives and limited resources in each setting

and responsibilities for protecting and enhancing the health of both individuals and communities is needed. Training in public and risk communication across public health and health care should be viewed as critical leadership and preparedness attributes. Primary care physicians and local public health physicians remain indispensable partners in enhancing and protecting the public's health—and will be again in the next pandemic.

These authors' experiences also highlight clear successes when intentional partnerships were built between public health and primary care, as supportive individuals and organizations to each other. We provided services and created innovative technologies to support vulnerable individuals and communities and ultimately fostered collaboration that can build a foundation for future planning.

A few summary lessons of this chapter that could inform the future of public health, primary care and pandemic preparedness include:

Poor investment in public health infrastructure for decades and lack of health care inclusion in a public health modernization process contributed to misunderstanding of public health and health care roles in the pandemic.

Recommendation: Funding for public health and primary care should increase significantly to meet the aspirations of Public Health 3.0 and build a public health system for the twenty-first century. Public health and health care leaders should be intentional about collaboration and role sharing in the communities they serve.

Public health's transition to less direct clinical service provision and more assurance of health care services allowed for an increased chief health strategist role potential but more dependence on primary care to fulfill health care gaps in communities.

Recommendation: Primary care and public health leaders should collaboratively assess the capacity, scope, and need of clinical services in the communities they serve. Assessment should include readiness for public health emergency response and medical countermeasure distribution.

Clinical electronic health records, public health surveillance systems, and vaccine registries were not integrated in a functional manner that enabled data portability across systems. Investment in interoperability of technology was siloed.

Recommendation: Primary care and public health leaders should work together with information technology experts to enable data interoperability and portability across systems. State and federal funding should support such data system solutions.

A lack of communications infrastructure and standardized messaging across health care and public health systems led to primary health care systems being overwhelmed with handling individual patient questions and care coordination.

Recommendation: Health care and public health systems should invest in modern communication infrastructure and workforce. Health care and public health leaders should maintain skill sets in risk and crisis communications.

Technology-enabled primary care and local public health physicians can jointly tailor outreach to vulnerable populations.

Recommendation: Further investment and sustainability in technology and data systems aimed at tailored community outreach should be a part of both routine practice and emergency preparedness.

LHDs successfully implemented mass vaccination efforts and focused vaccination campaigns to vulnerable groups with dedicated staff, local health care partnerships, community-based organizations, and volunteers.

Recommendation: LHDs should maintain their expertise in vaccines and preparedness in medical countermeasure distribution and build upon the community partner relationships developed during the COVID-19 pandemic to further move toward Public Health 3.0.

Local public health physicians drew upon their clinical and public health expertise to synthesize information garnered from their clinical experience with COVID-19 patients, scientific literature, professional colleagues, and state, federal, and international health authorities to then make decisions, recommendations, and policies that impacted entire populations.

Recommendation: Local and state jurisdictions should invest in the role and workforce development of local public health physicians as key leaders who provide medical advice to public health departments, guide population health improvement, and liaise between health care and public health systems.

Family medicine training and practice blends well for local public health practice; preventive medicine and public health training provides a unique skill set and perspective that enhances local public health physician practice.

Recommendation: State and federal governments should increase funding for preventive medicine residency programs as a key effort in protecting and improving community health. Family medicine and preventive medicine residency programs should evaluate opportunities for synergy in training across each discipline.

Local public health physicians, health care workers, and public health professionals suffered moral injury during and after the pandemic response despite fulfilling their duties in caring for individuals and communities.

Recommendation: Public health, health care, and community partners should view successful partnerships not only to achieve optimal community health but as an opportunity to mitigate circumstances that may give rise to moral injury in their workforce.

References

1. World Health Organization. Primary care. https://www.who.int/teams/integrated-health-services/clinical-services-and-systems/primary-care.
2. U.S. Centers for Disease Control and Prevention PHPG. 10 Essential public health services. https://www.cdc.gov/public-health-gateway/php/about/?CDC_AAref_Val=https://www.cdc.gov/publichealthgateway/publichealthservices/essentialhealthservices.html. Accessed 05/05/2024.
3. Berwick DM, Nolan TW, Whittington J. The triple aim: care, health, and cost. Health Aff. 2008;27(3):759–69. https://doi.org/10.1377/hlthaff.27.3.759.
4. U.S. Department of Agriculture; Food and Nutrition Services. WIC: USDA's special supplemental nutrition program for women, infants, and children. https://www.fns.usda.gov/wic#:~:text=WIC%20provides%20free%2C%20healthy%20foods,virtual%20appointments%20in%20many%20locations.
5. Multnomah County. Program #40010B- immunizations clinic redesign. https://multco.us/file/40010b-19_proposed.pdf/download.
6. Oregon Coalition of Local Health Offficials. Public health modernization. https://oregonclho.org/local-health-departments/public-health-modernization.
7. Bodenheimer T, Ghorob A, Willard-Grace R, Grumbach K. The 10 building blocks of high-performing primary care. Ann Fam Med. 2014;12(2):166–71. https://doi.org/10.1370/afm.1616.
8. Greene K, Roth E, Fiscus M, Wilkniss S, Stevenson S, Tewarson H. Public health modernization toolkit: key commitments, priorities, and strategies to advance collaboration between public health and health systems. 2023. https://nashp.org/public-health-modernization-toolkit-key-commitments-priorities-and-strategies-to-advance-collaboration-between-public-health-and-health-systems/.
9. Wagner EH, Coleman K, Reid RJ, Phillips K, Sugarman JR. Guiding transformation: how medical practices can become patient-centered medical homes. 2012. https://www.commonwealthfund.org/publications/fund-reports/2012/feb/guiding-transformation-how-medical-practices-can-become-patient#:~:text=Under%20these%20principles%2C%20a%20PCMH%20would%20provide,of%20their%20care%20through%20performance%20measurement%20and.
10. Institute of Medicine Committee for the study of the future of public health. The future of public health. National Academies Press (US); 1988.

11. DeSalvo K, Wang Y, Harris A, Auerbach J, Koo D, O'Carroll P. Public health 3.0: a call to action for public health to meet the challenges of the 21st century. Prev Chronic Dis. 2017;14:E78. https://doi.org/10.5888/pcd14.170017.
12. de Beaumont Foundation and the Public Health National Center for Innovation. The futures initiative: the 10 essential public health services. Aligning the 10 essential public health services public health services. https://phaboard.org/wp-content/uploads/EPHS-Alignment-EPHSvsFPHS.pdf. Accessed 04/29/2024.
13. Oregon Health Authority. Public health modernization manual. Foundations capabilities and program for public health in Oregon. 2017. https://www.oregon.gov/oha/ph/About/TaskForce/Documents/public_health_modernization_manual.pdf.
14. Public Health Accreditation Board (PHAB). The foundation of public health services. https://phaboard.org/center-for-innovation/public-health-frameworks/the-foundational-public-health-services/.
15. Committee on Public Health Strategies to Improve Health Institute of Medicine. For the public's health: investing in a healthier future. National Academies Press (US); 2012.
16. Tikkanen R, Osborn R, Mossialos E, Djordjevic A, Wharton G. International profiles of health care systems. Commonw Fund. 2020;12:227.
17. American Medical Association. Trends in health care spending. https://www.ama-assn.org/about/research/trends-health-care-spending. Accessed 08/05/2024.
18. Alfonso YN, Leider JP, Resnick B, McCullough JM, Bishai D. US public health neglected: flat or declining spending left states ill equipped to respond to COVID-19. Health Aff. 2021;40(4):664–71. https://doi.org/10.1377/hlthaff.2020.01084.
19. Marmagas SW, King LR, Chuk MG. Public health's response to a changed world: September 11, biological terrorism, and the development of an environmental health tracking network. Am J Public Health. 2003;93(8):1226–30. https://doi.org/10.2105/ajph.93.8.1226.
20. U.S. Centers for Disease Control and Prevention. About CDC's Cities Readiness Initiative (CRI). https://www.cdc.gov/readiness/php/cri/?CDC_AAref_Val=https://www.cdc.gov/orr/readiness/phep/cri.htm. Accessed 05/10/2024.
21. Department of Homeland Security. DHS H1N1 after action report: executive summary. https://www.hsdl.org/c/view?docid=783079. Accessed 05/10/2024.
22. Lenert L, Sundwall DN. Public health surveillance and meaningful use regulations: a crisis of opportunity. Am J Public Health. 2012;102(3):e1–7. https://doi.org/10.2105/AJPH.2011.300542.
23. Centers for Disease Control and Prevention. https://www.cdc.gov/nssp/php/onboarding-toolkits/essence.html.
24. Oregon Health Authority. ALERT immunization information system. https://www.oregon.gov/oha/PH/PreventionWellness/VaccinesImmunization/alert/Pages/index.aspx.
25. Chrysler D. Public health decision-making tool. Network for public health law – mid-states region at the University of Michigan School of Public Health. https://www.networkforphl.org/resources/public-health-decision-making-tool/.
26. Waggoner C, Healy Boufides C, Chrysler D, et al. COVID-19 FAQs for Michigan local health departments. The Network for Public Health Law. https://www.networkforphl.org/resources/covid-19-faqs-for-michigan-local-health-departments/#executive-decision-making.
27. Department of Homeland Security; FEMA. National incident management system. https://www.fema.gov/emergency-managers/nims.
28. Nettleton WD. Interpreting SARS-CoV-2 diagnostic tests: common questions and answers. Am Fam Physician. 2021;103(8):465–72.
29. Royster J, Meyer JA, Cunningham MC, et al. Local public health under threat: harassment faced by local health department leaders during the COVID-19 pandemic. Public Health Pract (Oxf). 2024;7:100468. https://doi.org/10.1016/j.puhip.2024.100468.
30. Simons J. Vaccine ambassadors reach out to those hesitating to get COVID-19 vaccination. https://www.secondwavemedia.com/southwest-michigan/features/Vaccine-Ambassadors-reach-out-to-those-hesitatin-to-get-COVID-19-vaccination-060821.aspx.

31. Simons J. Battle Creek NAACP session with experts offers info for those leery of COVID-19 vaccination. Southwest Michigan Second Wave's. https://www.secondwavemedia.com/southwest-michigan/features/Battle-Creek-NAACP-session-with-experts-offers-info-for-those-leery-of-COVID-19-vaccinat-021021.aspx.
32. Wells K. State releases race data for vaccinations, but nearly half of it is missing. Public media from Michigan State University. https://www.wkar.org/health/2021-02-24/state-releases-race-data-for-vaccinations-but-nearly-half-of-it-is-missing.
33. Remley K. Be first, be right, and be credible: translating lessons from crisis communications. J Public Health Manag Pract. 2019;25(2):208–9.
34. Cleveland Police Historical Society, Adams MM. 1918 Influenza pandemic in Cleveland. https://www.clevelandpolicemuseum.org/historical/1918-influenza-epidemic-in-cleveland/.
35. Regional Disaster Preparedness Organization. https://rdpo.net/.
36. Tan R. In an era of quarantine, crisis hotlines face growing. Washington Post. https://www.washingtonpost.com/local/crisis-hotline-quarantine-coronavirus-mental-health/2020/03/23/632e2d7c-6abe-11ea-9923-57073adce27c_story.html.
37. Keeter S. People financially affected by COVID-19 outbreak are experiencing more psychological distress than others. Pew Research Center. https://www.pewresearch.org/short-reads/2020/03/30/people-financially-affected-by-covid-19-outbreak-are-experiencing-more-psychological-distress-than-others/. Accessed 15 Apr 2020.
38. Mehrotra A, Ray K, Brockmeyer DM, Barnett ML, Bender JA. Rapidly converting to "virtual practices": outpatient care in the era of Covid-19. NEJM Catal Innov Care Deliv. 2020;1(2). https://doi.org/10.1056/CAT.20.0091.
39. Sinha S, Kern LM, Gingras LF, et al. Implementation of video visits during COVID-19: lessons learned from a primary care practice in New York City. Front Public Health. 2020;8:514. https://doi.org/10.3389/fpubh.2020.00514.
40. Lin S, Sattler A, Smith M. Retooling primary care in the COVID-19 era. Mayo Clin Proc. 2020;95(9):1831–4. https://doi.org/10.1016/j.mayocp.2020.06.050.
41. Perlis RH, Ognyanova K, Uslu A, et al. Trust in physicians and hospitals during the COVID-19 pandemic in a 50-state survey of US adults. JAMA Netw Open. 2024;7(7):e2424984. https://doi.org/10.1001/jamanetworkopen.2024.24984.
42. Mello MM, Gostin LO. Public health law modernization 2.0: rebalancing public health powers and individual liberty in the age of COVID-19. Health Aff. 2023;42(3):318–27. https://doi.org/10.1377/hlthaff.2022.01292.
43. Sexton V, Dale J, Bryce C, Barry J, Sellers E, Atherton H. Service use, clinical outcomes and user experience associated with urgent care services that use telephone-based digital triage: a systematic review. BMJ Open. 2022;12(1):e051569. https://doi.org/10.1136/bmjopen-2021-051569.
44. Rushton S, Boggan JC, Lewinski AA, et al. VA evidence-based Synthesis Program Reports. Effectiveness of remote triage: a systematic review. Department of Veterans Affairs (US); 2019.
45. Santos JJ, Chang DD, Robbins KK, et al. Answering the call: medical students reinforce health system frontlines through Ochsner COVID-19 hotline. Ochsner J. 2020;20(2):144–5. https://doi.org/10.31486/toj.20.0065.
46. De Sá Dias Machado MB. On the frontlines, behind the computer screen. Acad Med. 2020;95(11):e10–1. https://doi.org/10.1097/acm.0000000000003601.
47. Meaden CW, Ramdin C, Ruck B, et al. The Poison Center as a pandemic response: establishment and characteristics of a COVID-19 hotline through the New Jersey Poison Center. Clin Toxicol (Phila). 2021;59(12):1228–33. https://doi.org/10.1080/15563650.2021.1905163.
48. Song R, Choi YS, Ko JY. Operating a national hotline in Korea during the COVID-19 pandemic. Osong Public Health Res Perspect. 2020;11(6):380–2. https://doi.org/10.24171/j.phrp.2020.11.6.06.
49. Navarrete-Reyes AP, Avila-Funes JA. Staying in a burning house: perks and perils of a hotline in the times of COVID-19. J Am Geriatr Soc. 2020;68(5):E10–1. https://doi.org/10.1111/jgs.16479.

50. Matthewson J, Tiplady A, Gerakios F, Foley A, Murphy E. Implementation and analysis of a telephone support service during COVID-19. Occup Med (Lond). 2020;70(5):375–81. https://doi.org/10.1093/occmed/kqaa095.
51. Wang J, Wei H, Zhou L. Hotline services in China during COVID-19 pandemic. J Affect Disord. 2020;275:125–6. https://doi.org/10.1016/j.jad.2020.06.030.
52. Margolius D, Hennekes M, Yao J, et al. On the front (phone) lines: results of a COVID-19 hotline. J Am Board Fam Med. 2021;34(Suppl):S95–s102. https://doi.org/10.3122/jabfm.2021.S1.200237.
53. Cheng A, Angier H, Huguet N, et al. Launching a statewide COVID-19 primary care hotline and telemedicine service. J Am Board Fam Med. 2021;34(Suppl):S170–8. https://doi.org/10.3122/jabfm.2021.S1.200178.
54. Cheng A, Hart K, Baron A, et al. Unbiased care, unequal outcomes: a nursing telehealth intervention reveals systematic inequities in COVID-19 care delivery. BMC Nurs. 2024;23(1):622. https://doi.org/10.1186/s12912-024-02270-8.
55. Clackamas County. 2021-05-28 Clackamas County COVID-19 vaccine equity plan. Clackamas County. https://statelibraryor.recollectcms.com/nodes/view/186675.
56. Diaz K. Health departments lean on GIS mapping to track COVID-19. https://www.govtech.com/health/health-departments-lean-on-gis-mapping-to-track-covid-19.
57. Anthens E. 'X' marks the spot: officials map a route out of the pandemic. New York Times. https://www.nytimes.com/2021/08/01/health/coronavirus-vaccination-maps-geospatial.html.
58. Brown School of Public Health. New analysis shows vaccines could have prevented 318,000 deaths. https://globalepidemics.org/2022/05/13/new-analysis-shows-vaccines-could-have-prevented-318000-deaths/.
59. Norman SB, Maguen S. Moral injury. https://www.ptsd.va.gov/professional/treat/cooccurring/moral_injury.asp.
60. D'Alessandro AM, Ritchie K, McCabe RE, et al. Healthcare workers and COVID-19-related moral injury: an interpersonally-focused approach informed by PTSD. Front Psych. 2021;12:784523. https://doi.org/10.3389/fpsyt.2021.784523.

Chapter 5
When Things Don't Go as Planned: Family Medicine Residency Training During COVID-19

Brittany McAdams, Cynthia Chen-Joea, Rodika Coloka-Kump, Kathryn Holt, and Maria Montanez Villacampa

Our family medicine residents have been fantastic throughout this entire pandemic. As the patient need/availability shifted from clinic to COVID units, our residents followed them. They worked in the COVID units wearing the space suits, managing patients on vents, and having the difficult discussions with families when patients die. They have been forced to sacrifice some important educational experiences and have hardly complained a peep. They understand the gravity of the situation and have risen to the challenges.

Introduction

The COVID-19 pandemic created significant challenges for all members of the health care workforce. This chapter will speak to the challenges faced by resident physicians, a group that must balance the dual and sometimes conflicting roles of learner and physician. In the best of times, residency is one of the most unique times of a physician's career. For the first time in their medical careers, primary care

B. McAdams (✉) · K. Holt
Department of Family Medicine, Oregon Health & Science University School of Medicine, Portland, OR, USA
e-mail: mcadamsb@ohsu.edu

C. Chen-Joea
Charles R. Drew University of Medicine and Science Department of Family Medicine, Los Angeles, CA, USA

R. Coloka-Kump
Family Medicine Residency Program-NYMC at Saint Joseph's Medical Center, Yonkers, NY, USA

M. M. Villacampa
The University of Texas at San Antonio, San Antonio, TX, USA

A. Cheng et al. (eds.), *Primary Care in a Public Health Emergency*,
https://doi.org/10.1007/978-3-032-12487-6_5

resident physicians become the primary physician responsible for their patients, developing longitudinal relationships and gaining autonomy as they progress in their training. However, residents also work long hours, rotate through diverse learning environments, frequently change work teams, and are in a state of perpetual learning. Many residents are living far from family and extended friend networks. All of this makes residents vulnerable to large scale disruptions in workplace protocols, increased patient care burdens, and communicable disease.

During the COVID-19 pandemic, sponsoring institutions struggled to adapt their educational programs to meet the needs of residents, to expand their clinical services to meet the needs of their patients, while also reducing the risk of COVID-19 transmission. Simultaneously, the stress and workload increased. Residents are typically the primary physician point of contact for hospitalized patients and work long hours. They were therefore exposed to severe illnesses which posed intellectual challenge, psychological stress and risk of personal illness. Educational programming also faced significant disruptions with bans on in-person gatherings, cancellations of elective cases, restrictions on travel to away institutions, and redeployment of staff to care directly for COVID-19 patients.

This chapter focuses mainly on the pandemic experience of family medicine residents because, in contrast to other specialties, most family medicine residents work in primary care settings after graduation. This chapter will draw on the experiences of the authors either as residents or working closely with residents during the pandemic, as well as the published literature on residency education during the COVID-19 pandemic. Additional insight came from qualitative interviews with family medicine physicians who were resident doctors at Oregon Health & Science University during the COVID-19 pandemic about how their residency experience was affected by the pandemic. We will also provide some recommendations about how to mitigate these impacts in future crises. Our authors are from programs in Oregon, Texas, New York, and California to reflect the different experiences residents had based on their location.

Background

Residency training is the first step a physician takes after medical school to gain clinical training and specialization in their field of choice. Residency programs in the US vary from 3 to 8 years depending on the specialty, with longer program lengths found in surgical subspecialties such as neurosurgery. After residency, physicians may complete fellowship training programs to gain additional sub-specialization in areas such as cardiology, critical care, or surgical fields. The majority of the primary care workforce graduates from a three- or four-year residency program in family medicine, pediatrics, obstetrics and gynecology (OB GYN), or internal medicine. Residency training is a form of a working apprenticeship; residents are licensed physicians working under the supervision of attending physicians. The majority of residents' day-to-day work involves direct patient care in either a clinic or hospital setting. The levels of direct or indirect supervision of residents may vary based on their level of training. Work schedules are often set around 2–8-week rotation blocks in related medical specialties and environments. Residents frequently change work locations and teams to allow learning in different settings such as the clinic, the emergency room, the hospital inpatient setting, and the operating room. Working hours are often long, with residents scheduled for up to 80-hour work weeks for multiple weeks in a row.

Residents are the backbone of the hospital physician workforce at thousands of hospitals across the country. They are often the doctors in the hospital overnight, responding first to new consults from the emergency room and serving as the primary point of contact for nursing teams. In addition to working in inpatient hospital and emergency department settings, primary care residents spend a substantial amount of clinical time in a primary care outpatient clinic, functioning as primary care doctors for thousands of patients.

In March 2020, there were 144,988 residents and fellows in the United States, distributed among 12,092 programs nationwide, with the greatest percentage of residents training in traditional primary care specialties, specifically internal medicine (20.2%), family medicine (9.5%), and pediatrics (6.4%) [1]. Shortly after the onset of the pandemic, the Accreditation Council for Graduate Medical Education (ACGME, the national accreditation organization for resident and fellowship programs) released several position statements providing guidance to programs on how to best balance the needs of hospital systems and the ongoing safety and protection of learners. While recognizing the historic and unique circumstances surrounding the COVID-19 pandemic, the ACGME reaffirmed that programs must continue to (a) protect work hour requirements, (b) provide appropriate training in treatment and infection control protocols to any residents caring for COVID-19 patients, (c) continue to provide appropriate supervision for the level of education of a resident or fellow, and (d) fellows should continue to function in their core specialty [2].

Clinical Duties and Learning Environments

The remainder of this chapter will focus primarily on the pandemic experiences of family medicine residents, starting first with the clinical impacts. Family medicine training is primarily based in hospital, emergency department, and outpatient clinic environments with some time also spent in other settings (e.g., doing home visits, supporting community sports teams, rounding in nursing homes, working at community health fairs). The first year of residency is called internship and typically involves alternating time between an outpatient continuity clinic and rotating through the major medical disciplines. Many interns spend time learning on non-family medicine teams such as OB GYN, emergency medicine, internal medicine, pediatrics, and critical care. Hospital teams usually consist of a first-year intern, a second- or third-year senior, and a supervising attending faculty physician. Senior residents continue to rotate on hospital teams while spending increasing amounts of time in the outpatient clinic, honing their skills as primary care physicians providing ongoing, longitudinal continuity of care for panels of patients. Residents learn primary management of their outpatient panel including responding to patient phone calls and electronic messages, following up on test results, communicating with specialists, and completing paperwork. Much of this work is done asynchronously while rotating on other services, or during evenings and weekends. A primary learning point during family medicine residency is learning how to balance direct clinical care hours with the volume of this asynchronous workload. This chapter will describe the pandemic's impact on family medicine residents in a broad array of clinical settings.

Family Medicine Residents Doing Inpatient Medicine

The pandemic affected all parts of the medical system—straining and highlighting deficiencies in the health care infrastructure in the United States. Family medicine residents working in the hospital came face-to-face with this strain and cared for some of the sickest patients with COVID-19. At baseline, inpatient rotations can be challenging and involve long hours and care of complex patients. The pandemic exacerbated this experience for residents given the severity of illness, impact on the population and effect on the health care system. Residents experienced the moral distress of trying to provide patients with safe, equitable care in hospitals that were overflowing with patients. This made it challenging to get patients the proper care they needed and deserved.

New York was one of the hardest hit areas of the country early in the pandemic. In Yonkers at St. Joseph's Medical Center, all off-site rotations were temporarily suspended, and the residents' schedules were restructured to cover the inpatient services. Additional residents were added on each shift on the inpatient medical units, intensive care unit (ICU), and emergency department (ED) while ensuring adherence to duty hours regulations. Podiatry residents were integrated into the family medicine inpatient teams to help care for the substantial increase in the inpatient census. Bed triage was an enormous challenge as the hospital reached maximum capacity. Personal protective equipment (PPE) shortages required rationing and reuse of N95 masks and gowns in the first several weeks of the pandemic. Daily outreach was provided to ensure that residents had at least minimum PPE to feel safe.

Due to differing state public health recommendations and regional variation in population density, rates of severe COVID-19 illness were highly variable with some regions experiencing high volumes while other parts of the country (e.g., the Pacific Northwest) avoided some of the initial overwhelming waves. Residents in Oregon hospital systems were spared during the first waves of the pandemic and even experienced lower than average patient census as elective procedures were delayed or canceled. However, residents reported that after this initial lull, both the number and acuity of patients they cared for in the hospital increased. Even between COVID-19 spikes, the number of patients in the hospital reached unprecedented levels as patients who had been avoiding medical care came in with decompensated chronic conditions. Later in the pandemic we began to see the consequences of delayed preventive care and chronic disease management (e.g., higher numbers of patients being diagnosed with late-stage cancers).

In California, COVID-19 was devastating from the start. The initial lockdown contributed to a low hospital census in the early weeks, but hospitals very quickly were overrun by patients with severe COVID-19 infections as the virus spread. Residents were faced with caring for patients in ambulances or in tents outside of the hospital ED due to lack of space and beds. Resources for physicians and patients became scarce as the sheer number of patients at any point in time far outweighed anything the country had prepared for. Supplies of commonly used medications for pain or blood pressure were low. Hospitals ran out of crucial, lifesaving machinery and items such as blood products or ventilators. One co-author clearly remembers a colleague describing the horrific scene in the ED of a patient admitted for a gastrointestinal bleed who needed to undergo a massive transfusion protocol. The patient never received blood and died in the ED.

Outside of disaster scenarios, hospitals in the US are generally able to manage all patients who seek care. Triage protocols are available for disaster scenarios. Typically, these protocols are applied during events of a limited duration, such as natural disasters. During the COVID-19 pandemic, at one hospital in California, it became customary practice to assign a Sequential Organ Failure Assessment (SOFA) score for every patient admitted to the hospital. A SOFA score assesses several organ systems in the body and assigns a score based on the function or rate of failure of that organ. The higher the SOFA score, the higher the likelihood of mortality. While it is commonly used for ICU patients to track their progress, during the pandemic it became something physicians used (1) to determine how quickly a patient may decompensate and unintendedly (2) to triage ventilators. The unspoken consensus was that patients with the lowest SOFA scores may be more likely to receive ventilators upon rapid decompensation since they are more likely to recover if given the chance. This life-or-death decision, sometimes occurring multiple times per day during the peak COVID-19 period, was difficult for any physician, but especially for residents who were just starting to learn clinical medicine. This intense triage mentality persisted for at least 6–9 months until the ventilator shortage gradually eased, marking a turning point in managing the crisis.

When ICUs were full, the medical floor and ED rooms ended up having to try to provide intensive level care without the same resources. As one Oregon resident said, "People were boarding in the ED [admitted to the hospital but without a room on a medicine floor] still on day 3 of hospital admission, and they were crumping [slang for quickly decompensating] and they needed pressors, which we were doing through peripheral lines until we could get a fellow down to the ED who could place a central line." Family medicine residents typically do short rotations in an ICU as part of their training, but many do not routinely provide ICU level care during residency. During the pandemic, these residents managed respiratory support with high-flow oxygen and ventilators, titrated medications for blood pressure support, and tried to keep patients stable until an ICU bed opened. Residents reported feeling their attendings were less knowledgeable about ICU-level care, so with the ICU overwhelmed, residents relied on their short rotations for knowledge on how best to support patients. Residents were also pulled from other rotations to help cover inpatient and ICU rotations as colleagues got sick and the volume of patients increased. At some hospitals, residents were also leading oversized teams with patients that far outweighed their normal ACGME set capacity and census. In some cases, family medicine and internal medicine residents were leading teams with residents from multiple specialties with little experience caring for patients on a typical medicine ward. The vast majority of residents did not receive any overtime compensation or days off in exchange, although most residents viewed this as a duty to their patients and colleagues.

In addition to working overtime, feeling overwhelmed and experiencing heightened moral distress, the shortage of PPE was profound. With the emergence of universal mask mandates in March 2020, hospitals nationwide faced an abrupt crisis in available PPE including surgical masks, N-95 respirators, face shields, and gowns. For many residents, PPE was initially entirely unavailable due to limited stock. In April 2020, 50% of New York City residency program directors reported residents across all specialties having to work with suboptimal PPE, with 99% of residents reporting reuse or extended use of their masks [3]. As the supply of hospital-grade PPE gradually dwindled nationwide, non-medical grade PPE became more commonly used as some protection was better than nothing at all. Historical norms of medical learner hierarchy often dictated in-person care of patients and usage of limited PPE. Some hospitals created protocols to accommodate ACGME rules and regulations while rationing PPE. For example, at some institutions, only one resident physician could enter the room to see the patient while others on the team cared for the patient from afar. At other places, all residents entered the room but each resident was allowed one set of PPE per day. Others had residents refrain from seeing patients in person altogether during the surge to protect them from unknown exposures with suboptimal PPE. By mid-2020, most family medicine residents nationwide reported feeling safe about the amount of PPE available at their institution, though notably 15.2% of residents still did not feel the availability of PPE was adequate to keep them reasonably safe from contracting the virus [4].

Family Medicine Residents Doing Outpatient Medicine

A core part of a family medicine residency is working as a primary care physician (PCP) for a panel of patients in a longitudinal continuity clinic. At least 40 weeks a year must involve providing care to a panel of patients in the family medicine clinic, with no more than eight interrupted weeks in a row. In 2020, family medicine residents were expected to complete 1650 in-person patient encounters in their longitudinal outpatient clinic by the end of residency. It is in continuity clinics that residents learn the majority of outpatient medicine, build significant mentoring relationships with faculty, and develop longitudinal relationships with patients. The scope of outpatient family medicine is very broad, including care of newborns, pregnant women, and elderly adults. Many people affectionately call family medicine the specialty that cares for patients "from cradle to grave." In addition to the inclusive age range, the scope of practice is broad and comprehensive. Care provided also expands to meet the needs of patient subpopulations and communities being served. For example, in recent years, many family medicine residency clinics include gender-affirming care, full spectrum reproductive health care, and substance use treatment as a standard part of their outpatient training. As a family medicine resident advances in their training, they gain more independence when physically seeing patients in clinic and managing administrative duties, and their panel size grows. By the final year of training, individual residents see 20–24 patients per day and manage hundreds of patients as part of a continuity panel.

In the first few months of the pandemic, 81.5% of family medicine residents experienced a decrease in their clinical activity. Reportedly, 52.7% of family medicine residents were reassigned medical duties outside their previously assigned duties. Of those reassigned, most were somewhat or very comfortable with this decision despite most of these reassignments being nonvoluntary. An estimated 10% were asked to work in a different specialty than family medicine or their previously assigned rotation [4]. By early 2021, 50% of surveyed family medicine residents were concerned they would not meet necessary graduation requirements for total number of outpatient visits at their home continuity clinic, and 41% reported feeling less prepared for the next stage of their career [5]. These feelings were magnified in the Northeast and South compared to the West, likely reflecting the increased disease burden and clinical care disruption in these regions.

One of the most significant impacts the pandemic had on outpatient training was the rapid expansion of telehealth and sharp increase in the number of virtual visits. Before the COVID-19 pandemic, providing medical care virtually, often referred to as telehealth or telemedicine, was an emerging field not yet integrated into residency education; primary care residents were not allowed to care for patients via video or phone visits. This quickly changed with the emergence of COVID-19. By June 2020, telehealth services had been implemented or expanded at virtually all family medicine residency programs nationwide, and residents were quickly starting to care for patients using video platforms and phone visits. This shift proved that many medical appointments, including follow-ups, consultations, and even some diagnostics, could be effectively conducted virtually. It challenged the traditional in-person model and demonstrated the potential for greater flexibility, accessibility, and efficiency in health care. While most residents were participating in virtual visits, only about half of residents nationwide were reporting that they had received formal training on best practices for telehealth visits by summer 2020 [4].

The response to increasing virtual access has been mixed. A survey of family medicine residents at three programs in different regions and practice settings found that while some residents praised increased access to care and flexibility for patients, others felt that virtual care was often substandard and could erode the patient-physician relationship [6]. Internal medicine and family medicine residents in Georgia felt that telemedicine decreased visit time, improved clinic time management, and reduced anxiety/nervousness about contracting COVID-19 in the early part of the pandemic [7]. Of note, increased virtual access may have also increased access to care for many patients who have difficulties with transportation or physical disabilities. It also promoted creativity around in-home monitoring of chronic diseases such as diabetes and hypertension.

In Yonkers, NY, during the early pandemic, the outpatient clinic was primarily treating patients by telemedicine and staffed by pregnant residents. In March and April 2020, the Yonkers continuity patients were too afraid to come into clinic. As in other parts of the state, elective procedures, well visits for adults and children, chronic medical condition follow-up visits, and even prenatal care essentially stopped. If patients had complaints, they scheduled telemedicine visits to address them. However, in this population health care disparities play a significant role. Many patients, especially geriatric patients, did not have access to telemedicine and did not seek medical care to minimize their COVID-19 exposure risk. Virtual medicine was implemented as a necessity in Yonkers, NY, but neither residents nor patients found this interaction as effective or as rewarding as direct patient-physician encounters, and it was phased out as patients started to return to the clinic.

A trend noted by residents in Oregon was the change in patient expectations of PCPs' virtual availability over the course of the pandemic. As clinics shifted to provide more virtual care, patients began to send more patient portal messages, which had increased by 157% of pre-pandemic levels by December 2020 [8]. Managing this increased volume of messages and other in-basket management tasks mainly happens between scheduled patients in clinic or before or after scheduled clinical duties, which was an additional stressor for residents already working 40–80 hours of scheduled time per week.

Depending on location, the types of patients that residents saw in clinic changed as well. Some clinics set up "respiratory clinics" to direct all patients with respiratory symptoms so that they could be seen by providers with adequate PPE and potentially infect fewer clinicians. This meant that some residents saw fewer standard respiratory symptoms and associated complications, such as ear infections, bacterial sinus infections, eustachian tube dysfunction, and classic childhood viruses.

One family medicine residency clinic in San Antonio, Texas, noticed a marked decrease in pediatric visits, in particular the well child visits for Texas Health Steps and vaccinations. Parents expressed concerns about bringing healthy infants and young children to a primary care facility full of waiting patients with upper respiratory symptoms. The vaccination rate therefore decreased prompting the department to open a pediatric clinic for well child visits/vaccinations after hours on specific Saturday mornings throughout the pandemic. This was quite successful with parents feeling more comfortable bringing children to an empty clinic that had been cleaned thoroughly between visits, therefore minimizing exposures.

Another aspect of training that was different during the early years of the pandemic was in counseling patients about vaccines. In some places, patients were frustrated about the early shortages of vaccines and clamoring to get vaccinated as soon as possible. In other places, there were high rates of vaccine hesitancy. For example, in Texas the political atmosphere surrounding COVID-19 vaccines inevitably exposed residents to conversations that required mindful practice of motivational interviewing skills, as well as de-escalation behavioral techniques when vaccine recommendations were met with conflict. Anecdotally, these interactions provided unique learning opportunities but were also a source of stress and frustration that adversely affected residents' wellness. Residents in Oregon were initially very motivated to convince patients to vaccinate against COVID-19. When their efforts were met with mixed results in patient uptake (and sometimes hostility), residents reflected on the challenging balance between prioritizing public health and patient autonomy. Some reported becoming more apathetic about the need to convince patients about the merits of the vaccine over time. From a public health perspective, more vaccinated patients in a population reduces the transmission and severity of the disease. Patient autonomy describes the right of the individual to determine what treatments or medical recommendations they undergo, including whether to accept or refuse vaccination. Many residents reported initially being highly motivated to engage patients in conversation around vaccines, strongly recommend them, and try to debunk vaccine misinformation or conspiracies. However, over the course of the pandemic, residents reported reducing the amount of time and energy they spent discussing vaccines with patients who did not seem open to conversation. Some Oregon residents reported that earlier in the pandemic it felt like a moral failing on the resident's part if they were unable to convince a patient to get vaccinated but that they had to make peace with their inability to change some patients' minds given the amount of time and emotional energy required to have those discussions multiple times per day. In some populations with high vaccine skepticism, residents reported offering vaccination and to answer any questions, and if a patient refused, they dropped the subject to preserve rapport. Their pragmatic view was that the risk of alienating the patient was higher than the chance of persuading them to get vaccinated, so the best thing for the patient was to preserve the patient-provider relationship.

Family Medicine Resident Rotations

Family medicine residency clinical training encompasses participating in several required core rotations as well as seeking out elective and other non-core experiences. Early in the pandemic, the most disrupted rotation was geriatrics and the least disrupted was ICU, without significant variation among type of program or community size. Disruptions to geriatrics curricula were likely influenced by senior living facilities closing to outside providers and visitors to protect their at-risk residents. Other rotations with higher amounts of reported disruption were surgery and family medicine outpatient clinic sites, reflecting the impact of stay-at-home orders and cancellation of elective surgeries. Surveyed family medicine residency program directors were not significantly concerned that early curricula disruptions would negatively impact overall accreditation, though there was some variation by region with increased concern in the Mid-Atlantic (New York, Pennsylvania, New Jersey) and East North Central regions (Wisconsin, Michigan, Ohio, Indiana, Illinois) [9].

In a national survey done in early 2021, 83% of surveyed residents reported that the pandemic had a negative impact on their training with 59% reporting a decline in hands-on procedural experience, 61% reporting having missed a scheduled rotation (usually due to facilities not accepting residents at that time), and 34% were still reporting a reduction in clinical volume at the end of 2020 [5]. In Oregon, there were immediate disruptions in rural health rotations with residents pulled from a rural general surgery rotation and rural primary care rotation from March—May 2020 until clarity could be reached on travel safety and exposure risk. Additional disruptions were seen at off-site training locations including local Planned Parenthood clinics, county underserved clinics, and high school health centers (located in schools closed to in-person instruction). Oregon residents reported feeling the biggest impact to elective training occurred in sports medicine, advanced reproductive health care, and geriatrics. They felt they were able to obtain adequate training either during or shortly after residency but that true mastery of those skills felt delayed.

Educational Didactics and Changes in How Residents Interacted Outside of Clinical Rotations

While family medicine residents spend the majority of their time in clinical environments simultaneously caring for patients and advancing their skills as new physicians, they also spend some time participating in didactic teaching sessions and other non-clinical environments. COVID-19 propelled the virtual mediums for didactic learning to new heights. National data show that virtual classrooms and video conferencing rapidly became the primary residency education didactic method of teaching in the immediate first stage of the COVID-19 pandemic [4]. Virtual learning provided a way for attending physicians and residents to connect despite being forced to quarantine or remain separated. These environments allowed learning to continue in ways that did not expose individuals to COVID-19 and also reduced the need to spend time and money traveling to a distinct location. Initially, benefits of virtual learning were applauded. For example, in a national survey of family medicine residents and faculty in May–June 2020, two-thirds of respondents reporting wanting to see distance learning options continue long term after the pandemic [4]. However, by early 2021, only 26% of family medicine residents nationally felt that virtual didactics were superior to in-person learning, with 63% of respondents reporting the pandemic had an overall negative impact on their didactic activities [5]. Many found the extended virtual sessions to be exhaustive and tedious. Many advocated for a return to "normalcy" and increased interpersonal connection, especially as new COVID-19 variants became milder and less deadly.

There were both advantages and disadvantages noted by residents who commented about the virtual educational environment. Some residents liked being able to watch lectures and learn in the convenience of their own home, often saving time on commuting or money on food. Residents also liked the increased flexibility inherent in virtual didactics with the ability to watch lectures while on off-service rotations or while at home taking care of children. Alternatively, they noted the difficulty of discussing sensitive topics in a virtual forum and the awkwardness and uncertainty associated with learning virtual lecture etiquette. Some also experienced challenges when sessions dedicated to supporting resident well-being (e.g., Balint or support groups) were conducted virtually. In addition, varying levels of technical experience contributed to differences in lecturer comfort with the medium and subjectively affected the quality of some lectures.

In some cases, virtual offerings and formats sprang up almost organically. For example, in New York during the early months of the pandemic, a self-study curricula was designed with a combination of assigned review articles, modules, webinars, and question sets to allow for patient care and resident rest. It was quickly evident that residents were looking at all of the sources to understand COVID-19, the impact of the pandemic, and how to best manage their patients. A network of shared resources and guidelines became a regular "didactic." Video didactics were implemented in addition as the COVID-19 admissions started to diminish and other patients remained apprehensive about coming to the ED. Ultimately, hybrid didactics were developed where attendance could be either in-person or remote, allowing each resident the choice of how they prefer to learn. In a state with some of the most restrictive requirements for schools and didactic learning, residents in Oregon spent many months in a virtual learning environment and had varied thoughts on whether paying attention and staying engaged with lectures was easier or more difficult than in-person lectures.

Another significant expansion in virtual interactions in family medicine residency programs centered around the annual residency application cycle, which happens each year between September–March. Historically, fourth-year medical students have spent thousands of dollars traveling to interview in person at residency programs across the country. With increasing competitiveness for limited residency spots, many medical students were starting to apply to dozens of programs and sometimes completing upwards of 20–30 in-person interviews. Over 50% of medical students have historically also chosen to participate in visiting rotations to improve their chances of matching into a desired residency program. While these in-person interviews and rotations were often a significant financial burden for medical students, they did offer students an opportunity to gain insight into a future program and expand networking opportunities [10].

Due to the COVID-19 pandemic, the 2020–2021 recruitment cycle was completed entirely virtually. Three years later, many residency programs have maintained at least some component of virtual interviews with perceived benefits in the realms of convenience, time savings, cost savings, and environmental footprint. The primary drawback identified by recent studies has been difficulty in programs and applicants assessing each other to find a good fit [11]. Programs and applicants have evolved alternate ways to address this drawback with some programs offering a "second look" and some residency applicants choosing to visit high interest programs on an alternate day. Virtual socials also provide a more in-depth look for potential applicants by chatting with residents and faculty in a more casual manner.

Home Life and Wellness

The impact of the COVID-19 pandemic on resident wellness evolved throughout the pandemic. In an early national survey (May–June 2020), 16.8% of family medicine residents and 24.5% of faculty screened positive for higher emotional distress, and 39.7% of residents and 35.4% of faculty screened positive on a single-question burnout questionnaire. The most identified stressor at that time from both groups was concern for their families' health. Both groups identified that the pandemic had provided some positive elements to combat burnout including more time with loved ones, increased sense of shared purpose/camaraderie with colleagues, and more time for self-directed learning. For those with high burnout, institution-provided well-being support services were helpful, and education on how to properly use PPE improved perceptions of safety [4].

Different from the national trend, residents in Yonkers, NY, were not reporting burnout. In fact, in Yonkers, a burnout survey was given at multiple intervals in the first year of the pandemic, and no residents reported symptoms of burnout. In retrospect, residency administration reflected on hospital and community support for the residency program and the medical staff being an infusion of energy. There was a steady supply of donated meals, snacks, PPE, scrubs, self-care products, and free educational resources and meditation apps. A wellness curricula was developed which encouraged self-care and relaxation. Most importantly, there was an unprecedented sense of collaboration and support among the residents themselves, a true team environment.

An updated national survey of family medicine residents later in the pandemic utilized a more comprehensive burnout scale and demonstrated an increased burnout burden. During January–February 2021, 52% (n = 119) of respondents met the threshold for personal burnout, 59% (n = 134) for work-related burnout, and 29% (n = 65) for client-related burnout. In this study, there were not statistically significant differences in burnout based on region of the country or training year [5].

In our experiences, there were many reasons for the increase in resident burnout in most areas of the country. Ongoing high inpatient census numbers, delayed care leading patients to present at more advanced disease states, and an overwhelmed system where referrals and surgeries were delayed and hard to access for patients on their continuity panels contributed to resident burnout and a sense of moral injury. Family medicine residents often rotate through other departments and are stretched to learn a broad scope of medicine. When the pandemic began, some programs deployed residents even more broadly, and they were sent to areas of the hospital or community that were not on their schedules. Their skills often did not match the surgical or intensive care needs utilized at bedside, leading to feelings of strain and inadequacy. In addition, some residents struggled with being in primary patient-facing roles of the medical system without having much ability to affect how well the system was functioning. Some residents also expressed frustration with the broader systems in place in our country that, in their opinion, worsened an already challenging situation.

Family medicine residents become very adept at human connection and communication in their training; however, they were called upon to provide even more communication than usual during the early months of the pandemic which took a toll on their mental health. For example, when families were not allowed to be with patients at bedside, residents were often tasked with making daily calls to family members to inform and explain their loved ones' health status and complete end-of-life discussions. Though an important task, this contributed to resident burnout as they held daily the emotional struggles of families unable to be with their loved ones as well as their anger and frustrations with a system struggling to deliver positive outcomes. End-of-life discussions are part of residency training, however residents during the pandemic engaged in these discussions more often than in previous years. These sicker patients also had more frequent "codes" involving the need to perform chest compressions and other heroic measures to bring them back to life, which was especially impactful to residents earlier in their training. They were also delivering this care to sick and infectious patients while having limited access to appropriate PPE.

As with most people in the population, residents were experiencing social isolation. Residency is a unique time in life when many people move across the country, away from friends and family, to complete their residency training. Residents often live alone or with other residents who have demanding work schedules and are seldom at home. Being in a new city and being unable to physically meet up socially with friends, family, co-residents and program faculty caused residents significant stress and increased their sense of burnout. Attempts to connect virtually were often difficult, so many residents got most of their social interaction from work. A broad survey of primary care and surgical residents in the US and Canada in November 2020 found that residents saw a reduction in dating frequency and social event attendance because of the pandemic. This was greater among the primary care residents compared to surgical residents [12]. The limits on in-person interaction caused residents to have increased feelings of isolation and loneliness.

Coupled with the social isolation that blanketed the country, residents work and learn in hospitals and clinics. Most, if not all, residents were worried about contracting COVID-19 and then spreading it to their loved ones. As one Oregon resident said, "I remember just feeling so scared and anxious and then also worrying that I was going to catch this disease and bring it home to my partner and potentially, you know, kill my partner." Many residents avoided visiting family members for years during the pandemic to attempt to mitigate risk. Some residents reported feeling those outside of medicine were not able to understand what they were going through, which made it difficult to share their experiences with close friends and family members. Some residents felt a sense of betrayal when seeing their friends and family go to concerts or on trips that increased their risk of contracting or spreading COVID-19 to others.

Most residents are young adults, and many have young children or are actively planning to have children soon. Like many non-physician parents nationwide, residents with children faced unique challenges during the COVID-19 pandemic. In a 2022 survey asking recent parenting residents in Oregon about the impact of COVID-19 on their families, residents shared a heightened fear of spreading illness to family and vulnerable kids, increased challenges with childcare and daycare closures, and isolation from parenting support networks. One resident shared, "Being a parent, during COVID, in residency has been the most difficult and isolating experience I would say of my life." For another resident, "I constantly worried early on of my ability to work effectively, keep myself safe, keep my family safe, and not miss work due to exposures and sickness. That was really, really hard to navigate that season." A few residents did share that the change to virtual didactics allowed more time at home with family, which they perceived to be a positive change. One remarked, "I spent more time at home, which allowed more time with kids, but also made work more difficult at times (trying to negotiate work and childcare at home)."

Beyond Family Medicine Residencies

This chapter is not meant to fully capture the experience of all resident physicians during the pandemic; to do so could require a book unto itself. However, we would be remiss not to acknowledge the pandemic's impact on residents from non-primary care specialties, particularly regarding clinical duties which can vary substantially between specialties. A systematic, international review in November 2020 described broad themes of how the COVID-19 pandemic impacted residency training in both surgical and non-surgical fields. The most common effect was decreased clinical activity and potential failure to meet the program's training requirements, particularly in surgical specialties during the months in which elective cases were suspended at most hospitals. Positive themes included implementation of virtual learning tools, expansion of telemedicine and more time for self-study. Notably, this international review found minimal literature on the impact on internal medicine residents, and there was no mention of family medicine programs [13].

Other surveys of non-family medicine and non-primary care program directors during the early phase of COVID-19 echoed the themes noted above, including concerns about suspension of surgical procedures, redeployment of residents to help directly with COVID-19 care, decreased contact time with patients, use of virtual didactics, and broad concerns about residents not meeting required case numbers [9]. Most of this literature was collected and published in 2020–2021, reflecting the immediate impact of the first 3–6 months of the pandemic but not yet capturing longer-term impacts on graduation rates or professional competency post-training.

Interventional cardiology fellows in New York reported an immediate drop in procedural numbers (typically cardiac catheterization lab procedures) with one fellow reporting that their "training [was] thwarted right at the time we would normally be gaining more independence. All potential job prospects and impending offers are on hold" [14]. In May 2020, thoracic surgery residency program directors also reported temporary pauses on elective procedures at all their institutions, with 83% of residents having transitioned to a non-standard schedule, and some impact on overall case volumes for junior and graduating trainees. At three programs, thoracic surgery residents were reassigned to non-surgical services to help with the care of COVID-19 patients [15]. A group of urology program directors surveyed at the end of March 2020, reported an average of 50% reduction in weekly clinical hours, and 26% of programs had already started redeploying their residents to other fields. Sixty percent of programs were concerned that residents would not meet minimum case requirements due to the pandemic [16]. Similar concerns about reduced case volumes were also reported in pediatric gastroenterology fellowship programs [17] and oral and maxillofacial surgery (OMFS) residencies [18].

In radiology, outpatient imaging volumes decreased more than 70%, and inpatient volumes decreased as much as 50%. Along with reduction in total imaging cases, radiology residents also faced redeployment, with an estimated 46% of redeployed residents being sent to clinical departments outside of radiology and worse perceived morale among these programs [19].

Some procedural residents faced increased risk of exposure to contracting COVID-19. Anesthesia residents in New York City appeared to be at higher risk of contracting COVID-19 compared to their local peers in internal medicine and pediatrics [3]. OMFS residents also faced increased risk of exposure to COVID-19 due to the nature of the surgeries and exams they perform and the risk of aerosol generation from the respiratory tract. Notably over half the OMFS programs also reported shortages of PPE, particularly N95 respirators [18]. Some pediatric gastroenterology programs described altering clinical duties for fellows who were pregnant, had other health conditions, had childcare needs, or had spouses working ED or ICU shifts [17].

Residents, like most health care workers, are considered essential workers with very few work-from-home options. Residents with young children depend on reliable childcare, including on evenings and weekends. Often, residents are in households where both parents work outside the home. For example, at our institution in Oregon, over 50% of recent resident parents have full-time working spouses, and over 50% rely on a center-based daycare for childcare. In the spring of 2020, many daycares reduced hours, changed illness policies, or shut down completely in response to the pandemic. National childcare data demonstrates that daycare supply and availability has still not yet returned to pre-pandemic levels with ongoing variation by state. As in most places, Oregon residents were navigating the early years of the pandemic with dwindling options for childcare. Oregon estimates showed a drop of 36% in the number of childcare employees from February to April 2020 (which was midrange for national data), and this number was still down 12% in June 2022, in the bottom bracket nationally. Oregon was also one of only 11 states that showed a net decrease in number of childcare programs statewide after the pandemic [20]. Disruptions in the childcare industry leave resident parents reliant on spouses, extended family members, expensive in-home paid care, or forced to use limited sick days while asking coworkers to cover their clinical duties. Although there are now work hour restrictions on how many hours residents should be working during a given time period, resident work hours are more unpredictable than in many other professions with less certainty about when they will complete a clinic session or complete rounds in the hospital setting.

Data is still emerging about resident parents and their unique experiences during the pandemic. There is no national data available on how the pandemic impacted male versus female resident parents differently. However, a 2021 JAMA article described experiences of work-family conflict and mental health symptoms by gender among non-resident physician parents during the COVID-19 pandemic. Among this cohort study of 276 physicians, during the pandemic, mothers were more likely than fathers to be "responsible for childcare or schooling and household tasks...to work primarily from home and to reduce their work hours." Female physicians were also more likely to lose childcare during the COVID-19 pandemic and were twice as likely to voluntarily reduce their work hours during the pandemic compared to men [21].

Considerations for Future Pandemics

When looking ahead to future pandemics, residency programs must have sufficient systems in place to cover critical services, protect resident physical and mental health, prioritize in-scope resident training, and continue to provide high-quality patient care. Residency programs need to have established on-call ("jeopardy") systems with enough depth to support multiple residents being out for extended periods. We recommend residencies consider a formal "extended leave coverage" policy in addition to their routine sick call jeopardy policy to cover the multi-day absences we saw during COVID-19 illness and quarantines. The residents available for this extended leave coverage would likely be assigned to an outpatient or elective rotation while staying available to cover critical rotations. At our residency in Oregon, the extended leave coverage rotation has continued to provide back-up coverage when residents are out for extended personal or family leave (such as pregnancies, mental health leaves, and family deaths or illnesses). We have found it helpful for senior residents (rather than interns) to be assigned to this coverage block as they have more familiarity with the variety of services we cover, are more likely to have the required badge access at partnering institutions, and can step into either a senior or junior role. A consideration could also be to coordinate with other residency programs in the area to share coverage responsibilities and resources. This could include agreements for temporary exchange or support from nearby programs. Due to ACGME regulations, exceptions may be considered for financial incentives for potential resident exchange programs during future pandemics.

Residency programs should be prepared for their residents to be managing very sick patients on standard floors while awaiting ICU space and need to know the upper scope of the inpatient faculty who will be supervising their residents. If attendings are not comfortable managing BiPAP, high-flow nasal cannula and starting pressors on peripheral lines, we recommend considering dedicated continuing medical education (CME) sessions and simulation training, and understanding what ICU consult resources are available at your institution. Programs may also consider adapting assessments to include evaluations and expectations related to pandemic-specific scenarios, such as management of critically ill patients.

Procedural training programs need to be prepared for cancellations of elective cases and the impact this will have on resident case numbers. ACGME recommends residency programs utilize competency-based assessments of residents and fellows (rather than relying entirely on traditional time-based or volume-based measures) and has provided a framework for assessing core competencies. Examples of alternate forms of assessment include in-training exams, faculty feedback, direct observation, and multisource feedback models such as a 360° evaluation [22]. If residency programs are not already utilizing a competency-based framework, we recommend a transition to including these kinds of evaluations prior to the next pandemic. We also recommend an ongoing robust investment in simulation resources including computer-based simulations, standardized patients, mannequin patient simulators, cadaver labs, mock codes, and emerging virtual reality simulators.

Support for residents extends to helping them with essential needs outside of work, especially when they have limited time for shopping, cleaning, car maintenance, and other tasks. For example, in San Antonio, early on in the pandemic supermarkets were not able to meet demand of supplies for extended periods of time. Our resident physicians and first responders were unable to find necessary goods after work, increasing stress and deteriorating well-being. Our institution reached out to the major supermarket HEB and created a program for first responders at the university hospital. After enrolling, our pickup orders were prioritized to ensure we could obtain necessary goods. This was very helpful for morale and overall well-being of our providers. We recommend institutions proactively seek out relationships with local entities that can establish similar programs in other areas.

Incorporating pandemic-related training as part of residency curricula may be a crucial consideration for the future, given the challenges faced during COVID-19 and the likelihood of future global health emergencies. Residency programs should allocate specific time for clinical simulation training that focuses on pandemic-related scenarios, including triage, resource allocation, and the management of critically ill patients with severe respiratory conditions like those seen in viral pandemics. This type of hands-on training can better equip residents and attendings to manage high-acuity patients in ED or non-ICU settings, where overflow from critical care units may become necessary.

By 2021, most family medicine residency programs had already adapted their residency curricula to include didactic training on COVID-19 resources, guidelines and policies, with a minority of programs expanding this training to include contract tracing, health literacy, and communication skills. It will continue to be important for family medicine residency programs to include training on public and population health, particularly as it relates to pandemic preparedness and critical aspects of crisis management. These modules should include training on contact tracing, outbreak response, health literacy, and communication skills to ensure physicians are prepared to engage with the public and manage community-level health crises. To further enhance preparedness, residency programs could offer training in population health, pandemic response frameworks, and ethical decision-making in resource-limited settings. One proposed idea would be to create a certificate of added qualification (CAQ) in public health training which would allow family physicians to gain additional expertise in public health training. Embedding this kind of certification within residency programs would require programs to continue to recruit and maintain faculty with a public health credential, such as a Master of Public Health (MPH) [23]. An alternate idea is to embed public health competencies—such as crisis leadership and interagency coordination—into the curricula for all residents, allowing residents to understand the broader societal impact of pandemics and their role in public health interventions. These steps will not only prepare residents for the clinical demands of future pandemics but will also empower them to play a key role in preventing and managing large-scale public health emergencies. To maximize efficiency, residencies could partner with local departments of public health or communication public health organizations to help create this type of curricula.

Resident training in communication is a high priority at all times and became even more critical during the early years of the pandemic. This training should be more clearly integrated into the curricula in preparation for future pandemics. During pandemics, physicians should focus on delivering clear, timely, and compassionate information to both medical teams and patients. Residents need to be adept at managing patient expectations, especially when addressing delays or changes in care due to resource constraints. Training should also include skills for combating misinformation by providing accurate, evidence-based updates.

Telemedicine training should be a core part of the residency curricula, given its critical role during the COVID-19 pandemic and its increasing importance in future health care delivery. As in-person visits were limited, telehealth became essential for maintaining continuity of care while minimizing infection risk. Residents must be trained not only in the technical aspects of using telemedicine platforms but also in effectively conducting virtual consultations, managing patient assessments remotely, and triaging cases based on urgency. This training should also focus on fostering strong patient relationships, even in virtual settings, while ensuring clear communication and high-quality care. Incorporating telemedicine into residency programs will prepare future physicians to adapt to changing health care environments, providing flexible and accessible care during pandemics and beyond.

Many institutions have stronger virtual didactics now compared to pre-pandemic, which often allows more residents to participate in lectures and provides a degree of flexibility for those with young children or responsibilities at home. Virtual meetings are also now more commonplace, increasing the ability for people to form connections and utilize the perspectives of others. We recommend that residency programs continue to utilize virtual didactics as a part of a blended in-person and remote curricula, prioritizing virtual sessions for topics that do not depend on robust discussion.

We also acknowledge that virtual sessions are not as well suited to certain sensitive or emotional topics. In future pandemics, we recommend attempting to restart in-person small group sessions as soon as possible for curricular elements such as support groups, intern orientation, Balint groups, and resident retreats. Offering ways for residents to connect with each other and their program faculty can help with combating isolation and burnout and will need to be weighed with the risk of potential infection exposure.

In late spring 2020, ACGME published a virtual course and corresponding guidebook for promoting resident and fellow well-being during the COVID-19 pandemic with a dual focus on strategies for promoting well-being during the pandemic and responding to illness and death due to COVID-19. One key recommendation is for all residents and supervisors to be trained in Psychological First Aid (PFA), an evidence-informed approach to reducing stress and promoting recovery for individuals affected by trauma or disasters. Links to training resources are available in the guidebook. Additional recommendations include ensuring ready access to telemental health for residents and fellows, setting up virtual support for quarantined and self-isolating residents, being prepared for daily communication between leadership and trainees, offering temporary sleeping accommodations for residents who need to reduce exposure to family members, monitoring residents for compassion fatigue, and considering virtual resident and fellow peer support groups facilitated by a trained mental health professional. One model offered is CopeColumbia, a guide for virtual peer support groups to address stress and emotional consequences of COVID-19. Finally, the course provides specific recommendations on how programs can respond when a resident, fellow, or colleague becomes ill during a pandemic, or faces the death of a family member or peer. We recommend that all residency program directors be familiar with this salient and comprehensive publication prior to the next pandemic. You will find at the end of the document a COVID-19 Program/Institutional Well-Being Worksheet that provides a framework for programs to self-assess their current programming, identify necessary areas for growth, and document action plans [24]. To build on these recommendations, integrating physician coaching and other proactive well-being resources can further enhance resilience and support during crises. Formal coaching can provide residents and fellows with personalized tools to manage stress, enhance emotional intelligence, and navigate professional challenges. These programs complement the guidebook's strategies, ensuring a holistic approach to physician well-being. By prioritizing coaching, mental health resources, and proactive measures, residency programs can better prepare for future pandemics while fostering a supportive environment for residents and fellows to thrive. It is our hope that by taking proactive steps now, all programs will be better prepared during the next pandemic to protect their residents and fellows while continuing to provide high-quality patient care.

Focusing on resilience and adaptability in residency training is essential for preparing physicians to navigate the challenges of future pandemics. Resilience training should equip residents with the emotional and mental tools to manage stress, uncertainty, and the demands of working in rapidly changing environments. This can be achieved through workshops on mindfulness, stress management, and emotional intelligence, fostering coping strategies that help prevent burnout and enhance well-being. Equally important is cultivating adaptability in clinical practice, encouraging residents to develop a flexible mindset. This involves learning to adjust care based on evolving resource constraints, fluctuating patient volumes, and shifting public health directives. By embracing change and maintaining a focus on high-quality patient care, even under pressure, residents can become more effective in delivering care during health crises. Building these capacities will ensure that future physicians remain resilient and adaptable in the face of unpredictable health care challenges.

Conclusion

While the pandemic was challenging and stressful for those in health care and residency, there were positive changes and lessons learned that can be applied to the future. Many residents reported the pandemic made them feel more confident in their ability to adapt in rapidly changing health situations and handle stressful work. Some residents compared changing and adapting to the pandemic to potential future disasters related to climate change. The pandemic has made them feel more prepared to help patients in future crises and adapt their practice to become more flexible as needed. Many residents now have experience with providing virtual care in a way that was unthinkable before the pandemic. This creates much more flexibility both for providers and for patients with health conditions that affect their mobility, or social and financial situations that make it difficult for them to regularly travel to their doctor's office.

The pandemic also highlighted the importance of residents in the health care system and that many institutions rely on them to function. In a stressed health care system, the needs of patients and hospitals were often at odds with the need for residents to have enough time for learning and consolidating knowledge. Residents gain valuable knowledge and skills during their residency but are also providing a critical service for hospitals and are deserving of rights and protections.

The COVID-19 pandemic was an unprecedented event for which no hospital system or residency was fully prepared but demonstrated that, when necessary, even large systems can adapt quickly and creatively to solve challenges. Residencies were put in the challenging position of balancing patient and health care system needs with the need to educate resident physicians. If similar situations occur in the future, residencies can use the lessons from this pandemic to inform their responses. With increased globalization, the chance of another worldwide pandemic is unfortunately not as low as we would wish. However, with the lessons learned during COVID-19, we can face any future events with a dedication to serving our patients and helping to train future generations of doctors.

References

1. Accreditation Council for Graduate Medical Education. Accreditation Council for Graduate Medical Education resource data book: Academic year 2019–2020. https://www.acgme.org/globalassets/pfassets/publicationsbooks/2019-2020_acgme_databook_document.pdf.
2. ACGME reaffirms its four ongoing requirement priorities during COVID-19 pandemic. 2020. https://www.acgme.org/newsroom/2020/4/acgme-reaffirms-its-four-ongoing-requirement-priorities-during-covid-19-pandemic/.
3. Breazzano MP, Shen J, Abdelhakim AH, et al. New York City COVID-19 resident physician exposure during exponential phase of pandemic. J Clin Invest. 2020;130(9):4726–33. https://doi.org/10.1172/jci139587.
4. Awadallah NS, Czaja AS, Fainstad T, et al. The impact of the COVID-19 pandemic on family medicine residency training. Fam Pract. 2021;38(Supplement_1):i9–i15. https://doi.org/10.1093/fampra/cmab012.
5. Upadhyay S, Flora R, Rajaee A, Ugiliweneza B, Iles AM. Training of family medicine residents in the first year of the COVID-19 pandemic. J Family Med Prim Care. 2023;12(5):996–1002. https://doi.org/10.4103/jfmpc.jfmpc_1777_22.
6. Ngo SB, Clark PJ, Parr SE, et al. Moral injury during the COVID-19 pandemic: a Delphi model survey of family medicine residents. Int J Psychiatry Med. 2022;57(4):293–308. https://doi.org/10.1177/00912174211054385.
7. Mills K, Peterson A, McNair M, et al. Virtually serving the underserved: resident perceptions of telemedicine use while training during coronavirus disease 2019. Telemed J E Health. 2022;28(3):391–8. https://doi.org/10.1089/tmj.2021.0112.
8. Holmgren AJ, Downing NL, Tang M, Sharp C, Longhurst C, Huckman RS. Assessing the impact of the COVID-19 pandemic on clinician ambulatory electronic health record use. J Am Med Inform Assoc. 2022;29(3):453–60. https://doi.org/10.1093/jamia/ocab268.
9. Fashner J, Espinoza A, Mainous AG III. COVID-19 disruption to family medicine residency curriculum: results from a 2020 US programme directors survey. Fam Med Community Health. 2021;9(3):e001144. https://doi.org/10.1136/fmch-2021-001144.
10. Domingo A, Rdesinski RE, Stenson A, et al. Virtual residency interviews: applicant perceptions regarding virtual interview effectiveness, advantages, and barriers. J Grad Med Educ. 2022;14(2):224–8.
11. Lochner J. Virtual residency interviews in family medicine. Fam Med. 2022;54(10):765–6.
12. Farr S, Berry JA, Berry DK, et al. The impact of the COVID-19 pandemic on resident physicians well-being in the surgical and primary care specialties in the United States and Canada. Cureus. 2021;13(11):e19677. https://doi.org/10.7759/cureus.19677.
13. Chen SY, Lo HY, Hung SK. What is the impact of the COVID-19 pandemic on residency training: a systematic review and analysis. BMC Med Educ. 2021;21(1):618. https://doi.org/10.1186/s12909-021-03041-8.
14. Gupta T, Nazif TM, Vahl TP, et al. Impact of the COVID-19 pandemic on interventional cardiology fellowship training in the New York metropolitan area: a perspective from the United States epicenter. Catheter Cardiovasc Interv. 2021;97(2):201–5. https://doi.org/10.1002/ccd.28977.
15. Coyan GN, Aranda-Michel E, Kilic A, et al. The impact of COVID-19 on thoracic surgery residency programs in the US: a program director survey. J Card Surg. 2020;35(12):3443–8. https://doi.org/10.1111/jocs.14954.
16. Rosen GH, Murray KS, Greene KL, Pruthi RS, Richstone L, Mirza M. Effect of COVID-19 on urology residency training: a nationwide survey of program directors by the Society of Academic Urologists. J Urol. 2020;204(5):1039–45. https://doi.org/10.1097/ju.0000000000001155.
17. Mallon D, Pohl JF, Phatak UP, et al. Impact of COVID-19 on pediatric gastroenterology fellow training in North America. J Pediatr Gastroenterol Nutr. 2020;71(1):6–11. https://doi.org/10.1097/mpg.0000000000002768.

18. Brar B, Bayoumy M, Salama A, Henry A, Chigurupati R. A survey assessing the early effects of COVID-19 pandemic on oral and maxillofacial surgery training programs. Oral Surg Oral Med Oral Pathol Oral Radiol. 2021;131(1):27–42. https://doi.org/10.1016/j.oooo.2020.08.012.
19. Robbins JB, England E, Patel MD, et al. COVID-19 impact on well-being and education in radiology residencies: a survey of the association of program directors in radiology. Acad Radiol. 2020;27(8):1162–72. https://doi.org/10.1016/j.acra.2020.06.002.
20. Crouse G, Chertner R, Chien N. The impact of the COVID-19 pandemic on the child care industry and workforce. Office of the Assistant Secretary for Planning and Evaluation, U.S. Department of Health and Human Services. https://aspe.hhs.gov/sites/default/files/documents/a6108c6a08b6bc61732f50c2d3220f83/covid-19-child-care-industry.pdf.
21. Frank E, Zhao Z, Fang Y, Rotenstein LS, Sen S, Guille C. Experiences of work-family conflict and mental health symptoms by gender among physician parents during the COVID-19 pandemic. JAMA Netw Open. 2021;4(11):e2134315. https://doi.org/10.1001/jamanetworkopen.2021.34315.
22. Accreditation Council for Graduate Medical Education. Guidance statement on competency-based medical education during COVID-19 residency and fellowship disruptions. https://www.acgme.org/newsroom/2020/9/guidance-statement-on-competency-based-medical-education-during-covid-19-residency-and-fellowship-disruptions/.
23. Sanders M, Fogarty CT, Morley CP, et al. Training family medicine residents to address the COVID-19 pandemic: a national survey of program directors. Fam Med. 2022;54:343–9.
24. Konopasek L, Rackley SJ, Jones W, et al. Guidebook for promoting well-being during the COVID-19 pandemic. Accreditation Council for Graduate Medical Education (ACGME). https://dl.acgme.org/learn/course/guidebook-for-promoting-well-being-during-the-covid-19-pandemic/guidebook/guidebook-for-promoting-well-being-during-the-covid-19-pandemic.

Chapter 6
Medical Student Education During and After the COVID-19 Pandemic

Sean Robinson, Austin Morgan, Richard Moberly, and Rebecca Cantone

I think a lot of us worried about 'What is the impact this is gonna have on medical training?' We just started taking clinical students again this spring, because we could barely keep our own people going. We couldn't spare extra time or attention or space. We were distancing ourselves for a long time, but thinking about two years' worth of students who couldn't get clinical placements in our area was really concerning.

Introduction

In an effort to flatten the curve of infection, on March 17, 2020, the Association of American Medical Colleges (AAMC) issued a pivotal recommendation with far-reaching implications: all medical students were to be removed from in-person education [1]. As explored throughout this book, health care providers witnessed unprecedented demand for COVID-19 testing, severe illness, and skyrocketing hospitalizations. Following the AAMC's recommendation to remove students from in-person activities, the timeline for return varied across the nation from April to August 2020. During the peak of these restrictive educational practices, between April and May 2020, nearly 94% of US medical students were not involved with direct patient care [2]. This was an unprecedented departure from the norm in medical training. The return to clinical education depended largely on the ability to secure personal protective equipment (PPE) for students. Students' ability to access PPE was inconsistent. While some students gained access to PPE within 8 weeks [3], others were unable to obtain PPE even a year later [1, 4]. Smaller and rural health care institutions were often left to fend for themselves; larger institutions

S. Robinson (✉) · A. Morgan · R. Moberly · R. Cantone
Department of Family Medicine, Oregon Health & Science University School of Medicine, Portland, OR, USA
e-mail: robinsse@ohsu.edu

A. Cheng et al. (eds.), *Primary Care in a Public Health Emergency*,
https://doi.org/10.1007/978-3-032-12487-6_6

swallowed up the PPE supply. Differences in beliefs regarding the origin of COVID-19, what caused people to contract the virus, and whether there was a need for universal vaccination against COVID-19 may have inhibited better coordination among health care systems early in the pandemic [5].

Educators advocating for students faced difficult tradeoffs between their duty to protect students by following AAMC guidance and removing students from in-person clinical experiences versus wanting students to continue being immersed in these robust educational environments. Meanwhile, clinician educators in various practice environments struggled to prioritize students in the face of competing challenges. Frontline health care workers, who do double duty as clinical educators, faced intense personal and professional stress, including anxiety about infecting family members, exhausting shifts with limited staff and PPE, constantly evolving protocols, and the emotional weight of caring for dying, isolated patients [6]. On August 14, 2020, the AAMC formally recommended a return of students to clinical learning with guidelines on direct in-person activities, with the caveat that these recommendations should not override individual decisions made by academic health centers given regional differences and other special circumstances. Internationally, multiple health organizations issued similar guidance, and unique models were developed to have students live and rotate together in their clinical experiences to achieve social learning augmented by virtual work. For the next year, between August 2020 and January 2021, there was regional variation in how educational activities were happening and what restrictions were placed on students. Most medical schools shifted back to pre-pandemic activities and norms by January 2021 when vaccines became available. As students gradually returned to in-person activities, we recognized deficiencies in learning outcomes. We asked: how could we swiftly make up for lost educational ground?

Years later, medical schools across the country continue to grapple with the impacts of the COVID-19 pandemic. It is now apparent that medical education was forever changed by the pandemic, and permanent changes to educational delivery have been seen. We will outline a few of these transformative changes, including virtual learning, transition to residency, wellness and team dynamics, national pressures, widening inequities, and new avenues for innovation. It should not be forgotten that any changes to allopathic (MD) curricula for most US medical schools are monitored by the Liaison Committee on Medical Education (LCME), and any changes need to work within the LCME standards (there is a similar process for osteopathic or DO curricula), which add more stress to a rapidly changing landscape.[1]

[1] The LCME (Liaison Committee on Medical Education) accredits medical schools in the US and Canada that grant the MD degree, while the DO degree is accredited by COCA (Commission on Osteopathic College Accreditation). We do not address COCA standards in this chapter.

Disruptions to Traditional Medical School Learning Approaches and Modalities

Medical educators collaborated nationally as they adjusted their curricula. Curricula committees adopted agile work styles to account for rapid environmental changes. They partnered with the LCME to ensure changes to the curricula would adhere to any accreditation standards set.

Educators relied on new technology to achieve their goals. Some schools had already adopted the foundations of virtual education and hoped for greater standardization as more schools adopted virtual education. Unfortunately, many educators were not familiar with the established virtual options or did not have the budget to pay for subscriptions. Other schools took it upon themselves to find better solutions. New companies created programs with free trials of educational solutions. Consequently, greater variability, rather than standardization emerged [7]. Leaders in virtual education platforms and resources continued to gain higher membership with others offering free temporary access for students who did not have other options [8].

Educational groups collated curricular options that could be done asynchronously, online, and/or shared previously published educational models that did not rely on in-person learning with 'ready to use' materials for instructors tasked with changing their curricula [9]. Unfortunately, many of these free resources, such as the AAMC iCollaborative, have been removed from online access since the public health emergency was declared over. These lessons learned have shown the importance of improving the access to limited educational resources, highlighting the ongoing need for sustainable, high-quality online educational platforms.

Changes to the Preclinical Years

The preclinical years typically begin with community-building activities that build connectedness through a shared professional identity with each other and with school faculty. In 2020, students started medical school without in-person classes and welcome events. Students and faculty alike faced unfamiliar, isolating experiences. Schools scrambled to replace the essential rites of passage with virtual alternatives, but even the best efforts could not fully replace what was lost.

Prior to these abrupt changes, educators had already observed a gradual decline in class participation [10]. Positive perceptions for virtual curricula in the preclinical years mirrored a global trend [11, 12]. Educators were concerned about the impact on student experience, learning outcomes, and well-being. Studies of the changing patterns of engagement with medical education reported a mixed impact on student experience, student well-being, and satisfaction [13]. Similarly, studies comparing online-only versus hybrid educational experiences had shown contradictory impact of on students' mean final grades.

With COVID-19, required all-day lectures were eliminated, and many activities became optional. Some students appreciated that COVID-19 made it more socially acceptable to not attend lectures, watch materials online after delivery, and utilize other resources, but many students would have preferred to have the social interaction and clinical exposure in person [14]. Students saved time and money by not travelling for coursework, exams, and meetings. Parents and caregivers could perform their duties external to medical school while studying from home. However, internet access became a necessary, possibly incremental, expense [11, 12].

The most significant negative impacts of virtual education were seen in teaching clinical skills in the first two years. Most in-person, hands-on demonstrations were replaced with instructional videos, and interactions with real-life patients were replaced by standardized patient actors, often virtually. Students reported a decrease in confidence of their skill acquisition [15]. Over time, schools became more adept at remote teaching and assessments, but ongoing concerns about achievement persist [16]. Additionally, the lack of exposure to clinical experiences in the preclinical years slowed their decision making about their desired medical specialty.

An additional layer of concern emerged as educators' engagement mirrored student disengagement. Interpersonal relationships had drawn many educators into teaching and the loss of face-to-face interactions harmed morale [16].

Changes to the Clinical Years

Virtual education clearly detracted from the clinical phase of medical education. The clinical phase of training requires interactions with real patients in real clinical settings. Educators expect students to develop their clinical skills, learn how to work on a team, and choose a medical specialty. Students in the midst of their clinical years when the pandemic hit were shifted into virtual-only clinical rotations at a critical juncture of an extremely short (e.g., 12–24 months) phase of training. The loss of in-person clinical interactions was profound. The lack of PPE delayed return to face-to-face education. As previously mentioned, PPE availability for students was inconsistent, raising concerns about the management of non-COVID-19 respiratory illnesses as well [17, 18]. Some schools fought, and earned, an early return of their students as necessary members of the health care workforce, ensuring that future providers training in these environments received all aspects of their traditional clinical training. Others were not able to return students to in-person learning because their clinical years relied heavily on community partners too taxed with heightened patient care demands and too few resources (PPE being one example), which left them unable to train students. Within health systems, the ability of students to return to in-person rotations varied depending on the clinical specialty's role in the health care system. For example, at Oregon Health & Science University (OHSU), surgeries were canceled due to the need to preserve operating rooms for urgent cases, shift staffing to frontline locations, and preserve PPE. Medical schools were creative in maintaining rotations outside of the medical school's health system. To avoid drawing from a community clinic's PPE supply, some institutions, such as ours, sent students with PPE secured by the medical school.

Many students were eager to contribute in medical or non-medical settings but faced concerns about infecting their relatives and patients, limited access to PPE, or legal risks due to gaps in knowledge and training [18]. Other students feared contracting or spreading COVID-19 [17]. Medical educators had mixed opinions about returning students to full patient care, isolating students from COVID-19 positive patients.

Creative solutions emerged to accommodate students when clinical experiences were not available. In the early months and years of the pandemic, students administered vaccines, staffed call centers, and provided childcare for health care workers whose children's schools and daycare facilities had closed [19]. At OHSU, we created the "COVID-19 Inquiry Group." In this new elective, students worked with faculty to research evidence-based accessible answers to complex questions related to COVID-19. Learners and faculty worked together and gained knowledge on quickly changing information. They provided a valuable resource to health care providers and community members [20]. The findings of the group were shared through a COVID-19 hotline and OHSU's website, which was used by patients and clinicians [20]. This model of accelerated learning equipped students with invaluable experiences and essential skills necessary for their future roles as health care providers. These skills of quickly finding literature resources to answer questions coupled with collating and presenting answers in a concise fashion will uniquely prepare them to combat similar public health challenges, offering lasting benefits for future generations.

Numerous changes to clinical rotations were required. For instance, some educators developed virtual rounds to engage students in clinical care safely from home [21]. The United Kingdom led novel 'social bubbles' of 12-week face-to-face clinical placements, reverting to the apprenticeship model, to combine seminars, clinical care, quality improvement, and research together [22]. Clinical rotations in the US also combined asynchronous learning at home with shortened in-person rotations to fit more students into fewer clinical placement slots. Didactics during the clinical years remained virtual as well and slowly transitioned back to in-person learning [12].

Educators met unique challenges returning students to in-person training in rural settings. Rural training is essential to promote recruitment into high-need rural areas and provides distinct learning because of the unique needs of rural communities [23, 24]. Rural training experiences have been limited for years before 2020 due to deteriorating health care infrastructure in rural America. The pandemic compounded the shortage of placement opportunities due to increased demands on health care workers, surges in patients seeking care in 2020, staffing deficits, and insufficient federal relief to mitigate worsening budget deficits at rural clinics [25]. In some rural communities, people feared that students from urban areas would spread COVID-19. One practitioner noted, "In this pandemic, there are many patients who are asymptomatic, and young patients are spreading their infections in urban areas. So, medical trainees can be transmitters of the infection even in rural areas. That is why at first, we did not welcome medical trainees." [24]

The challenges in the clinical years resulted in diminished experiences working with patients. Students experienced fewer direct patient interactions and started them later. Delays heightened anxiety for some students and steepened the learning curve during an already complicated transition from the preclinical to the clinical years.

School administrators faced increased challenges during this time because student performance lagged behind national standards which were not changed. From a national perspective, increased variability in medical school curricula and learning outcomes created concern about the integrity of our medical education system [26].

To adapt, some schools implemented competency-based promotion criteria and time-variable curricula. These changes allowed advanced learners to graduate early to join the workforce and delayed learners to spend more time improving clinical skills and gaining confidence [27, 28].

The impact of the pandemic lingers on. As mentioned above, specialties were differently affected due to their roles in the health care system. For example, some specialties were "sidelined" while others were working furiously around the clock. Students, of course, noted these disparate effects and specialty perceptions shifted. One study showed these shifts were driven by concerns that students could not explore specialties or obtain letters of recommendation due to prolonged suspension of clinical rotations [29]. One study found that 11.6% of students changed their top specialty choice, [30] while another observed no clear pattern to changes in specialty [31]. Educators aware of career choice implications from changing student experiences proposed virtual advice to offset these shifts [32].

Residency Transition

Medical school educators have a responsibility to prepare students for residency by holding students to performance standards. The pandemic forced educators to make changes to a proven medical education program and to adjust standards for pragmatic reasons. Educators made necessary tradeoffs between quality and workforce volume needs with only a partial understanding of the implications.

Virtual rotations, decentralized student evaluations, and delayed deadlines for completing the residency application process were necessary [33], but significant concerns remained about competency and the burden that might be placed on residency educators.

As will be discussed in Chap. 5, residency was impacted positively and negatively, too. For example, the residency application process changed from in-person to virtual interviews, offered minimal away rotations for students to experience potential residency programs or find their 'fit,' and created a perceived need by applicants to increase the total number of programs applied to. However, virtual residency applications reduced carbon emissions and improved equity for those who could not afford travel.

Wellness and Team Changes

Student Mental Health

As with many groups within and outside of health care, the pandemic increased anxiety and stress among medical students [2, 34–37]. Many students missed significant milestones, including undergraduate graduation ceremonies, medical school welcome events, and Match Day celebrations. Multiple studies cited unfavorable impacts on the medical school community, preparation for intern year, isolation, and communication [38, 39].

Although some students experienced improvements in sleep duration and quality while learning from home [39], heightened anxiety became widespread [2, 34–36]. Medical schools quickly recognized the crucial need to implement changes to improve student health and sustain a positive outlook among this next generation of health care practitioners. These challenges mirrored those faced by other education programs and are likely to persist for many years post-pandemic [40].

Other facets of wellness were also affected, such as financial strain [27]. Extra expenses such as higher cell phone bills, costs of reliable internet, and perception of home background environments may have limited participation inequitably or forced students to acquire additional debt.

To improve wellness, multiple projects and studies emerged [41, 42], including virtual wellness and learning communities to improve peer connectivity and personal wellness [43]. The lack of professional identity formation combined with actual limitations in training made building skills to help navigate imposter syndrome even more important. Without in-person conferences or activities, students missed opportunities to connect with like-minded individuals for specialty discernment, networking, and presenting work nationally. Interest group activities waned without faculty able to excuse themselves from additional clinical duties or unable to find campus locations appropriate for large gatherings. Clinically, this created confusion in identifying what ‘normal’ is for their educational experiences, patient interactions, and clinical systems.

Medical Educator Mental Health

As discussed above, medical educators struggled with the balance of education, safety, and new competing demands as well. Those advocating for students faced tremendous pressures from health care systems to remove students, posing challenges to effectively prepare students, balance infectious spread, and demonstrate equal experiences to accrediting bodies. Contract negotiations and deprioritization of education in larger health care delivery systems led to educators needing to advocate for their learners and secure the pathways of future health care providers. Clinician educators faced these same challenges, while simultaneously being asked to pick up additional clinical hours, risk their own health, and risk transmission to loved ones. These compounding stressors were worse for those in generalist or frontline clinical fields with already higher rates of burnout and emotional exhaustion than proceduralists and those performing elective services who remained paid despite canceled work [44]. The stark inequities in what was demanded of faculty in different professional roles were further exacerbated by inequitable pay structures. Extra work in most medical schools did not come with additional remuneration for those continuing to work both roles double time while their social support and promotion opportunities waned with cancellations of conferences, funding, and collaborations.

Staff and Teams

Mental and physical health impacts from the pandemic hit staff in medical education settings just as hard [45]. Advocacy for increased flexibility and salaries emerged, but little is known about non-medical personnel on which the education of medical students relies. While not studied, administrative teams struggled with the new realities such as shifting to virtual meetings, barriers in work-life balance, lack of childcare, inconsistent work hours, and loss of in-person interaction. The relationships and collaborations that usually prevent burnout or isolation were gone.

Admissions, student affairs, and curricular teams also faced personal burnout and stress trying to define what qualified as sufficient experience before, during, and after medical school in a shutdown world. Challenges with deadlines, medical college admission tests and reduced in-person volunteer and shadowing experiences not only limited the criteria on which to select future medical students but has lasting impacts on those trainees [46]. Test centers offering licensing exams continued to close with little notice, further placing stress on administrators trying to ensure their trainees were prepared and were completing all required steps for success in the future.

National Pressures

In January 2021, the United States Medical Licensing Examination (USMLE) changed their Step 1 test to pass/fail, while increasing the passing threshold. This increased the risk of failure and loss of ability for residencies to stratify applicants, recognizing this was not the purpose of this test. This put additional pressure on the

USMLE Step 2 Clinical Knowledge exam, leading students to shift their focus away from clinical care and onto successful test taking strategies during their clinical rotations. Due to only one contracted testing center, many students faced testing cancellations or limits on scheduling from office closures and insufficient staff during COVID-19. The Step 2 Clinical Skills examination was also adjusted due to COVID-19, requiring it to be offered online and then leading to its permanent cancellation [47]. This then removed the ability for schools and international programs to ensure a requisite level of competency in clinical skills before starting intern year. Additional work to verify medical graduates can safely work with patients is in process and should be encouraged to continue in a standardized way.

Many medical schools shifted to pass/fail or more flexible grading systems due to increased pressure from students and lack of significant stratifying data from evaluators [48]. This change helped stressed preceptors in discriminating subtle differences between multiple grades but also limited the ability for course directors to accurately represent their students on the Medical Student Performance Evaluation [26] for their future residency placements. Fortunately, national guidelines were developed to label rotations that were affected due to COVID-19 [26]. At the same time, competency-based medical education was increasing, and the focus on skills, over grades, felt more important.

Throughout this time, multiple institutions continued to work toward accreditation with benchmarks set by an educational organizing body. Schools were held to requirements of student satisfaction in a world where students, faculty, and staff all felt dissatisfied with the shift in their curricula from their ideal. While simultaneously advocating for excellent education and student safety, students were less and less engaged, and thus less satisfied. For instance, improvements in curricula, student spaces, advising, or other accreditation requirements may have significantly improved, but the students were not on campus to experience these positive changes, and thus continued to report dissatisfaction which led to accreditation concerns. Similarly, comparability between rotations and sites was another standard that had challenges as smaller institutions, community health clinics, and rural networks faced additional lack of PPE, funding, and sufficient staff and providers for patient care.

Parallel Inequities

During the COVID-19 pandemic, there was a heightened focus on social and systemic drivers of health and racism. Students were very astute in acknowledging and bringing focus to these important issues [49]. Students themselves faced some of these inequities, with increased isolation, challenging access to virtual learning, racial trauma, and inequitable residency experiences [38]. At some institutions, greater recognition of these inequities led to increased uptake of curricula about social and structural determinants of health, race, and racism in education [38].

The political polarization surrounding the vaccine, masking, and isolation, quarantine, and social distancing recommendations likely had an impact on students as well. While there is limited data, many schools experienced personal or religious vaccine hesitancy of students that opposed institutional regulations, as pointed out in Kabul, Afghanistan [50]. This introduced yet another new challenge, as students were prevented from returning to school when requirements for vaccination were in place. Acceptance and guidance varied between clinical environments, adding confusion to many students' already stressful experiences. Mask mandates and varying patient uptake added additional infectious risk to students, especially those who were immunocompromised or were vulnerable due to other health diagnoses that they were concerned about disclosing for fear of discrimination or stigma. Streamlined accommodations aligned with the Americans with Disabilities Act were needed. Finally, prevention and treatment guidelines continued to evolve along with widely variable uptake of these guidelines, causing medical confusion and disagreement between providers and students alike.

Opportunity to Innovate

As with any crisis, innovations were developed across the globe. Table 6.1 summarizes specific strategies implemented to offset restricted learning during the pandemic that may offer valuable insights for educators in the future. Countless other advancements emerged worldwide, likely shaping the ongoing evolution of medical education delivery.

Learning Points and Suggestions for Future Pandemics or Crises

Medical educators can draw valuable lessons from the COVID-19 pandemic to prepare for future crises. Our recommendations are listed below:

- **Leverage Established Frameworks:** Consult existing frameworks designed to manage change before creating new ones [51].
- **Advocate for Learners' Needs:** Emphasize the importance of learners in health care's future, especially given the increased percentage of health care professionals retiring at early ages. This includes ensuring access to PPE and broad patient care experiences.
- **Strengthen Student Health Resources:** Provide robust health and wellness resources for students, particularly when in-person support is limited.
- **Engage National Leadership:** Advocate for national guidance on medical student education during crises to ensure consistent support and direction as well as equity across regions.

Table 6.1 Selected strategies implemented to offset restricted learning during the COVID-19 pandemic. This table highlights innovative approaches adopted by medical education programs in response to pandemic-related disruptions. Strategies reflect adaptations in curricula delivery, clinical skills training, assessment, and learner support. These examples may inform future developments in medical education delivery

Innovation	Effects
Students trained to give COVID-19 vaccines	Early exposure to clinical care and patient interaction Development of communication skills and informed consent procedures
Virtual small group learning	Reduced infection risk Addressed caring for family members and/or children during shutdowns Lowered transportation costs and carbon emissions Managed inequities related to home environments, transportation challenges, and associated costs
Shortened clinical rotations with asynchronous component	Reduced burden on rural or community clinics Promoted self-directed learning Standardized topics covered
Free online learning or online resources with institutional paid subscriptions	Augmented learning opportunities Reduced educator demand, allowing clinician-educators more time to serve patients Lowered costs for hiring and training faculty
National organizations publishing free online curricula	Free resources for schools with financial challenges Supported faculty promotion through shared contributions Uptrained faculty lacking expertise in essential topics
Telehealth (covered in detail in Chap. 9)	Prepared students to use new digital interfaces Taught 'soft skills' for building rapport via video Practiced assessment of illness severity and triage for determining the need for in-person visits
Students helping with discovery and public health	Immersed students in communication skills through care/call centers Enhanced rapid evidence review skills Provided public health experience through contact tracing Developed research skills Strengthened social connections for vulnerable populations Fostered interdisciplinary collaboration and networking with researchers and practicing clinicians
COVID-19 inquiry group (Robinson 2020)	Offered elective course credit Enabled collaboration with faculty Facilitated review of current literature Provided networking opportunities with public health officials and clinicians

- **Adapt Quickly to Shifting Needs:** Establish flexible learning models that allow for studying and practicing with in-person, hybrid, and online-only learning curricula.
- **Define Communication Standards:** Develop a clear communication plan and philosophy regarding in-person vs. online expectations, considering when hybrid models are equitable or pose challenges for participants.
- **Promote Agility in Curriculum Committees:** Embrace curriculum flexibility while adhering to accreditation standards.
- **Address Resource Inequities:** Offer safe and private study spaces, assistance with internet and phone costs, and flexible attendance options without requiring students to disclose connection quality or home environment.
- **Expand Access to Learning Materials:** Ensure online and downloadable resources are free or low-cost (or institutionally covered) and accessible to all learning styles.
- **Support Clinician-Educators:** Reduce pressure on clinician-educators by involving additional faculty or specialists in delivering high-quality education.
- **Foster Equity Among Educators:** Ensure collaborative equity across clinician-educators in different specialties to enhance resilience during crises.
- **Adjust Accreditation Standards:** Allow flexibility in accreditation, especially when student satisfaction levels correlate with extraordinary health care circumstances.
- **Enhance Simulation-Based Learning:** Invest in virtual and in-person simulation centers to maintain hands-on training if clinical sites become unavailable.
- **Encourage Interprofessional Learning:** Foster collaboration and learning across health care professions to enhance crisis response.
- **Refine Assessments for Virtual Learning:** Continue developing rapid, effective assessment tools for online learning environments to facilitate timely feedback and student growth.
- **Promote Public Health Literacy:** Emphasize epidemiology and public health literacy within the curriculum.
- **Coordinate with Graduate Medical Education (GME):** Collaborate with GME to improve transition processes and support competency-based, time-variable graduation for future residents.

References

1. Association of American Medical Colleges. Updated interim guidance for medical students' participation in patient care during the coronavirus (COVID-19) outbreak. https://www.aamc.org/news/press-releases/updated-interim-guidance-medical-students-participation-patient-care-during-coronavirus-covid-19. Accessed 29 Mar 2024.
2. Harries AJ, Lee C, Jones L, et al. Effects of the COVID-19 pandemic on medical students: a multicenter quantitative study. BMC Med Educ. 2021;21(1):14. https://doi.org/10.1186/s12909-020-02462-1.

3. Goldenberg MN, Hersh DC, Wilkins KM, Schwartz ML. Suspending medical student clerkships due to COVID-19. Med Sci Educ. 2020;30(3):1273–6. https://doi.org/10.1007/s40670-020-00994-1.
4. Peery-Wolf A, Gupta S, Raja A. A year into the pandemic, vulnerable communities still don't have access to PPE. https://www.aamc.org/news/year-pandemic-vulnerable-communities-still-don-t-have-access-ppe. Accessed 29 Mar 2024.
5. Rebmann T, Alvino RT, Mazzara RL, Sandcork J. Rural infection preventionists' experiences during the COVID-19 pandemic: findings from focus groups conducted with association of professionals in infection control & epidemiology (APIC) members. Am J Infect Control. 2021;49(9):1099–104. https://doi.org/10.1016/j.ajic.2021.06.008.
6. Novilla MLB, Moxley VBA, Hanson CL, et al. COVID-19 and psychosocial well-being: did COVID-19 worsen u.s. frontline healthcare workers' burnout, anxiety, and depression? Int J Environ Res Public Health. 2023;20(5):4414. https://doi.org/10.3390/ijerph20054414.
7. Southworth E, Gleason SH. COVID 19: a cause for pause in undergraduate medical education and catalyst for innovation. HEC Forum. 2021;33(1–2):125–42. https://doi.org/10.1007/s10730-020-09433-5.
8. Aquifer. COVID-19 response: free access extended to new programs. https://aquifer.org/covid-19-response-free-access-extended-to-new-programs/. Accessed 29 Mar 2024.
9. MedEdPORTAL. MedEdPORTAL's response to COVID-19. https://www.mededportal.org/covid. Accessed 29 Mar 2024.
10. Murphy B. Why some medical students are cutting class to get ahead. https://www.ama-assn.org/medical-students/medical-school-life/why-some-medical-students-are-cutting-class-get-ahead#:~:text=People%20study%20better%20at%20different,needed%20to%20learn%20the%20material.%E2%80%9D. Accessed 29 Mar 2024.
11. Reinhart A, Malzkorn B, Döing C, Beyer I, Jünger J, Bosse HM. Undergraduate medical education amid COVID-19: a qualitative analysis of enablers and barriers to acquiring competencies in distant learning using focus groups. Med Educ Online. 2021;26(1):1940765. https://doi.org/10.1080/10872981.2021.1940765.
12. Binks AP, LeClair RJ, Willey JM, et al. Changing medical education, overnight: the curricular response to COVID-19 of nine medical schools. Teach Learn Med. 2021;33(3):334–42. https://doi.org/10.1080/10401334.2021.1891543.
13. Lee BE, Zlotshewer BA, Mayeda RC, Kaplan LI. Impact of online-only instruction on preclinical medical education in the setting of COVID-19: comparative analysis of online-only vs. hybrid instructions on academic performance and mental wellbeing. Med Sci Educ. 2022;32(6):1367–74. https://doi.org/10.1007/s40670-022-01650-6.
14. Johansen PM, Celentano L, Wyatt AT. The influence of COVID-19 on medical student resource preferences. Cureus. 2022;14(8):e28593. https://doi.org/10.7759/cureus.28593.
15. Saad S, Richmond C, King D, Jones C, Malau-Aduli B. The impact of pandemic disruptions on clinical skills learning for pre-clinical medical students: implications for future educational designs. BMC Med Educ. 2023;23(1):364. https://doi.org/10.1186/s12909-023-04351-9.
16. Gaur U, Majumder MAA, Sa B, Sarkar S, Williams A, Singh K. Challenges and opportunities of preclinical medical education: COVID-19 crisis and beyond. SN Compr Clin Med. 2020;2(11):1992–7. https://doi.org/10.1007/s42399-020-00528-1.
17. Rolak S, Keefe AM, Davidson EL, Aryal P, Parajuli S. Impacts and challenges of United States medical students during the COVID-19 pandemic. World J Clin Cases. 2020;8(15):3136–41. https://doi.org/10.12998/wjcc.v8.i15.3136.
18. Michno DA, Tan J, Adelekan A, Konczalik W, Woollard ACS. How can we help? Medical students' views on their role in the COVID-19 pandemic. J Public Health (Oxf). 2021;43(3):479–89. https://doi.org/10.1093/pubmed/fdaa271.
19. Bauchner H, Sharfstein J. A bold response to the COVID-19 pandemic: medical students, national service, and public health. JAMA. 2020;323(18):1790–1. https://doi.org/10.1001/jama.2020.6166.

20. Robinson S, Angier H, Pierce K, et al. Responding to community questions during a pandemic: development of a COVID-19 inquiry group. 2020. COVID-19 collection. https://deepblue.lib.umich.edu/handle/2027.42/154809.
21. Buba M, Dulude C, O'Donnell R, et al. Virtual family-centered rounds: a quality improvement initiative to adapt inpatient care during COVID-19 using a human-centred participatory design approach. BMC Pediatr. 2023;23(1):289. https://doi.org/10.1186/s12887-023-04091-1.
22. Stout RC, Roberts S, Maxwell-Scott H, Gothard P. Necessity is the mother of invention: how the COVID-19 pandemic could change medical student placements for the better. Postgrad Med J. 2021;97(1149):417–22. https://doi.org/10.1136/postgradmedj-2021-139728.
23. Okayama M, Kajii E. Does community-based education increase students' motivation to practice community health care? - a cross sectional study. BMC Med Educ. 2011;11(1):19. https://doi.org/10.1186/1472-6920-11-19.
24. Ohta R, Ryu Y, Sano C. The uncertainty of COVID-19 inducing social fear and pressure on the continuity of rural, community-based medical education: a thematic analysis. Healthcare (Basel). 2021;9(2):223. https://doi.org/10.3390/healthcare9020223.
25. Oster N, Patterson D, Skillman S, Bianca F. COVID-19 and the rural health workforce: the impact of federal pandemic funding to address workforce needs. 2022. https://familymedicine.uw.edu/chws/publications/covid-19-and-the-rural-health-workforce-the-impact-of-federal-pandemic-funding-to-address-workforce-needs/.
26. Association of American Medical Colleges. May 2022 MSPE guidance for disruptions related to COVID-19. https://www.aamc.org/media/55136/download?attachment. Accessed 29 Mar 2024.
27. Kaul V, Gallo de Moraes A, Khateeb D, et al. Medical education during the COVID-19 pandemic. Chest. 2021;159(5):1949–60. https://doi.org/10.1016/j.chest.2020.12.026.
28. DeWitt DE. Fighting COVID-19: enabling graduating students to start internship early at their own medical school. Ann Intern Med. 2020;173(2):143–4. https://doi.org/10.7326/m20-1262.
29. Byrnes YM, Civantos AM, Go BC, McWilliams TL, Rajasekaran K. Effect of the COVID-19 pandemic on medical student career perceptions: a national survey study. Med Educ Online. 2020;25(1):1798088. https://doi.org/10.1080/10872981.2020.1798088.
30. Lee KE, Lim F, Silver ER, Faye AS, Hur C. Impact of COVID-19 on residency choice: a survey of New York City medical students. PLoS One. 2021;16(10):e0258088. https://doi.org/10.1371/journal.pone.0258088.
31. Esposito A, Patti L, Laumbach S, Polvino D, Butler L, Heinert S. 92 The impact of the COVID-19 pandemic on medical student residency specialty selection. Ann Emerg Med. 2021;78(2):S43. https://doi.org/10.1016/j.annemergmed.2021.07.094.
32. Moberly R, Schneider B. The OHSU OASIS program: reinventing career advising in undergraduate medical education (for students). 2024.
33. Liesman, D. R., Pumiglia, L., Kemp, M. T., & Alam, H. B. (2020). Perspectives From Rising Fourth Year Medical Students Regarding Strategies to Counteract the Effects of COVID-19 on Medical Education. Journal of Medical Education and Curricular Development, 7. https://doi.org/10.1177/2382120520940659
34. Rahiman HU, Panakaje N, Kulal A, Harinakshi, Parvin SMR. Perceived academic stress during a pandemic: mediating role of coping strategies. Heliyon. 2023;9(6):e16594. https://doi.org/10.1016/j.heliyon.2023.e16594.
35. Jaishankar D, Dave S, Tatineni S, et al. U.S. medical student experiences during the COVID-19 pandemic: a national survey. Acad Med. 2021;96(11s):S207–8. https://doi.org/10.1097/acm.0000000000004272.
36. Ukwuani S, Kloosterman N, Hammack-Aviran C, Davidson M, Finck L. Qualitative assessment of medical student concerns about the COVID-19 pandemic: a multicenter study exploring medical student perspectives. Acad Med. 2021;96(11S):S206–7.
37. Bughrara MS, Swanberg SM, Lucia VC, Schmitz K, Jung D, Wunderlich-Barillas T. Beyond COVID-19: the impact of recent pandemics on medical students and their education: a scop-

ing review. Med Educ Online. 2023;28(1):2139657. https://doi.org/10.1080/10872981.2022.2139657.
38. Walters M, Alonge T, Zeller M. Impact of COVID-19 on medical education: perspectives from students. Acad Med. 2022;97(3s):S40–8. https://doi.org/10.1097/acm.0000000000004525.
39. Winn AS, Weaver MD, O'Donnell KA, et al. Interns' perspectives on impacts of the COVID-19 pandemic on the medical school to residency transition. BMC Med Educ. 2021;21(1):330. https://doi.org/10.1186/s12909-021-02777-7.
40. Schwartz KD, Exner-Cortens D, McMorris CA, et al. COVID-19 and student well-being: stress and mental health during return-to-school. Can J Sch Psychol. 2021;36(2):166–85. https://doi.org/10.1177/08295735211001653.
41. Guo AA, Crum MA, Fowler LA. Assessing the psychological impacts of COVID-19 in undergraduate medical students. Int J Environ Res Public Health. 2021;18(6):2952. https://doi.org/10.3390/ijerph18062952.
42. Cherak SJ, Rosgen BK, Geddes A, et al. Wellness in medical education: definition and five domains for wellness among medical learners during the COVID-19 pandemic and beyond. Med Educ Online. 2021;26(1):1917488. https://doi.org/10.1080/10872981.2021.1917488.
43. Ahlers CG, Lawson V, Lee J, et al. A virtual wellness and learning communities program for medical students during the COVID-19 pandemic. South Med J. 2021;114(12):807–11. https://doi.org/10.14423/smj.0000000000001330.
44. Seda-Gombau G, Montero-Alía JJ, Moreno-Gabriel E, Torán-Monserrat P. Impact of the COVID-19 pandemic on burnout in primary care physicians in Catalonia. Int J Environ Res Public Health. 2021;18(17):9031. https://doi.org/10.3390/ijerph18179031.
45. Burrowes SAB, Casey SM, Pierre-Joseph N, et al. COVID-19 pandemic impacts on mental health, burnout, and longevity in the workplace among healthcare workers: a mixed methods study. J Interprof Educ Pract. 2023;32:100661. https://doi.org/10.1016/j.xjep.2023.100661.
46. Dowd B, McKenney M, Elkbuli A. The impact of COVID-19 pandemic on medical school admissions: challenges and solutions. J Surg Res. 2021;258:213–5. https://doi.org/10.1016/j.jss.2020.08.072.
47. Achike FI, Christner JG, Gibson JL, et al. Demise of the USMLE Step-2 CS exam: rationalizing a way forward. J Natl Med Assoc. 2023;115(4):385–91. https://doi.org/10.1016/j.jnma.2023.05.003.
48. Mostafa SA, Ferguson R, Tang G, Ashqer M. An analysis of the COVID-19-induced flexible grading policy at a public university. High Educ Policy. 2023:1–34. https://doi.org/10.1057/s41307-023-00315-2.
49. Casola AR, Kelly EL, Smith K, Kelly S, de la Cruz MS. Impact of the COVID-19 pandemic on medical students' perceptions of health care for vulnerable populations. Fam Med. 2023;55(2):89–94. https://doi.org/10.22454/FamMed.2022.940208.
50. Azimi M, Yadgari MY, Atiq MA. Acceptance and hesitancy toward the Covid-19 vaccine among medical students in Kabul, Afghanistan. Infect Drug Resist. 2023;16:457–61. https://doi.org/10.2147/idr.S389582.
51. Sullivan C, Quaintance J, Myers T, Rogers B, Gaddis M, Pirani N. A framework to support medical students' professional development during large-scale societal events. Acad Psychiatry. 2023;47(4):422–7. https://doi.org/10.1007/s40596-023-01795-5.

Chapter 7
Response of a Connected Community Health Center: Meeting the Health care Needs of Patients and Community While Providing a Unique Medical Student Educational Opportunity

Alissa Goldberg, Jessy Silfer, Chad Garven, Robin Gotler, and Kurt C. Stange

> *Across the country, primary care was the real frontline of the pandemic response – not the intensive care unit, not the emergency department – but the practices that used their investment in knowing patients and the community to do whatever was needed. [This practice] like so many others innovated and abided every day amidst tremendous uncertainty. I don't know that the response will ever be fully appreciated, except by the many whose lives were saved or made better, but I'm glad that you are going to tell the story.* —CHC Family Physician

The devastation of the COVID-19 pandemic resulted in pain, cultural turmoil, and millions of lives lost [1]. However, it was also a time when activism and innovations shined [2, 3]. Untold numbers of primary care clinicians leveraged creative solutions to keep underserved communities safe, informed, and cared for [4].

To fully understand how primary care responded to the needs of the United States' most underserved communities during the pandemic, it is important to understand the response by frontline community health centers (CHCs). This is the story of how one multi-site CHC in Cleveland, Ohio, responded to the pandemic: its innovations, challenges, and lessons for those caring for underserved communities in times of public health crisis.

Authors Alissa Goldberg and Jessy Silfer have contributed equally to this work.

A. Goldberg · J. Silfer
Case Western Reserve University School of Medicine, University Program, Cleveland, OH, USA

C. Garven
Case Western Reserve University School of Medicine, Center for Community Health Integration, Case Western Reserve University, Cleveland, OH, USA

Cleveland Clinic, Middleburg Heights Family Health Center, Cleveland, OH, USA

R. Gotler · K. C. Stange (✉)
Case Western Reserve University School of Medicine, Center for Community Health Integration, Case Western Reserve University, Cleveland, OH, USA
e-mail: kcs@case.edu

A. Cheng et al. (eds.), *Primary Care in a Public Health Emergency*,
https://doi.org/10.1007/978-3-032-12487-6_7

Context

Cleveland, Ohio, is a health care hub, home to Cleveland Clinic, University Hospitals, MetroHealth, and the VA health systems, and their residency training programs. Case Western Reserve University (CWRU), also located in Cleveland, has nursing, physician assistant, social work, and dental programs as well as three medical schools: two traditional 4-year medical schools and a 5-year physician investigator program in partnership with the Cleveland Clinic.

In spite of its wealth of medical facilities, Cleveland is littered with public health disparities and barriers to care for the most vulnerable. The city is a mix of mansions, modest homes, warming and cooling centers frequented by unhoused individuals, and every living situation in between. Refugees, asylum seekers, and immigrants have made their home among long-time Clevelanders proud of the city's reputation for grit and determination. Cleveland has a history of racial, social, and economic discrimination that is well known among local communities and community leaders, many of whom use this history as a springboard for improvement and motivation to work towards equity [5].

Gathering Perspectives from the Frontline

We set out to understand how changes at a high-functioning CHC in response to the COVID-19 pandemic affected community health, vulnerable patient populations, and the CHC workforce. We did so by interviewing CHC staff and clinicians, community members and organizers, public health leaders, and students and educators from local health professional schools. Our research and writing team included two second-year medical students, a bioethicist/medical historian with qualitative methods expertise, a primary care physician-scientist, and a primary care physician-informaticist.

Participants for this qualitative study were recruited from the study team's professional networks. To increase the participant pool, we contacted additional key players who were mentioned in interviews.

Each interview began with open-ended general questions, such as, "Can you walk us through what happened at [the CHC] in the first few months of the pandemic," followed by prompts to draw out more detail, including, "What was the general atmosphere of the practice like?" Questions then drew out the breadth of relevant interviewee experience during and after the pandemic. Data collection continued until further interviews yielded no substantial new findings.

The student investigators read and reread interview transcripts, assigned codes to commonly occurring categories of information, and noted evolving study themes and specific supporting quotations from participants. The entire study team discussed these preliminary results and, to help refine themes, team members challenged emerging ideas and searched for confirming and disconfirming information.

Selected participants were contacted for follow-up to reflect on and refute preliminary findings, leading to further distillation of the study's results.

Below we present themes from our analyses with an eye toward transportable lessons for primary care practices, community partners, and health care system leaders looking to equitably and effectively care for their patients and communities before, during, and after a crisis.

The CHC Ecosystem: Deep Roots and Many Branches

The CHC's response to the pandemic can be understood as a deeply rooted and highly branched tree living in a mutually supportive grove (See Fig. 7.1). The roots depict the CHC's foundational concepts and values; the branches represent pandemic era innovations, and the fruits of the tree exemplify changes made in the wake of the pandemic that continue to shape the CHC's care for its communities.

The Roots

Founded in 1980 as a storefront practice and transitioning to a federally qualified health center in 2000, the CHC spent decades developing its roots including a clear vision, pragmatic approach, and extensive community connections.

Need Breeds Creativity and Pragmatism

> *[The CHC is] a more nimble organization... Our lack of resources often makes us a little bit more innovative... we don't have to move an entire hospital system to get behind a new initiative.*
>
> —CHC Senior Leader and Clinician

The CHC's origin story is one of humble and resourceful beginnings. It began as a single private practice site with two practitioners caring for patients in a former "biker bar." To meet the needs of their underserved population, the practice became a Federally Qualified Health Center (FQHC). As an FQHC, they could apply for grants and funding, allowing a new mindset and new projects to develop. Some interviewees described this mindset as, "No money, no mission." The availability of funds and ongoing new projects required the workforce to continually adapt. This sense of ongoing change was felt strongly in a small practice where, "... resources-wise, we don't have the same infrastructure built up around us the way a hospital system or some of the old historical primary care networks would otherwise provide," a clinician and former senior leader explained.

Over time, the practice grew from one site to seven sites, increasing its reach to meet the demands of Cleveland's distinct and dispersed vulnerable populations.

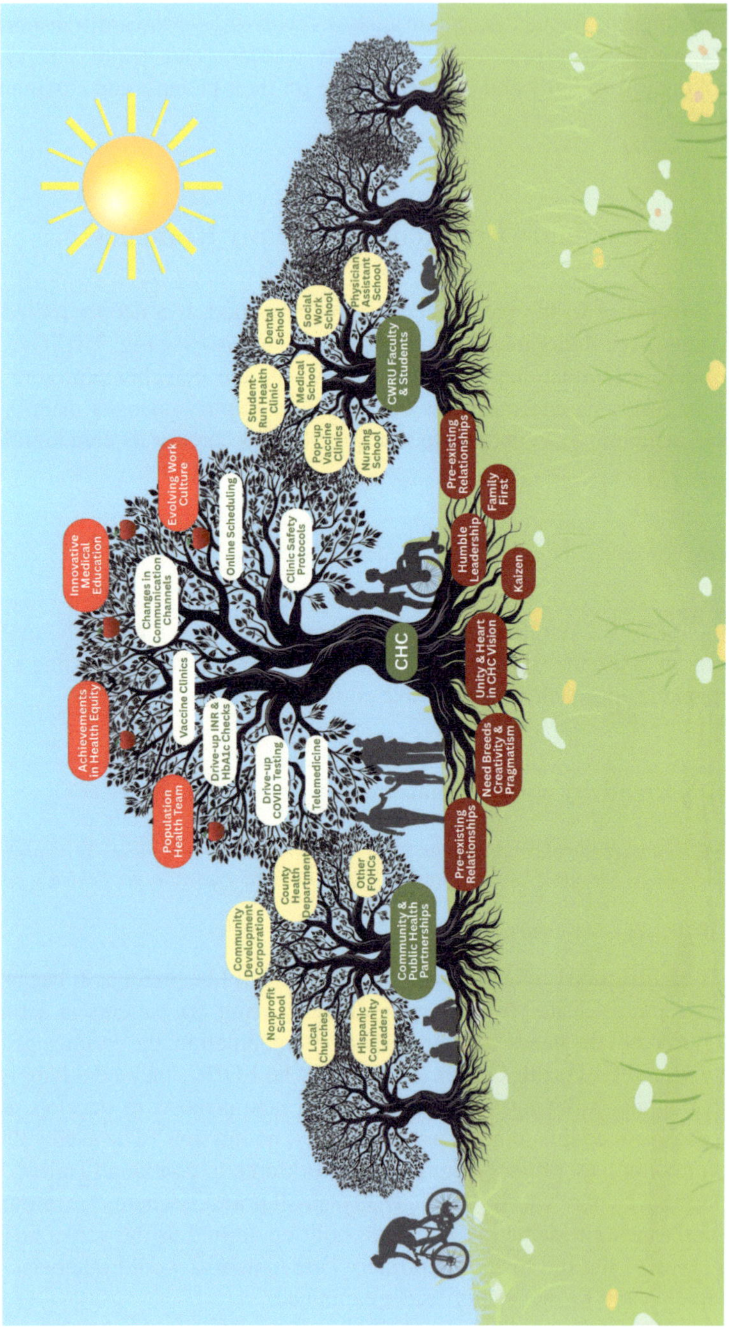

Fig. 7.1 CHC's Supportive Grove. (Source: Authors)

With growth, and with the flexibility required to serve patients with complex backgrounds, conditions, and needs, the CHC retained a commitment to creative problem solving. They sought to apply creativity not only to patient care but also to operational issues. This included recognizing the value of data and developing a partnership with a data sharing and practice improvement collaborative [6]. They developed a CHC practice-based research network to generate new knowledge to care for underserved patients and advocate for policy changes to serve them, and they created a storytelling initiative to give voice to the uninsured and used those voices to advocate for the Affordable Care Act.

When the pandemic hit, there was a new need for creative yet pragmatic solutions: how to provide patients with resources and services in a time of lockdown. The CHC decided to build on their knowledge of their patient populations. Using their patient registries, they called to check on vulnerable patients with chronic illnesses. A senior practice clinician knocked on the doors of patients from immigrant families to ensure they felt safe and knowledgeable about pandemic protocols, later explaining, "It's always important for…community health centers to stay at that forefront level...our role is really to be a voice and an eyeball to make sure the communities that we serve are getting…the care that they need." A crucial pandemic innovation, the development of a telemedicine system, came together quickly, over the course of a long weekend, thanks to the efforts of a CHC physician-informaticist (see the Telemedicine section, below).

CHC leadership took a flexible approach to roles during the pandemic, offering a voluntary temporary furlough to staff who preferred to lock down or had personal needs to attend to. The furlough both reduced overhead costs and resulted in a committed workforce. It also required continuous adaptation, as many remaining staff members took on multiple new roles.

Later in the pandemic, the CHC redefined what a care provider looked like by relying on health professional students to lead vaccine distribution at an on-site Student Run Health Clinic and to conduct patient outreach when telehealth was initiated. A senior leader described students as part of the clinical "tribe" and therefore ready and able to take active roles. According to another clinician and senior leader, "That Student Run Health Clinic became a vaccine hub for the [surrounding] neighborhood [in a] way that I don't think we'll ever be able to measure, which is to say they were doing hundreds of those a week for months."

Unity and Heart in CHC Vision

> *Community health centers are always full of people that are not just there to be clinicians, but they're there to be advocates...that's kind of a prerequisite to working at one, you have to have that passion...COVID was just an example of why all of that is important.*
> —CHC Senior Leader and Clinician

A broad smile from a front desk worker, a cheery "Hello" or "Hola" from a call center agent, a hug from a clinician, the quiet confidence exuded by a senior leader who leans in when speaking; these expressions are not superficial but exemplify the workforce's collective commitment to the CHC's mission.

CHC work tends to draw and unify those who are mission-focused, as a clinician described: "I do believe that that is what leads us all, when everybody is very clear what the mission is and everybody is trying to swim in the same direction. You're either resonating with that and you want to be there or you very quickly find your way out…." The CHC's mission and vision were important guideposts during the pandemic. As a CHC clinician and senior leader explained, "[The] administration [asked]…what do we need to be helpful to the community? It's not about...are we getting reimbursed.... So whenever I would go to somebody...and say, 'Hey, I think we should do this' or...'I think we should...go to this place or this place to do vaccines,' the answer was always, 'Okay, well, let's see, how do we make that happen?'...having a group of like-minded individuals committed to… bringing care to areas that are primary care deserts...that makes it much easier to get buy-in..."

In our interviews, we found that the staff, managers, clinicians, and leadership, all of whom were instrumental in the pandemic response, shared the organization's vision. Beginning in January 2021, staff and clinicians gave up their Saturdays to work at daylong vaccine clinics despite the fear and uncertainty associated with catching the disease. They described standing in the CHC's parking lots dressed in full PPE in the rain, sun, heat, and cold. One site manager described staying late each day to make sure testing samples were properly collected, packaged, and transported for assessment. What was the secret to the smooth operation? The site manager explained, "Honestly...you could run this very successfully if you had the right people in place, and that's what our goal was...to make sure...those that were going to help us through this had it…in their hearts as much as everybody else did. Then we knew that we would be successful."

The same vision that drew staff and practitioners to work at a CHC led the workforce to continue providing necessary primary care throughout the pandemic.

Humble Leadership

> *First and foremost is that there is just nothing like a high performing team… You have to trust one another. And if you make decisions together you have to support those decisions.*
> —CHC President and CEO during the pandemic

A Philosophy of Respect

Few employees of the CHC today reflect on the pandemic without noting the leadership's exemplary behavior. When describing senior leaders, one physician used phrases such as "goodwill," "extremely caring and available," and "awe-inspiring," stating that "our medical leadership was right there with us." In a time of extreme uncertainty and anxiety, leaders supported their CHC "family." While the pandemic may have highlighted this quality, the foundation had been laid long before. In the

CHC's early development, a former leader applied Family Systems Theory to Organization with the idea that "a structure that nurtures the nurturers can result in optimum effectiveness and efficient use of health care dollars." A belief that care and respect from leadership will trickle down to staff, patients, and their families was an important part of the CHC's philosophy.

Trust and team-building were valued as corollaries to the emphasis on respect. A leader explained that, at the time of the pandemic, they had "a stable team that [she] trusted who worked well together," and that they were used to making quick decisions while supporting one another. Trust in the team was noted by a nursing student participating in the Student Run Health Clinic vaccine clinic nearly a year into the pandemic. She explained, "They really allowed us to be a part of this... They were willing to listen... They were willing to make changes and they trusted our opinions... It was not a question of if we could do it together, but how we are going to do it together." While health professional students are often perceived as lower members of the medical hierarchy, at the CHC they were respected team members.

Listening

The importance of listening to others was intrinsic to the leadership culture. A longtime leader reflected that, before the pandemic, she would "check on each nurse pretty much every day," making sure they had the support they needed. She continued this practice during the pandemic, going from room to room daily and holding Zoom meetings to "just talk about what was happening and how they were managing their stress and what things...could be done a little bit differently to make it easier for them."

The result was not only attending to colleagues' feelings but also uncovering ideas for improvement. This approach was mirrored by younger leaders as well. One such leader described the CHC as "a place where we really try to do as best we can an all-hands-on-deck approach when something happens... 'What are your thoughts about this?' ... a lot of people had an opportunity to give their experience and their thoughts on [the pandemic response]." She emphasized the importance of listening to feedback and changing plans accordingly. While leadership positions allow some to have power over others, in this case power was harnessed to gather insights from all members of the CHC community.

Uplifting

CHC leaders worked to uplift and encourage those around them. When the pandemic began, the CHC president felt that "the more brainpower we had to be able to take complex concepts and then translate it for our staff and for the community, the better." She identified two energetic and public health-trained young leaders and brought them into senior management, describing her mindset as, "Get these two brilliant young docs in here!" One of those new leaders, in turn, worked to uplift colleagues by encouraging them to make decisions: "the nurses, the MAs, the providers – they know what their patients need. It's just about supporting them in that, removing barriers when you can …giving organizational support… [and] Let's see what happens." This approach also extended to student volunteers. A nursing student described three leaders who, "really, really, really – I cannot stress this enough – lifted us up and instilled confidence in us. Instilled joy." She often heard CHC leaders say, "You guys are making a difference and this is helping so many people," "I'm so proud of you," and "We're doing great work together."

Communication and Transparency

When the pandemic struck, the CHC immediately began communicating with patients and staff. "We were very aware of the fear in the community and the contagion of the illness that we knew so little about," the president/CEO explained, "but also the contagion of fear."

Clinicians reached out to patients, explaining what was and was not known and asking about concerns. They practiced what one senior leader called "unapologetic transparency," i.e., identifying and articulating the information they did not have. Thus, CHC leaders kept coworkers and patients informed even when information was limited. One leader's strategy was "using your medical knowledge to distill [information] in a way that people can understand… bringing a little bit of the basics, a little bit of humor to it … [explaining]…what's in the locus of the community's control, your individual control, your family's control, and giving people that information so they felt like they had something to do." She focused on giving advice about masking and grocery visits rather than virus statistics.

More formally, the CHC set up what some called "Vaccine Town Halls," virtual meetings in which community members could ask questions about the pandemic. They also established accessible communication channels with members of local ethnic community groups in the Hispanic, Vietnamese, and Nepali communities, among others, to exchange questions and information. One leader said that she welcomed questions from anyone in "whatever format," in hopes of removing barriers.

When the practice established social distancing, virtual communication within the CHC became essential. They held twice daily all-manager calls that included site leaders, senior managers, department heads, and anyone in a management role who wanted to join. These calls addressed rapidly changing protocols and related internal operations. Leadership also consistently sent out email updates to staff and, quarantining in her home attic, the president sent weekly videos summarizing the most up-to-date information and continually restating the CHC's priorities, "Our strategic plan is that we're going to have high-quality care and good financials." In spite of the repetition, she believed that "sometimes… managing well and leading is like parenting. You say the same basic things over and over again. You can't say them enough." The communications department reported that as many as 80% of staff watched the videos.

According to a clinician, internal communication efforts had their intended consequences, "I think our leadership team's ability to stay focused on what they knew and what they didn't know, and the importance of taking care of all of us was exemplary and as reassuring as it could be in a situation of such huge uncertainty."

Presence

It is interesting to note that goodwill toward CHC leaders was influenced by their physical presence. Many senior leaders, whose duties were not dependent on being on site, worked from home during the pandemic. Given the CHC's longstanding tradition of monthly in-person meetings and office sharing, this created a sense of emotional as well as physical distance for some staff: "Non-clinical leadership felt very far away from us." One leader, aware of this, would "occasionally go out to the sites…and… just thank everyone for giving up their Saturday."

Kaizen: An Atmosphere of Continuous Improvement

> *We're always looking at ways to improve. That's huge for [the CHC] as a whole, and I'm not just talking about one department, but as a whole... We're always looking at ways of improving services for our patients, our community.*
> —Patient Services Manager

The CHC had a longstanding tradition of Kaizen, a Japanese approach to continuous improvement [7]. Over time, the CHC's resource limitations and service to high-need communities contributed not only to an ethos of creativity and adaptation; they also motivated practice improvements. Prior to the pandemic, for example, the CHC worked to close population health gaps by leveraging the work of nurse care navigators. Another project sought to improve patient access to financial benefits.

During the pandemic, especially early on, the need to improve CHC operations was compounded by the crisis: the nature of the disease was unknown, public health guidance changed daily, and fear was rampant. In keeping with its commitment to Kaizen, the CHC was prepared to make quick adjustments to meet the moment and stay open and operational. This was exemplified by the operations of the Patient Service Center (PSC), the CHC's centralized call center. Before the pandemic, PSC staff answered phone calls, with a goal of answering 90% of calls in the first minute, scheduled appointments, and started the medication refill process. In March 2020, as the shutdown began, call volume doubled and the intensity and duration of conversations with patients increased as people dealt with COVID-19 symptoms and fears. Call waiting times soon rose from 5 minutes to 30 minutes, increasing PSC staff stress and patient frustration. The CHC hired more PSC staff and created several improvements, described by a PSC supervisor, "we…[put messages] in our phone menu to let our patients know 'We apologize. The wait may be longer than usual'…. We added additional mailboxes because there [were] so many [messages] that we weren't able to tackle. If someone was calling only for a vaccine, we had a voicemail that we set up so that they didn't have to wait in the call queue and [could] just leave their information." The PSC also re-evaluated their workflows related to non-COVID-19 calls, i.e., calls from existing and new patients about primary care and acute care issues. PSC staff began determining whether an in-office or virtual visit was most appropriate for patients based on their symptoms. This required keeping PSC staff up to date on CDC COVID-19 guidance and establishing communication channels with senior leaders, who consulted on these decisions. Given the PSC's increased communication needs and disparate locations, with some staff in the office and others working from home, the PSC supervisor instituted more frequent staff check-ins, "We created daily huddles...Weekly touchdowns! 'What's working?' 'What's not working?' 'Let's hear from you guys.' … and because of [their] feedback we were able to improve immediately… 'Okay, this isn't working,' or 'We need to change this.'" Finally, they regularly monitored phone data to ensure that call wait times decreased.

After the pandemic subsided, the practice's call volume remained higher than pre-pandemic levels. The practice's openness to improvement and the PSC's ability to change quickly has allowed the call center to maintain the increased call volume.

Pre-existing Relationships

You don't start passing out business cards in a crisis…that's not the time when you first get to know people.

—Preventive Medicine Resident quoting the County Health Commissioner

The CHC cared for, tested, and vaccinated thousands of community members during the pandemic. A key to this extensive capacity was their strong pre-existing relationships with other health care institutions, community organizations, local public health leaders, and health professional students.

The CHC was highly connected to other CHCs prior to the pandemic, in part through meetings such as the National Health Center Week hosted by the Ohio Association of Community Health Centers and through their development of the Safety Net Providers' Strategic Alliance, a regional practice-based research network [8, 9]. According to a senior leader, local CHC leaders met regularly to discuss their experiences as "health centers in a hospital dominated community." Eventually representatives from hospitals joined these meetings. The CHC also worked with a regional health improvement collaborative that included FQHCs, public health partners, and clinicians on quality improvement efforts to improve chronic disease care and the social drivers of health [10]. The collaborative met virtually during the pandemic, as the CHC and other FQHCs worked together on an equitable and effective COVID-19 response and on such issues as accessing PPE, establishing a website to help community members find care, creating COVID-19 testing protocols, and establishing workflows that optimized employee safety. Their solutions were shared with hospitals and public health departments to collectively care for underserved populations.

Pre-existing partnerships with community organizations, including churches, a nonprofit school, and a neighborhood development collaborative, were crucial to the CHC prior to the pandemic. Throughout its history, community organizers and the CHC's community engagement team played an important role in establishing the CHC as a trusted institution. During the pandemic, these relationships provided channels for disseminating accurate information to combat vaccine hesitancy and misinformation. Some of these community hubs also served as locations for vaccine clinics.

Distinct to this CHC was its direct links to the county health department. A CHC clinician was the county's medical director and the pandemic incident commander, and therefore, as one colleague described, "was in on all the higher-level public health decision making and information...we were particularly lucky to have that kind of...information." Another CHC clinician took a temporary pandemic furlough to lead the county's contact tracing efforts and mass testing and vaccination clinics in nursing homes, group homes, and juvenile detention centers. The relationship between the CHC and the county health department was furthered through their joint involvement in the health improvement collaborative.

The CHC had myriad preexisting relationships with graduate training programs in Cleveland, contributing to its ability to mobilize a student workforce. The local Student Run Health Clinic, run entirely by CWRU medical, nursing, physician assistant, social work, and dental school students, was supervised by a CHC physician who also helped lead the CWRU medical school clinical curriculum. During normal prepandemic times, first- and second-year medical students would be paired with physicians in the community for longitudinal training on clinical decision making. When the pandemic struck, completing these requirements became impossible. Simultaneously, however, the CHC needed people to call patients about the establishment of telemedicine. The faculty member was able to bridge these needs and pivot the medical curriculum to allow students to fulfill their clinical requirements by participating in patient outreach.

On Tuesday, January 19, 2021, the Student Run Health Clinic was preparing to open its first COVID-era Saturday clinic at the CHC when they learned that the CHC would be receiving COVID-19 vaccines and that many extra hands would be needed to provide injections. To fill the gap, the CHC brought in nursing students, many of whom were struggling to complete their required clinical hours. One nursing educator explained, "Leveraging the fact that we had an existing relationship [with the CHC] in place... the red tape of the agreements was done... if you're trying to introduce that red tape in that moment of crisis, it's not going to happen that quickly."

Just as the CHC drew support from its multiple connections, individual clinicians stressed the importance of their own professional networks. A CHC physician described the difficulty of finding readily available information during the challenging transition from virtual back to in-person care, and turning to colleagues for help, "I remember ...texting other leaders at health centers or [in] public health and [asking], what would you do if this was you? What do you think I should tell my team to keep them safest? ... We were all bouncing ideas off of each other." The physician recommended "working to…meet [with outside colleagues] when you're not in times of crisis…and establish relationships because we don't need to recreate the wheel."

Family First: Respect for Patients and Employees

> *They care about every single one of their patients.… They treat every patient like they're their family. And that's how all the staff at [the CHC] was.*
> —Student volunteer

The CHC's philosophy included treating all those who walk through its doors—patients and employees—as family. According to a former leader, "One of the things that made [the CHC] more responsive to the pandemic was a history of really trying to take care of our staff." Clinicians, for example, could choose the number of weekly hours to work. "A lot of community health centers just have revolving doors… we've always been very happy that that hardly ever happens with us."

The family-first philosophy permeated the practice, as many staff members emphasized the CHC's two top pandemic priorities: staff safety and patient safety. The CHC president and CEO emphasized the gravity of safety decisions, "[I] was very aware that if we didn't do our job right, that people would die." Another leader explained that decision making was based on the question, "Is this best in line with what our patients need and our staff need? And if the answer was yes, then, okay, how do we make it happen?" Protections for staff included a voluntary furlough, a halt in inpatient rounding at a local community hospital, and moving staff to individual offices. A clinician described feeling "attended to" by leadership, as opposed to being treated as "people who are just supposed to keep producing."

The Trunk and Branches: CHC Innovations

Strong established roots allowed the CHC to not only survive the intense and uncertain pandemic but also to innovate and thrive.

Telemedicine

In March 2020, days after the county went into lockdown, the CHC decided that clinicians would not see patients in person for the near future. They had not previously established a telehealth platform, but doing so suddenly became an urgent priority. A CHC clinician who was trained in electronic medical record (EMR) operations spearheaded the development of the CHC's telehealth system. During a round-the-clock weekend, the clinician (and friends and family) tested HIPAA-secure platforms by simulating visits and eventually selected one for use. The platform could integrate into the CHC's existing Epic EMR and did not require patients to download a separate application, an important factor since the CHC was unsure how many of its underserved patients had smartphones. The web-based platform was user-friendly, the clinician explained, while also "bridging those divides of the potentially more complex patients."

The system was quickly implemented, and with the help of first- and second-year medical students enrolled in a new pandemic elective, the CHC called patients to ensure that they were alerted to and scheduled for telemedicine visits. From April through fall 2020, the CHC provided 90% of its care through telemedicine. As a clinician/leader described, "We structured the [telemedicine] process to maintain as much of the same quality of care. Still making sure we were doing all the little things that we know are so important when you're bringing a patient into the clinic." With that in mind, patients were sent a link to access the telemedicine platform. After logging on, they met with a medical assistant who would verify their identification and ask relevant screening questions and then with their clinician.

Clinicians found that telemedicine visits were especially helpful in providing patient education for chronic care, sometimes serving as a remote home visit. One clinician described a diabetic patient who had his medications with him, "And he was sitting in his kitchen, and I said, well, why don't we go through your fridge? ... opening a fridge and getting an idea of what somebody was eating was very different. I had other patients where we're talking about their blood pressure, and they're sitting in their living room, and they said, oh, yeah, you did give me a blood pressure cuff a year ago. And...well, let's go find it. Let's walk through your closet...and let's get it out, and let's check it." Clinicians were seeing patients' homes for the first time and gaining new insights.

When patients were in acute pain, telemedicine fell short, with clinicians unable to conduct a physical exam and patients fearful of going to the emergency room where COVID-19 was rampant. Looking back, clinicians still wonder if diagnoses were missed.

The CHC's behavioral health team continues to see most patients virtually. However, there were limitations to virtual behavioral health. In some cases, it was difficult to gain a sense of patients' self-care virtually, and in other cases, patients hid aspects of their home that might signal a more severe mental health challenge. According to one behavioral health clinician, "Four years in...We struggle still to figure out who is an appropriate virtual visit...where we're talking more about emotional symptoms, where there's not an objective measure, should all of those [visits] be virtual, and how do you structure that...?"

Certain patient populations were also more challenging to serve with virtual care. For patients without smartphones, who were unable to participate in virtual visits, appointments took place by telephone. Older patients were more likely to have challenges initially using the virtual platform, although they often succeeded with assistance from a more technologically savvy family member or aide. Non-English-speaking patients, who faced language barriers and limited technology literacy, were also challenged by the telehealth call link.

Providing care for patients exclusively through telehealth early in the pandemic led to changes in clinicians' patient volume and workflows. Six weeks into the pandemic, the weekly number of patient visits exceeded the weekly visit volume one year before in 2019. One clinician described the increase in workflow, "At community health centers, no-show rate for visits is about 30%. It's a lot lower when [patients are] sitting on [their] couch…. what does access mean if the schedules now are full? We often talk about the virtual day of seeing 11 patients back-to-back…That's really hard in patient care too and the strain it created on providers and staff." In contrast, other clinicians said that a virtual day of care allowed the workday to end earlier, as there were fewer notes to take compared to an in-person visit. The no-show rate for behavioral health visits also fell, "from 30% to 10% and has stayed that way."

Telehealth had other unintended consequences as well. A behavioral health clinician explained that, prior to the pandemic, mental health and behavioral health were strengthened by being co-located at the practice. However, "If mental health is going to remain 75%, 80% virtual, now those providers and staff rightfully don't need to be on site. So now they're not co-located anymore. What does that do for the feel of the clinics and how we talk about and structure these clinics looks different?"

By spring 2021, as in-person care returned, approximately 30% of care was virtual. Today, clinicians still offer some virtual care each week, and the behavioral health team still provides 70% of its care virtually. The success of virtual care during the pandemic and its ongoing use suggest that the CHC designed and implemented a virtual platform that the CHC needed and that patients wanted.

Drive-Up COVID Testing

In April 2020, in the midst of providing virtual care, the CHC began providing COVID-19 testing. As one CHC site manager explained, "We actually went down a path that we never thought we would, and that was …going to the community to [conduct] testing, and eventually with vaccines… trying to implement something that is successful for the patients, meeting them where they're at." The CHC created daylong testing clinics and used a hospital system nearby to run labs and test specimens. The site manager continued, "We collaborated with them. …We'd have pop-up testing, but we predominantly did a lot of the testing at [one CHC site] in the back parking lot." As cars flooded in, the CHC numbered their parking spaces, 1–13, "so … we knew where we were going."

The site manager of the CHC's main testing site described the operation:

> We were in head-to-toe personal protective equipment. We had a face mask on, the shield…. gloves, everything. On a typical day we would have maybe one or two medical staff conducting the testing. And then a runner would go out to each of the cars and …check people in... because a lot of these weren't even our patients. They were just from the community. …We had a lot of new patients, so we're obtaining their insurance, their IDs, their information...then other staff members were putting together the supplies...the labels...the vials, the swabs, making sure everything was ready to go, and then countless numbers of

> bags...because you had to double, triple, wrap the specimen in the containers...And then the...provider, one or two of them would go out to the vehicles and get more information about when they were exposed. What symptoms are you having? Depending on the severity of their symptoms, we would have to … check blood pressures in the parking lot. We're listening to them, assessing them as best as we could, just to make sure they're breathing. Okay, their blood pressure is fine. They're stable versus having a horrible COVID virus, right?...So then...the medical team would go out, do the testing, do their assessments, grab the specimens...after we completed our testing...And then after we collected the specimen, we had to bag everything up...and that would take an hour...we had to print the orders out, and then you had to match the orders up with the patient specimen. We would have hundreds of specimens that we would have to go through, and — you're trying to go so quickly — that we didn't always have time to try to bag the order with the specimen. Sometimes we'd have to go back and do it after the fact, but we tried to stay on top of it by putting the order with the specimen, and...as the day...completed, we had to make sure all the orders were in the right bag... We might have been done testing at 4 pm, but we were probably there for a good couple of hours after making sure everything was correctly labeled...cause we knew how important it was for the patients to know whether or not they had COVID. And then, following it... we would send it all out. [The lab] would pick up the specimens. And about 48 hours later we would get the results. And [we] were making phone calls to all those positive patients and then going through all the education of what you needed to do now.

Testing sites held many challenges, including finding a lab to process the samples within a reasonable timeframe. Initially, the CHC used a phlebotomy company with a 1-week turnaround time, which wasn't suitable for the severity and infectiousness of the disease, and they did not have enough collection tubing or specimen containers. This prompted a switch to a hospital system lab, which required numerous virtual coordination meetings. The testing site, which had a small parking lot, had overflow traffic, and short time slots for testing made congestion worse. One clinician could not complete one car's worth of testing in the scheduled timeframe, "You had families of six coming in a vehicle… you're educating them, and you had the language barriers…. So we had to bring interpreters with us to the car, so that added a whole [other] timeframe. So we went from a…shorter appointment time slot to making it [longer] to allow for more time to educate, being able to get the car in safely, out safely and have [room] for the next vehicle to come in."

Lastly, testing clinics had a time intensive check-in process, with staff manually entering each patient's insurance and demographic information into a portal system. This required an increase in staffing from 3–5 staff members to 8–9. In the 4 years since the start of the pandemic, the CHC provided nearly 20,000 tests and administered more than 47,000 vaccines.

In spite of the challenges, testing clinics were successful: "We pulled it off amazingly...I had a great team there that was all on board. … through the snow, through the rain, through the heat, we were out there in the parking lot, testing patients and providing them with the education and resources they needed to keep themselves and their families safe … and at the same time trying to keep my staff safe, too."

Drive-Up INR and HbA1c Checks

From August to October 2020, the CHC held drive-up International Normalized Ratio (INR) and Hemoglobin A1C (HbA1c) checks. Similar to drive-up COVID-19 testing, the CHC used a parking lot at their largest site. The site manager described the set up, "We would have them line up [by the] employee entrance on the side of the building …, and we…mass texted all of our INR patients [with their scheduled time]... We had all of our equipment on carts. We had all of our [participating] staff gowned up, full PPE. We had all of our sharps containers [on carts]. The patient would drive up, and we had our INR machines. [Staff] would go up to the vehicle, they would poke [the patient's] finger, they would get their results, and …made sure the patient is fine, get their results, and then they would drive away. The provider would call them with their results, do any adjustments, if needed, to their medicine and their coumadin, and then that was their visit." The operation required five or six gowned employees, and a similar set up was also used for HbA1c checks.

Some staff were hesitant about reintroducing in-person interactions due to fear of catching COVID-19, and others were uncertain if this untested innovation would work. The site manager explained, "You …were kind of thrown into it. And it looks good on paper. Let's go try it…There's no practice session. You just really have to try it …. and at the time it worked."

Vaccine Clinics and A New Workforce: Students

On Saturday, February 23, 2021, CWRU's Student Run Health Clinic, which was located at the CHC, began administering vaccines to the community. After injecting fifty doses the first day, they went on to serve 200 patients every subsequent Saturday until August of that year, for a total of 20,587 vaccines administered. With this demand, the CHC realized that they would need more manpower, and they turned once again to students. Most nursing and medical students required training, so student leaders developed a training system; learners had to see three vaccines administered and then perform three supervised before working solo. The Student Run Health Clinic made other adjustments to the new workforce as well. For example, it proved to be difficult to provide each volunteer with an EMR login, so they created paper forms that students could fill out and deliver to the MA, who entered the patient data into the system. This gave the students a sense of agency, and the team revised the form regularly to maximize efficiency. Reflecting on the CHC's relationship with students, a nursing educator said, "I think part of what made the CHC so successful is that they were just willing. They were open to having students involved. So many of our other clinical partners put up barrier after barrier for involving our students and weren't necessarily willing to be creative on how we integrate students in."

After long months of relative isolation, for both students and patients, there was a sense of excitement. One supervisor commented, "It was the happiest clinic you've ever been in. You had all these super old people who were so thrilled to be there.

And you had students who had the time and were so excited to talk to people. And it was amazing every single time." In fact, the clinics became so popular that there was eventually an overabundance of volunteers.

At the same time, the CHC realized they could reach other populations by creating pop-up clinics off site. With the promise of more vaccines coming from the State of Ohio, they set up a vaccine clinic at a local multicultural church. Using the social networks of employees and community partners, they identified other community locations. Some community organizations heard about the pop-up clinics and requested their own. To meet this demand, student leaders at the medical, nursing, and physician assistant schools arranged for participation by eager student volunteers. A medical school leader explained that the CHC, "... would regularly update us, '[here's what] this month looks like,'... I would send out periodic emails about new upcoming vaccine sites.... I was able to create a master spreadsheet to make sure everyone had enough time to get their experience with volunteering."

To examine their success in reaching vulnerable populations with pop-up clinics, an analyst with a health improvement collaborative utilized the Social Vulnerability Index, a database that maps sixteen census variables to geographic locations and identifies communities who may be socially vulnerable in a disaster setting. The comparison of this data showed that the pop-up clinic locations matched locations of social vulnerability in Cleveland, demonstrating that they were able to reach populations that some of the larger health care systems did not. According to a member of the health improvement collaborative, a highlight of this period was "seeing people in communities that are more at risk for poor outcomes from COVID getting access to things that they should have equal access to."

The vaccine clinics had lasting effects on the CHC. Staff members who were involved in them reported feeling closer to other participating colleagues. One front desk employee recalled the Saturday clinics, "I think we became more close because it would be the same people every weekend. And…it felt like a family because we would see each other six days out of the week. And it was just nice to know that we were all there to help the patients... Our…CEO would be there and our VP would be there...the vibe was just amazing."

The vaccine clinics raised the profile of the CHC and attracted new patients, thus growing the CHC "family." According to Health Resources and Services Administration data, the CHC increased its patient size from 21,686 patients in 2020 to 22,399 patients in 2021, before decreasing to 21,057 in 2022 and rising again to 22,140 patients in 2023 [11]. Effective vaccine outreach and the ability to build on existing relationships with community partners and the student workforce contributed to this growth.

Changes to Internal Communication

Early in the pandemic, with meetings no longer occurring in person and staff working remotely or in separate office spaces, new methods of internal communication were needed. The CHC began using Microsoft Teams, allowing colleagues to instant message and call each other using audio-only or audio and video. The Teams calendar function allowed employees to know when their colleagues were busy and enabled more seamless patient scheduling.

Additionally, the CHC began using the Epic EMR's instant chat function to send protected patient information to one another. This was especially useful for PSC staff, who did not have access to patient charts. When the Epic chat function was implemented, the CHC developed a data-sharing system in which a PSC staff member was authorized to share with a patient any part of their record that the clinician put within quotation marks, allowing them to respond to patients inquiring about test results. No longer having to wait to connect to a provider, this innovation helped PSC staff respond to more patients more quickly, decrease call wait times, and better manage high call volumes.

Online Appointment Scheduling

An innovation introduced to decrease call volume was online appointment scheduling. A physician-informaticist developed an online appointment scheduling platform, which consisted of a Google form, and then analyzed the time stamps indicating when patients used the form to schedule appointments: "We had...analytics from this Google form about what time patients were scheduling their COVID testing, COVID vaccine. And it was like three in the morning, 11 p.m. All these non-traditional hours." The development of online scheduling allowed patients to schedule appointments at their convenience and helped reduce Patient Service Center call volume. The physician-informaticist continued, "You can schedule appointments online and we encourage it…more than 10 percent of our patient visits are scheduled online now across all [CHC] centers... Those are 10 percent of visits that are no longer calling in for appointments... we [had] a call center for a pre-COVID call volume [and we had] to adapt pretty quickly."

Clinic Safety Protocols

With patient and employee safety deemed a top CHC priority, safety measures were on display when in-person visits resumed. One such measure was the creation of a "rapid room," an area of the waiting room, walled by plexiglass, for patients suspected of having COVID-19. Patients were tested for COVID-19 in the rapid room prior to entering the clinic. Like most practices, the CHC also implemented temperature checks for patients before they entered the building. The sites also added buzzers on their outside doors. Arriving patients pressed the buzzer and stated their business into a microphone and camera. According to a former employee, this feature was added to avoid crowds in the waiting room: "They would confirm they had their appointment, they would make sure the room [was] clean, then they would buzz them in and get them checked in. So it was a way to streamline that process. [For] some of the sites, it was more for safety, because they had patients that were physically and verbally abusive towards staff. So, they kept it as a safe barrier."

The Fruits of the CHC's Labor

The CHC's efforts to innovate and stay operational for its patients during the pandemic led to lasting changes to the CHC's practice.

Population Health Team

One fruit of the pandemic is the CHC's population health team, which was established in February 2022. It conducts centralized outreach to patients for all sites, replacing the individual (and therefore inconsistent) outreach efforts of the seven sites. The team organizes routine outreach to patients for colorectal cancer, breast cancer, and cervical cancer screenings, hypertension and diabetes care, and COVID-19 and influenza immunizations. Gaps in these screenings are often tied to significant payer-based incentives in value-based care and therefore have significant financial implications for the organization. In addition, the team assesses patients' social determinants of health and pregnancy risk, conducts quality improvement projects, and is starting a food as medicine program allowing patients to pick up healthy food.

A key component of the population health team's success in reaching its outreach and performance goals reflects the nature of the CHC's pandemic response. The population health team manager explained that, "Patients have learned to trust [the CHC] and trust the providers and what they're saying. So I think that's pretty huge, especially during a pandemic. Who do you listen to? That's wonderful that we've been able to maintain our population and be able to answer those questions, especially for non-English [speakers] as well."

Achievements in Health Equity

A motivation for studying this CHC was its reputation for reaching Cleveland's underserved communities before and during the pandemic. One veteran clinician exclaimed, "I was extraordinarily proud of the practice and my colleagues [during the pandemic]. When you look at our vaccine numbers, our ability to [do] outreach into communities that...were not getting tested and not getting vaccines and not being seen in disparate ways all over the country, and also in Cleveland - we just did a good job, you know?"

A key strategy for reaching underserved communities was to keep the patients' needs in mind. A former senior leader stated, "I feel really proud ... that we built the organization from the patient's point of view. ... we were thinking a lot about not making it too hard for people to get what they needed." Another senior leader described the CHC's decision to not require insurance to receive a vaccine: "we wanted to vaccinate the community. If the community wasn't our patient, then they would have had to go through all that insurance. You know, the wallet biopsy. And we made a decision…early on that that's not what we were going to do."

The CHC relied on its pre-existing relationships with community partners and the county health department to vaccinate under-resourced populations. "[T]he vaccine clinic was just like a piece of art; it was amazing!...it just ran as smooth as silk. We were so efficient and our outreach was so good and we got the populations that we needed to get which nobody else in the city did; we were so far ahead of everyone else in any kind of minority group you can imagine, so it was something that we were all very, very proud of," said a senior leader. CHC personnel were particularly proud of providing outreach to a degree that they felt local hospital systems didn't achieve. "Seriously, the hospitals are going to do only a drive through and they're not going to do any community outreach!?" said a former senior leader. "…you guys, come on, you know that this is not going to help the City of Cleveland that well, because people don't have a car they can sit in for two hours on the line, not to mention the whole essential worker thing [and]...the unevenness of care." The senior leader had the opportunity to "speak truth to power" in a chance encounter with a local hospital CEO, and said, "I just want to let you know that the safety net organizations are not going to be able to take care of the [entire] community, we need the hospitals to be out in the community too." A month later, the hospital system started offering vaccines in the community.

Innovations in Medical Education

While many lamented the stall in medical education due to hospital and classroom shutdowns, the partnership between the CHC and the city's clinical students created unique opportunities for learning. Nursing students were able to count their work in CHC vaccine clinics as clinical hours. It became a core component of the public/community/population health classes, which normally required hours in the community. In addition, a nurse educator used the CHC's telehealth system to introduce students to virtual health practice using such tools as texting and phone calls: "They got a different experience and they got to learn how to use the different technology and they had a bit of patient interaction over the phone."

Later, vaccine clinics offered an ideal learning environment for vaccine administration due to the repetitive nature of the task: "I really love teaching vaccine clinics because students learn a skill and they get to practice it over and over and over again, which you don't get in the hospital because not every patient needs the exact same thing over and over again." Lastly, the communication between CWRU's School of Nursing and the CHC resulted in an ongoing trusting relationship which remains in place. "[They] …put out feelers like, 'Hey, we might be doing something, we might need some help.' And it's very easy for me to … say, 'Here are parameters, … I'll have students.'... I think it just became easy to … go back and forth."

Working at the CHC during the pandemic gave students insights into the broader inner workings of clinical decision making. A leader of the Student Run Health

Clinic said that her understanding of how health care systems work as a whole is much stronger now, something that her current colleagues have noted: "One of my clinical instructors... was like, 'Oh my gosh, you're always thinking about the bigger picture,' and I was like, 'Oh, I spent a lot of time thinking about [the] bigger picture and what this means for the health care system....' It gave me a huge perspective on... how access to care is important."

With the return to in-person CHC appointments and waning of telehealth, as well as the end of the vaccine frenzy, the CWRU School of Medicine curriculum returned to normal. For some fourth-year medical students, participating in patient outreach through CWRU's pandemic elective was a leadership opportunity: "I had the opportunity to mentor and teach a little bit, which I did not expect... once the first and second year students came, and were there for a few hours we got to just talk about medicine... I got to flex those muscles at the end of my fourth year, but it was because I got the option to work with other medical students." Other students found meaningful work during a time of uncertainty by working in the vaccine clinics: "It's nice hanging out with all the volunteers, getting to meet ... people in the community... It was one of my highlights during med school." For the CHC, it was evidence that students could be trusted partners. According to one CHC leader, "You're a medical professional from day one, you sign on, you put your white coat on, you take your oath, and there you go. Everyone needs to have opportunities to learn and grow. So we were really happy to have them part of our team."

For some students, the experience of working with the CHC had a lasting effect on their career paths. A nursing student explained, "It really made me want to work somewhere where patient care is so important, in a place where providers are such huge advocates for their patients." A medical student shared, "The experience really got me more interested in urban health... I do want to be able to work in an area where I am providing care for an underserved community as part of my normal patient population. When I was choosing a residency program, I wanted to make sure that a portion of the population that they were serving was Medicaid or uninsured patients."

Evolving Work Culture

As staff, patients, and the practice evolved during the uncertainty and fear of the pandemic, the CHC's work culture inevitably changed. Changes in the organization's culture began before the pandemic, especially as the CHC grew, leading to a sense of disconnection among some veteran staff members. With the growth of the practice to more than 250 employees, the original "family" closeness could feel diminished, despite the unifying experience of the pandemic and Saturday vaccine distributions.

Changes in physical proximity also affected organizational culture before and during the pandemic. CHC administration, including the human resources (HR) and quality improvement departments and the board of directors, were originally located physically in the practice, creating a close connection between leadership, management, and staff. Just prior to the pandemic, however, leadership moved to a separate administrative building, creating separation for the first time. As the pandemic hit, clinicians and some middle management and staff worked on site at the clinic, while administrators worked exclusively from home. When virtual meetings were held, the difference between who was calling from home and who was calling from the CHC office reflected the division between administrators and site staff. The virtual separation during the pandemic amplified the physical separation between leadership and those in the clinics. As the CHC transitioned back to in-person care, CHC administration was perceived by some employees as being removed from employees who had worked on the frontline (with the exception of those senior leaders who were also clinicians and highly accessible to staff as they helped lead the CHC through pivots and innovations).

During and after the pandemic, many staff members left the CHC. There was turnover among the leadership team, staff, and clinicians. Some turnover came as long-time employees retired. Other reasons for leaving appeared to relate to the challenges of the pandemic, the stress and complexity of working in a CHC, a desire for higher pay and more flexible work schedules, and a re-evaluation of career goals and personal values.

The CHC, like other FQHCs, has not been immune to the corporatization of health care as it has grown from a small grassroots organization to a multisite organization. The need for financial stability and a business model suited to the number of patients and communities they serve have contributed to the CHC's evolving culture. We found, however, that the majority of the CHC's workforce values and retains a sense of family and honors the CHC's original grassroots energy and efforts.

Limitations

There were limitations to our data collection process. We were only able to interview individuals who responded to our outreach attempts, and these were primarily individuals still working at the CHC. A few interviews took place in participants' place of work, which may have led to response bias with overly positive interview answers. The quality of the data collected was also impacted by the gap of four or more years between the onset of the pandemic and the time of the interviews. A majority of the analyses were conducted by the same individuals who conducted the interviews, and analyses were done in a nonblinded fashion, leading to potential bias in the analyses. Lastly, two members of the research team were also study participants, potentially contributing to response bias or conflict of interest.

Conclusions and Take-Home Lessons

In 2020, the pandemic turned our world upside down with uncertainties of how to exist and stay safe. While the media shared important stories of frontline workers in emergency rooms, loved ones dying of the virus, and severe disparities faced by minority and underserved populations, there was a worthy story that received less airtime: the story of community health centers striving to meet their neighbors' complex health needs.

Despite having limited resources, this multisite CHC in Cleveland continued to innovate, serve, and meet its commitment to health equity during a time of intense loss. Lessons from the CHC's formative pandemic experience can inform the next public health crisis and improve care during smaller crises and everyday joys. Lessons include the following.

- **Invest in relationships and maintain an improvement focus before a crisis hits.** The CHC's long-term commitment to relationship building and ongoing improvement played vital roles in their ability to meet the needs of vulnerable populations during a crisis. Relationships include those that are internal, with employees, and those outside the organization, with community leaders and public officials who know their community well. These connections provide a trustworthy pipeline for sharing information with the community in a time of crisis.
- **In a public health emergency, CHCs have invaluable proximity to and knowledge of vulnerable populations and their barriers to care and health**. CHCs have unique opportunities and responsibilities to act on behalf of underserved populations when a public health crisis strikes. It is therefore essential that they nurture trustworthy connections with their patient populations over time and provide culturally tailored care. Policymakers should support safety-net institutions and look to them for on-the-ground perspectives regarding the needs of underserved and vulnerable community members.
- **Lead with humility.** Action in crisis is most effective when leaders approach their tasks with humility, listening to the people and populations serving and being served. This requires recognizing and articulating uncertainty and listening to more knowledgeable others, i.e., those on the frontlines. Listening not only provides leaders with an important source of information, it also conveys respect and value, characteristics which can become embedded in the organization's culture. The result can be an organization with strong connections, an ethos of trust, and the ability to withstand and grow from crisis.
- **Encourage the workforce to be flexible in their roles and find creative solutions when pivots are required**. Engaging willing workers, including learners, can bring passion and determination to the work of an organization. Indeed, during the unprecedented COVID-19 pandemic, we were all learners. Applying that beginner's mindset to the daily work of an organization, as well as to a pandemic response, can lead to innovation, creativity, and adaptability.

Such lessons can be transported and reinvented in any health care, public health, or advocacy institution working to improve the health of underserved populations. This CHC's innovations and post-pandemic adjustments are a microcosm of the changes seen at FQHCs and health care institutions nationwide.

Acknowledgments This work was supported by a training grant from the National Institute on Aging, T32AG086098, and by research grants from the National Institute on Aging (R01AG074946) and the National Institute on Minority Health and Health Disparities (R01MD016389). The funders had no role in the study design, analysis, interpretation of the data, writing this report, or the decision to submit the report for publication.

The authors are grateful to the staff of the community health center and their student and community partners for their time in being interviewed and for their dedication to their patients and to the community they serve.

References

1. National Academies of Sciences, Engineering, and Medicine. Long-term health effects of COVID-19: disability and function following SARS-CoV-2 infection. The National Academies Press; 2024.
2. Kwiatkowski J. COVID-19–inspired health provider innovation and collaboration should continue. Milbank Memorial Fund Blog. https://www.milbank.org/2020/05/health-provider-innovation-and-collaboration-should-continue/. Accessed 31 Aug 2024.
3. Sharfstein JM, Lurie N. Public health emergency preparedness after COVID-19. Milbank Q. 2023;101(S1):653–73. https://doi.org/10.1111/1468-0009.12615.
4. Etz RS, Solid CA, Gonzalez MM, Britton E, Stange KC, Reves SR. Telemedicine in primary care: lessons learned about implementing health care innovations during the COVID-19 pandemic. Ann Fam Med. 2023;21(4):297–304. https://doi.org/10.1370/afm.2979. PMC10365867, https://www.ncbi.nlm.nih.gov/pubmed/37487734.
5. Gullett HL, Brown GL, Collins D, et al. Using community-based system dynamics to address structural racism in community health improvement. J Public Health Manag Pract. 2022;28(4):S130–7. https://doi.org/10.1097/PHH.0000000000001492.
6. Better Health Partnership. https://www.betterhealthpartnership.org/.
7. Goyal S, Law E. An introduction to Kaizen in health care. Br J Hosp Med (Lond). 2019;80(3):168–9. https://doi.org/10.12968/hmed.2019.80.3.168.
8. Madden MH, Tomsik P, Terchek J, et al. Keys to successful diabetes self-management for uninsured patients: social support, observational learning, and turning points: a safety net providers' strategic alliance study. J Natl Med Assoc. 2011;103(3):257–64.
9. Reichsman A, Werner J, Cella P, Bobiak S, Stange KC, SNPSA Diabetes Study Working Group. Opportunities for improved diabetes care among patients of safety net practices: a Safety Net Providers' Strategic Alliance (SNPSA) study. J Natl Med Assoc. 2009;101(1):4–11.
10. Tanenbaum J, Cebul RD, Votruba M, Einstadter D. Association of a regional health improvement collaborative with ambulatory care–sensitive hospitalizations. Health Aff. 2018;37(2):266–74. https://doi.org/10.1377/hlthaff.2017.1209.
11. Health center program uniform data system (UDS) data overview. Hrsagov Published 2023. https://data.hrsa.gov/tools/data-reporting/program-data?grantNum=H80CS00665. Accessed 2 Sept 2024.

Chapter 8
Establishing Community Testing and Vaccination Centers Within a Week: Two Case Studies from the Primary Care Medical Home

Sonja Likumahuwa-Ackman, Shelby Lee Freed, Brian Garvey, Emily Myers, Joe Skariah, and Johanna Warren

> *There was this kind of fear and anxiety about the unknown, and many changing circumstances, along with this very deep sense of purpose that 'This is the work that we are called to do, and we are prepared to do it, and we have the flexibility to go into the ICU or to go into the streets of our communities, and we can do all of that.' So, that's what we did—set up mass testing sites, mass vaccination sites, and then the monoclonal antibody infusion, and now Paxlovid. And so, we signaled to the community that we're here to serve them. And I think that patients turned to us because people knew that they could trust us to make good recommendations or judgment calls. I think that that was part of building community collaboration and trust during the period* —Primary Care Physician.

Introduction and Background

Primary care teams pivoted to serve the needs of their communities and patients throughout the COVID-19 pandemic. In the early months, this included providing COVID-19 evaluation and testing. Later, this included providing vaccines to patients and communities. This chapter will include two case studies that illustrate the day-to-day realities being faced by primary care and some of the lessons learned from these experiences. The first: standing up an outdoor testing site at an urban federally qualified health center (FQHC). The second: standing up a weekend/evening vaccine clinic in a busy rural health center (RHC; in partnership with county public health) that served an entire rural county. We focus on the lifespan of each initiative and the evolution of decisions that were made to respond to the dynamic pandemic. Primary care was on the frontlines of the pandemic and at the forefront of innovation. We had to keep delivering 24/7 primary care but had to do so in the context of

S. Likumahuwa-Ackman (✉) · S. L. Freed · B. Garvey · E. Myers · J. Skariah · J. Warren
Family Medicine, Oregon Health & Science University, Portland, OR, USA
e-mail: likumahu@ohsu.edu

A. Cheng et al. (eds.), *Primary Care in a Public Health Emergency*,
https://doi.org/10.1007/978-3-032-12487-6_8

a contagious virus circulating in the community and the need to keep patients out of emergency rooms and hospital intensive care units as much as possible. This work was consistent with one of the common mantras of primary care: right care, right place, right time. This chapter highlights the ways in which our primary care teams tried to take care of the most vulnerable members of our local community and, ultimately, how profoundly we as a country failed at achieving this goal. Our mission to serve and to meet community needs (as an RHC and FQHC) gave us the courage and motivation to act during a time of fear and uncertainty.

COVID-19 Testing and Respiratory Care Initiative (March 2020–March 2021)

The Richmond Family Medicine Health Center, a Federally Qualified Health Center at Oregon Health & Science University (OHSU), in Portland, Oregon
In March 2020, our urban FQHC needed to figure out how to continue seeing patients with respiratory symptoms. Our FQHC is unique in that it is embedded with OHSU's network of family medicine clinics and is a training site for OHSU students and residents. We knew our population well (low income, predominantly Medicaid insured, with a disproportionately high burden of chronic medical and mental health conditions), and knew they were at higher risk for adverse outcomes due to COVID-19. The clinic had not yet implemented telehealth systems that could enable virtual visits. We did not want to turn people away, and we did not want to close our doors. Among staff members who were the first point of contact for patients, there was uncertainty, fear, and weariness about symptomatic patients coming into the clinic.

Within hours of the first case of COVID-19 hitting our local community, one of our experienced nurse practitioners, Dr. Shelby Lee Freed, stepped up to create an innovative outdoor testing station. She had been working in FQHCs for over 10 years and knew the systems and stakeholders well, which helped facilitate the process. Two medical assistants, also certified emergency medical technicians (EMTs), stepped up to help. Their emergency medicine training helped with planning, organization, set up, and triage. They were instrumental to the development and operation of this innovation.

In the early days, Dr. Freed started evaluating patients who had any COVID-19-like symptoms in the clinic parking lot. She would bring her stethoscope, blood pressure cuff, and oxygen saturation/heart rate monitor so she could get vital signs, often placing these on top of a bush while she interviewed the patient. On a small piece of paper, she would write down vitals and a few short notes for documentation in the electronic health record (EHR) later. Within a few days, other clinicians were doing something similar. It became clear that the clinic needed to create a more widespread practice with guidelines and a system wrapped around to provide safe, patient-centered, evidence-based care. See Box 8.1 for more details regarding Dr. Freed and her experiences.

Box 8.1: Rising to the Moment
In the early days of the pandemic, Dr. Freed spent many late nights in the clinic helping to develop workflows and presentations on how the information would be disseminated and to help gain institutional support for ongoing efforts. Many family members of health care professionals are accustomed to their loved ones spending long days and late nights caring for patients, but with COVID-19 the tenor drastically changed, given the nature of the work and risk involved. COVID-19 related stories were becoming commonplace across the news, social media, and internet from places that had been struck hard both nationally and internationally creating the fear and uncertainty that would soon permeate our worlds. On March 22, 2020, Oregon Public Broadcasting came to Richmond's outdoor testing and respiratory clinic site to document what they called "history." Dr. Freed was asked, "What does it feel like to be a part of an historic event?" Not entirely grasping the enormity of the moment, Dr. Freed responded, "I think I'm just doing my job." Dr. Freed remembers having a lot of hard conversations at home with her husband thinking about their 3-year-old daughter, their elderly parents, and what the implications of her work were for their family. Knowing no one was necessarily asking her to develop this clinic, Dr. Freed's husband asked her, "Do you have to do this?" With little thought she responded, "Yes. I have to do this because I *can* do this." It was a brief but meaningful exchange that set the stage for the next two years.

Although OHSU opened two large-scale, drive-through testing sites for the greater Portland, OR, community in March 2020 [1], conducting nearly 55,000 tests between March and October 2020, the FQHC testing site continued to operate and provide access to patients who had difficulty accessing the mass testing sites. Many patients preferred these local sites because they did not have a car and relied on public transportation, could not easily take time off work, or did not want to drive to an unfamiliar location such as a sports stadium. Trust in their primary care medical home and their primary care team was also a big factor.

The FQHC outdoor testing site morphed into a testing and respiratory clinic. Over the two years it operated, it evolved and changed, eventually integrating back into the primary care clinic. The outdoor testing initiative kept the clinic doors open, maintained access for patients, kept staff as safe as possible, and quelled anxiety and fear at the clinic while maintaining dedication to the mission as an academic medical center. This section describes how it was done, key contextual factors, lessons learned, and community impacts.

Zoom In: The Nitty-Gritty Details

The Richmond Family Medicine FQHC serves over 17,000 individuals; approximately half are considered low income; 34% are of a racial or ethnic minority; 71% are uninsured or publicly insured, and over 50% have one or more chronic medical conditions.

When the clinic leadership realized that a standardized approach to providing clinical care in their parking lot was needed, they began meeting daily. Most meetings were attended by the medical director, quality improvement (QI) lead, clinic manager, template/scheduling manager, and the lead respiratory medical assistant (MA). Decisions needed to be made minute-by-minute, and there was often no time or opportunity to seek approval, so the group adopted a fast-paced style of moving forward and agreed to plead for forgiveness later, rather than ask for permission. At an early meeting, Dr. Freed was given the go-ahead to develop protocols for outdoor respiratory care, the latitude to adjust EHR templates, and the ability to create schedules for providers and MAs to accommodate this type of care. This was a change from traditional hierarchies at our institution favoring leadership positions for physicians over advanced practice clinicians, such as nurse practitioners (NPs) and physician associates (PAs).

Phase 1: Outdoor Testing

The first testing initiative utilized a 10 × 10 tent canopy in the clinic parking lot, as seen in Fig. 8.1. Over the next 9 months, two larger event tents were added to provide more covered space and protection from the weather. The day-to-day work was done by the clinic leadership team plus nurses, MAs, providers, front desk, reception, and scheduling. Anyone who had a positive COVID-19 test result was called by the clinic's community health worker (CHW) to see how the clinic could support

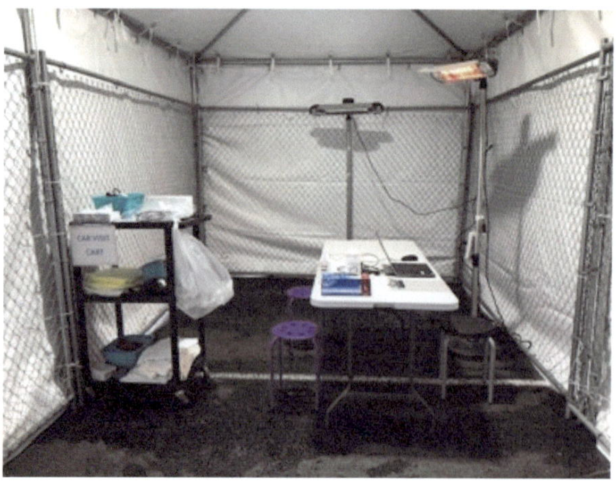

Fig. 8.1 Interior of the initial COVID-19 testing tent. This original photograph, taken by the author (SLF), shows the setup of the first testing initiative conducted under a 10 × 10 tent canopy designed to support safe and accessible specimen collection in the clinic parking lot

them at home or to obtain housing if they were unhoused and to provide them with other services (e.g., food, cleaning supplies, medication delivery).

During this time, the clinic leadership team consulted with their academic department, occupational health, and the university's infection control department frequently. There were innumerable daily emails and phone calls, as well as clinic, departmental, and institutional meetings with a constant flow of information. Dr. Freed worked with the chair of OHSU'S COVID-19 lab group, Dr. Johanna Warren, to develop and implement testing guidelines which were disseminated institutionwide. Changes to the guidelines were made as the evidence evolved, sometimes daily, for the better part of two years. The fluidity of the pandemic forced usual institutional structures and hierarchies to become more porous. One example is that Dr. Freed was able to join clinical leadership and institutional meetings to see how the rest of the organization was responding and how we could collaborate. Clinic leaders, including Dr. Freed, participated in the COVID-19 lab committee and primary care COVID-19 steering committee, which helped connect the local team to the larger institution more directly.

Protocols developed by the team covered scheduling, screening patients for respiratory symptoms, who should wear PPE, how to don and doff PPE, the role of the MA in taking vitals and documenting, how to obtain tests, and how to counsel patients. The initial staffing model was two providers and two MAs who could see 10–20 appointments per day or 50–100 people per week.

Phase 2: Indoor Testing and Respiratory Treatment

After 7 months of operating outdoors, the weather started to become colder and wetter. In October 2020, the testing moved from outdoors to an indoor space adjacent to and run by the clinic as part of our immediate care site. At this point, the role shifted from testing only to becoming a respiratory testing and care clinic. The structure and function of the respiratory clinic is described in more detail in Freed et al. 2022 [2]. This served as an institutional model for two other immediate care locations to become respiratory clinics and was plugged into an institutionwide initiative around respiratory care clinics in primary care settings. The overall goal of these innovations was to provide respiratory care services and testing regardless of insurance status, ability to pay, and whether people already had an established primary care provider.

Our FQHC testing team benefitted from being on the frontlines of the local community and connected to OHSU's larger system. For example, Drs. Freed and Warren worked closely together to manage protocols as well as develop and pilot test a point-of-care rapid testing algorithm, shown in Fig. 8.2, that were disseminated across ambulatory practices and the emergency department. For treatment, they met regularly with infectious disease leaders, who helped work through the different monoclonal antibody (mAb) and antiviral therapies and how they would be distributed in ambulatory care at the point when diagnoses were made. The team

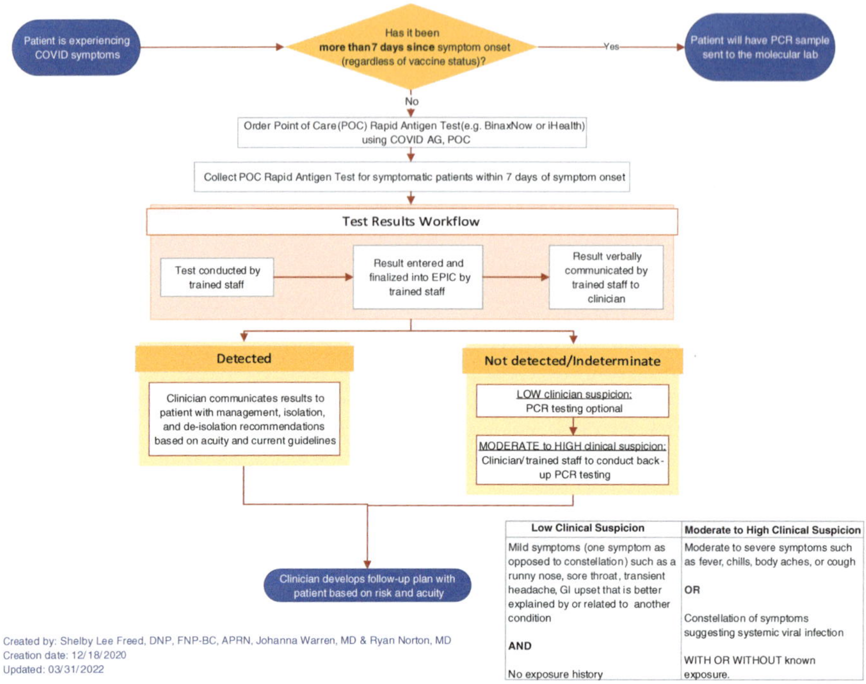

Fig. 8.2 Point-of-care rapid testing algorithm. Illustration of a clinical decision-making workflow designed to guide point-of-care rapid testing. Illustration created by the author (SLF, JW)

helped to distribute these protocols across the institution's primary care network and at immediate care sites.

Reimbursement to the FQHC for clinical services came from a variety of sources. As an FQHC, the clinic already had direct access to some federal and state funding. Other federal funding came by way of free testing and treatment until the end of the public health emergency. This was balanced with institutional support and funding that flowed from the state to all health care providers in the region. For our FQHC specifically, we relied heavily on Medicaid funding and some flexible funding streams to meet community needs. We also had some capitated funds that allowed us to be creative in meeting needs, an advantage we had compared to other settings reimbursed via fee-for-service mechanisms only.

Primary Care Values

As a patient-centered medical home (PCMH), the clinic already had a strong culture around process improvement and responsiveness to patient and community needs. The impetus behind outdoor respiratory care and, ultimately, the evolution of respiratory clinics at OHSU, was to be able to continue offering in-person care consistent with how we have always valued primary care. It significantly changed the *way* in which care teams were accustomed to operating. The clinic had to develop new workflows and models for care to continue delivering person-centered, high-quality, evidence-based care in a coordinated and integrated way.

Zoom Out: Broader Context and the Many Decisions Faced by the Team

It is important to remember the incredibly fluid and terrifying context of the first months of COVID-19. Knowledge was sparse; clinical guidelines and recommendations changed nearly daily. What were the questions that continuously had to be reviewed and answered to update testing guidelines? Instead of presenting details of the decisions made that were specific to COVID-19, here's a list of what we considered during this uncertain time, in the hopes that it will provide a helpful framework for future crises.

- Understanding how the virus is and is NOT transmitted. Who should be tested? Who should NOT be tested? What information and treatment are needed for patients who tested positive?
- Understanding the PPE available (particularly types and supply of masks) and how to acquire it and preserve it.
- Understanding what underlying medical conditions put people at higher risk than others.
- Understanding what testing modalities were available, in what quantities, what those test characteristics were (e.g., sensitivity and specificity), how to optimally swab patients (e.g., nasal, nasopharyngeal, serum antibodies), and how long the turn-around times were for actionable test results.
- Understanding isolation and quarantine recommendations and how they evolved.
- Understanding the evolution of local and national guidelines, appreciating differences in governance and politics that drove varying responses across the nation (and across our state).
- Understanding that social factors and mental health conditions also impacted risk, such as more crowded living spaces, people living at or below the poverty level, people working in service sector jobs and therefore unable to isolate or withdraw, and people with differing capacities to cope with the stresses of isolation.
- Understanding the important role of health care providers in determining when people were safe to return to work. For example, a negative COVID-19 test became the ticket back to "normal" life. Testing for COVID-19 was critical for those without paid time off; symptoms kept people out of work, impacting their housing, food, and health care access. A negative test meant returning to work.

Like so many aspects of the pandemic, access to health care and to accurate testing highlighted the fragile scaffolding of our communities.

- Understanding how trust and accountability played a role in our processes. The health care system and individual clinicians trusted the institutional, governmental, and public health sources as we took in and applied the evolving science and recommendations and were creative in adapting them to our communities' needs.

Bigger Contextual Factors and How We Handled Them

Changing Guidelines and Supplies

The fluidity and evolution of the landscape during the pandemic cannot be understated. Primary care was at the frontline of understanding and communicating the science as it evolved real-time to an emotional and fearful public and health care workforce. This was, and continues to be, *really* difficult. The level of fear and uncertainty was huge, with widely variable levels of risk tolerance throughout our health care teams. Some of the most consequential changes were: (1) guidelines ranging from no masks to all masking, and varying types of masking—from cloth to procedural to N95 masks; (2) supply chain shortages with initial pressure to conserve PPE which ultimately was resolved by a stable PPE supply; (3) perpetually changing testing guidelines, with various agencies updating guidelines—at the institutional, state, and federal levels. These guidelines determined who should be tested when, particularly when testing locations, labs, and supplies were very scarce. These types of changes resulted in a huge burden of stress at the clinic operations levels (e.g., we had 10 tests to use that day and 20 patients on the schedule, how do we decide who gets the test and who does not?).

There was wide variation in scarcity and surplus (e.g., for testing kits and lab capacity to process the tests and return results in a timely way). Although testing hesitancy wasn't an issue—as the people who came in wanted to be tested—the testing supplies and guidelines were challenging, i.e., the types of tests, the location to be swabbed, the timing of testing (days after exposure, etc.), the reliability (such as sensitivity and specificity) of the tests, the instructions for collection and storing of specimens, and how this changed over time, and messaging/expectations around all of it. There were important discussions at all levels (e.g., community, clinic, institutional).

To assist us, a clinical decision support document was developed and disseminated across the ambulatory setting. This tool was utilized by primary and ambulatory care teams including clinicians, clinic and call center nurses, and back office staff. It was updated regularly (sometimes daily, sometimes weekly) to reflect the changes in symptom presentation and testing supplies. Initial criteria were designed to test those at highest risk of adverse outcomes from the initial strains of the COVID-19 virus. As supplies became more available, we were able to broaden the criteria for testing and offer this to a wider range of the population. (See Resources at the end of chapter.)

Clinical Operations

All other functions of the clinic had to continue. Patients needed ongoing care. Telehealth was evolving rapidly and enabled our teams to temporarily shift much of our usual care services to virtual care. We learned we were able to address many health care needs without the traditional in-person clinic visit. It felt so good to have something to offer if clinicians had a phone or video visit with a sick patient who needed testing and care. Development of telehealth in primary care is one of the big upsides to the pandemic disruption. (See Chap. 9 for more details about telehealth in primary care during this time.)

FQHC clinic leadership had wanted to implement telehealth for a long time since many of our patients lacked transportation to get to medical appointments. Once we rapidly transitioned, our schedules were soon just as full with virtual appointments as they had been with in-person appointments, which was good for patients and for our visit volume overall. An important policy component that facilitated the transition to telehealth was Oregon's pioneering telehealth bill (HB 2508), which was passed and signed into law in May 2021. Oregon HB 2508 was the first in the nation to facilitate telehealth through payment parity compared to in-person visits [3].

Challenges Faced by Clinic Staff at Work and at Home

In addition to fears about exposure to COVID-19 at work, clinic staff faced new challenges at home (e.g., no available childcare, virtual-only schools, finding empty grocery store shelves when they needed to buy food for dinner after working a long shift). Clinic leadership created a rotation for Licensed Independent Providers (LIPs) and MAs to staff the clinic in order to make in-person obligations more equitable, but some people felt uncomfortable staffing the clinic in person. In response, clinic leadership created protocols based on evolving evidence and workflows which improved the comfort level of staff and providers. It was very important for all clinic staff to see that clinic leaders (including those with children and family members with high-risk conditions) were seeing and treating patients on the frontlines. This created a feeling that we were all in it together with the best available evidence and practices.

We could only care for the patients if we paid careful attention to how we cared for our staff. Understandably, this was a time of tension and conflict despite a shared mission. Social media played positive and negative roles. There was a lot of support from the community for our work voiced on social media. We also observed staff sending long, emotionally charged emails and posting criticisms on social media of clinic management for not being stringent enough about staff safety. Through this feedback, clinic leadership learned how to adapt workflows and communications to better reflect and address the safety of all staff—front and back office. The respiratory clinic and COVID-19 testing were held during regular clinic hours and integrated into day-to-day operations with all staff and providers participating, which reduced burnout.

Lessons Learned

In the early months, we did the best job we could with the tools we had at the time, adapting to knowledge at a blistering pace. We were so busy looking forward that we had no time to look back at how pandemics had been addressed in the past [4]. Over time, an informal playbook began to develop, though it was not simple; it was long, complex, and continued to evolve. Each year since 2020, we have looked back on our decisions and experiences and tried to build on them (e.g., when thinking about setting mask policies during respiratory season in the last three years). One important lesson learned and re-learned was that building relationships is key, and it is important to keep lines of communication open. For example, ongoing discussions need to happen with occupational health, infectious disease, hospital, and ambulatory operations leaders. Our coalition of hospitals around the state has been strengthened through our "Mission Control" teams, which collaborate on inpatient bed allocation [5]. We have a Chief Medical Officer forum across the state that continues to meet regularly. We have built (and are continuing to build out) our molecular lab for improved testing. And we have continued our deep conversations with communities.

We also learned that a healthy, resilient, multidisciplinary primary care system is needed in our country if we want to succeed with the next epidemic or pandemic. If we want to have people ready and willing to step up during crises, we need to invest in their training and education and we need to promote autonomy and professional development of all our clinicians so they feel engaged and connected and want to step into this work when it arises. This will require our nation to double down on many current efforts to strengthen primary care.

COVID-19 Vaccination Initiative (January 2021–June 2021)

The Scappoose Family Medicine Health Center, a Rural Health Center at Oregon Health & Science University (OHSU), in Scappoose, Oregon

> *I think rural physicians, especially rural primary care physicians, are very used to flexing and adapting to new circumstances very rapidly. We are used to working in a resource poor environment and so when the pandemic hit and we didn't have resources to care for people and we needed to do things differently, we were able to do that fairly quickly. So, I think that comes with being a rural person. You can't be a rural plumber and not be able to adapt to new situations; you can't be a rural electrician and expect to make a living if suddenly you can't install chargers or something. I think as a rural person you've got to be able to flex rapidly and work well in a resource-limited environment and work in an area that you know nothing about. That's what we were all doing early in the pandemic as we were working with something that we had limited knowledge about and limited resources; I mean, I've been doing that for 20 years. You see things you know nothing about all the time and you just figure it out.* —Primary Care Physician

As COVID-19 vaccines became available in December 2020, OHSU set up and supported community-wide mass vaccination sites at the Oregon Convention Center, the Portland Airport, and the Hillsboro Stadium, about 10 miles west of Portland. Together, these three sites administered more than 900,000 doses, approximately one-fifth of all the doses administered in the entire state of Oregon [6].

However, just as some populations faced barriers to the mass testing sites, many people were not able to easily gain access to the mass vaccination sites. One such population included community members in Columbia County, Oregon, located about 20 miles north of Portland. Columbia County had a population of just over 52,000 in the 2020 census [7]. The OHSU Family Medicine Scappoose clinic is a federally-designated Rural Health Center (RHC) located in the town of Scappoose. Pre-pandemic, in February 2020, the clinic had 85 staff and providers; in 2019 the clinic served 10,000 patients with 30,000 visits. The clinic is one of just a few sources of primary care in the county. To serve the community throughout the county, clinic leaders collaborated with Columbia County Public Health to plan and open weekend and evening vaccination clinics using the clinic space. Within two months, the model shifted to a separate space across the parking lot from the clinic. Throughout January—June 2021, the vaccine clinics engaged staff, providers, students and non-clinical volunteers, provided over 17,000 vaccinations, and responded to rapidly changing guidelines and vaccination scarcity and surplus.

In the first few weeks after the mass vaccine centers had opened, the Scappoose clinic primary care teams recognized their patients were not being served. Primary care needs to be an important part of any national vaccination strategy, especially in rural areas. Primary care teams are uniquely trusted by the communities they serve, and therefore able to overcome vaccine hesitancy and inequitable access to mass vaccination sites. Primary care teams are also able to quickly scale up or down outreach efforts like vaccine clinics as needed, and creatively reach people who are not being reached by other vaccination efforts. In a 2021 interview with Oregon Public Broadcasting [8] related to vaccine hesitancy, a family physician pointed out that for primary care providers (PCPs), the relationship with the patient and their family is what centers their experience in the health care system. When patients have strong connections to their PCP, the PCPs have status and trust that sets them apart, possibly, from the medical establishment. In other words, a patient may vehemently distrust a public health organization (such as the Centers for Disease Control and Prevention), but if their family PCP counsels them on the importance of a vaccine and leverages the relationship to allow them to explore their hesitancy in a safe space, rooted in trust, it is much more likely they will get vaccinated. Sometimes the clinic itself also benefits from that role. In Scappoose, clinic leaders saw this multiple times: families did not want to drive 20 miles into Portland for the mass vaccination sites because they did not trust the health care system as a whole, did not trust the government, or believed that the mass vaccination site was too far away; however, they *were* willing to line up at their clinic's doorstep and receive a vaccination by a trusted PCP.

Zoom In: The Nitty-Gritty Details

The initiative to provide vaccinations was rolled out over four distinct phases, as illustrated in Fig. 8.3. In Phase 1, we developed and piloted the vaccine clinic workflows; in Phase 2, we recruited volunteers and increased the vaccine clinic capacity to meet community demand; in Phase 3, we expanded access further and addressed vaccine hesitancy; and in Phase 4, we transitioned the separate vaccine clinic operating outside normal clinic hours and moved to vaccination in the regular clinic setting during regular clinic hours, while addressing significant burnout of staff and leaders.

The clinic utilized Plan-Do-Study-Act (PDSA) cycles throughout each phase. These typically were very rapid cycles, sometimes several in one day, to help with flow. The initial team that led the development of the vaccination initiative was composed of the Medical Director, Practice Manager, Columbia County Public Health (CCPH) Officer (also a physician at the Scappoose clinic), the Director of CCPH, a county commissioner, and a primary care development specialist from within the academic department.

Throughout the process, the clinic worked hard to be responsive to community needs. This meant that leaders ultimately were not just working with logistics leaders at the academic health center but meeting frequently with county leaders, public health officials, our local elected officials, our Medicaid Coordinated Care Organization (CCO), and others. The clinic also did extensive advertising and marketing outreach, with podcasts, billboards, etc. The billboard was created as a response to some crowdsourcing of information about vaccine hesitancy using the Next Door app. Working with a professor from Portland State University to analyze Next Door posts, we found that people who we were likely to influence were in a contemplative state for getting a vaccine. We also found that people were more likely to contemplate getting a vaccine if it was about protecting their loved ones and those they cared for. Based on this information, we developed a phrase for the billboards: Columbia County Cares (see Fig. 8.4). However, we did not measure the impact of the billboard on improving vaccination rates.

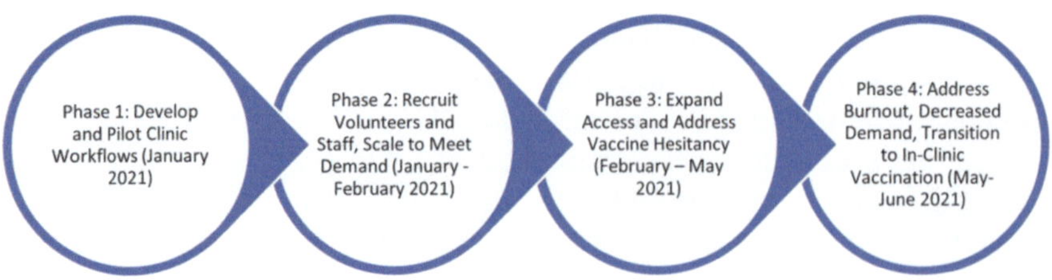

Fig. 8.3 Phased rollout of the COVID-19 vaccination initiative. This original figure, created by the authors, illustrates the four phases of the vaccination rollout

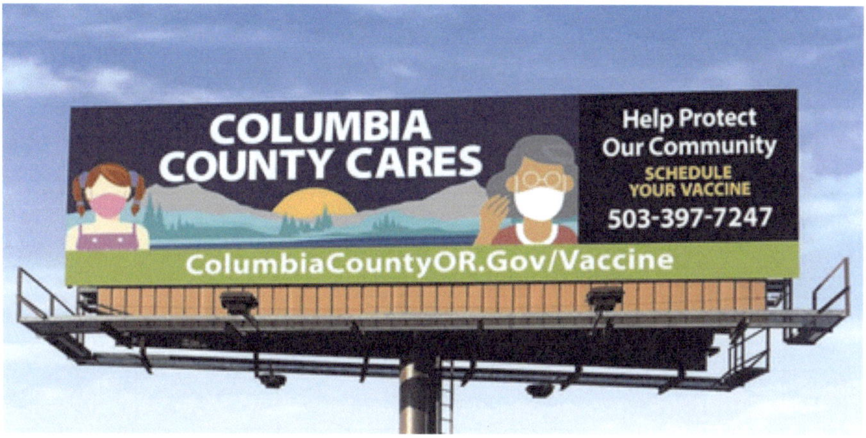
COLUMBIA
COUNTY CARES
Help Protect
Our Community
SCHEDULE
YOUR VACCINE
503-397-7247
ColumbiaCountyOR.Gov/Vaccine

Fig. 8.4 "Columbia County Cares" billboard messaging. A sample billboard featuring the campaign slogan *"Columbia County Cares,"* designed to appeal to community values and emphasize collective responsibility for health and safety. This message was informed by qualitative data suggesting that people were more motivated to vaccinate to protect others rather than themselves. The billboard photo was taken by the author

Phase 1: Develop and Pilot Clinic Workflows (January 2021)

Together with county health partners, we established a primary goal: vaccinate people in Columbia County, following public health's recommendations regarding vaccine prioritization, in a way that would not impact access to regular clinic care or operations.

We searched for examples of this type of vaccination site at a community clinic location and found very few. Therefore, through successive cycles of improvement, we developed a system that used three-person vaccinator teams—one vaccinator and two roomers or scribes (positions filled by MAs and outside volunteers). This model formed the operational core of our clinic's vaccine delivery strategy (see Fig. 8.5). Initially vaccinators were health care professionals, but OHSU held trainings for all interested employees to become vaccinators. We held two pilot clinics to test and scale the work and to rightsize flow and scheduling templates. After these pilot clinics were held, we developed a "rolling hills" approach to scheduling, to avoid extensive lines. The rolling hills approach was a technique we used where we would schedule and vaccinate a bolus of people at certain intervals throughout the day. It allowed us to get people in fast at the beginning of shifts but also allowed for us to catch up if there were delays. We did this by alternating the number of available slots at different time intervals, increasing the number of slots at peak hours and reducing the number of available slots by about one-third during the valleys. Having built-in "valleys" also let us do things like have a little extra time to clean up and prepare rooms, train new people, and transfer care responsibilities.

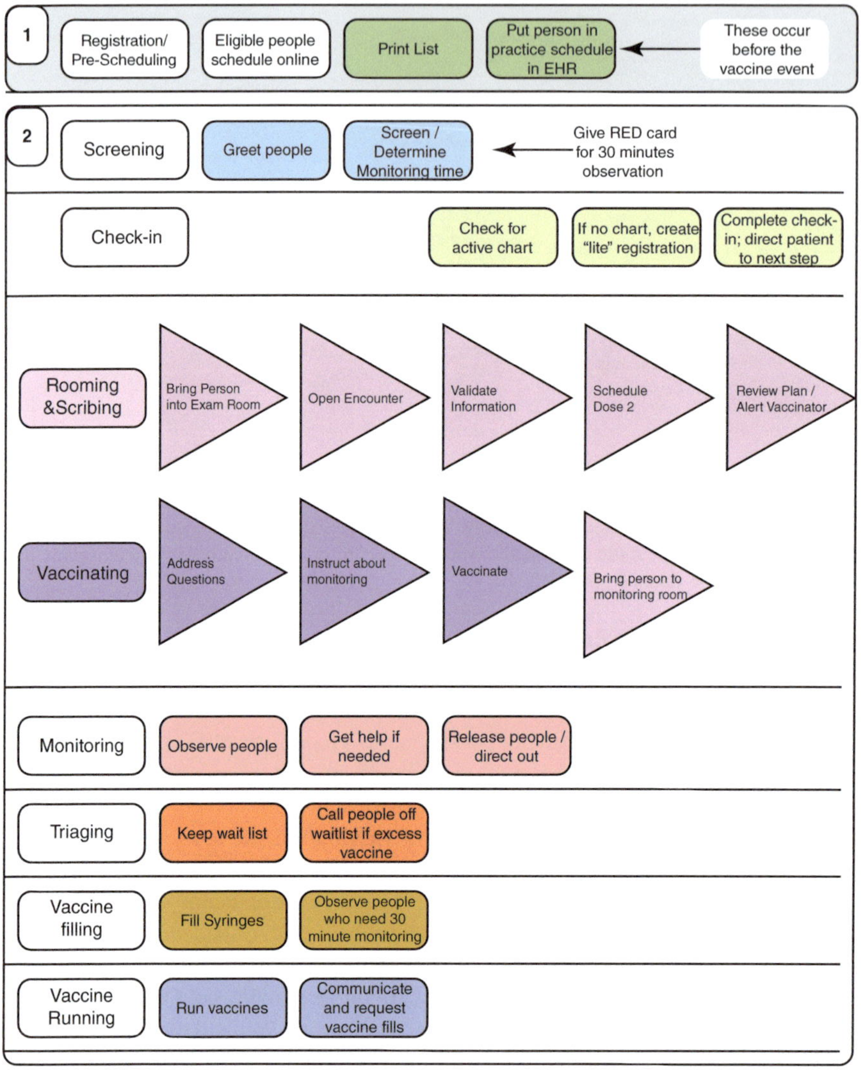

Fig. 8.5 Workflow for vaccine delivery. Illustration depicting the workflow developed for vaccine delivery. The operational structure was refined through iterative improvement cycles. Illustration created by the author

Phase 2: Recruit Volunteers and Staff and Scale to Community Demand (January–February 2021)

When we realized that we had a successful model for the clinic, we needed to look for outside volunteers (including medical students and residents) to help staff our operation. The vaccination clinics often would require 25–30 individuals working for 9 hours each weekend day. Our project coordinator developed brief training materials for each role. Each morning started with team huddles, followed by breakout groups to teach skills and verify competencies. We added daily IT support to help troubleshoot issues with our EHR and to get access for volunteers who were new to the system.

We created a plan with major stakeholders, which included pharmacy and IT support throughout our institution. Though the mass vaccination *model* developed for large parking lots and the convention center were in very different locations to ours, the foundational elements of pharmacy procurement, EHR setup, delegation protocols, staff training, and roles did apply. We had staff from our institutional IT team on site almost every day for the vaccination clinics. The leadership team worked with pharmacy to create our own revised protocol, but we borrowed ideas from other general vaccine protocols. All the setup and staff trainings were things we created as a team *ad hoc*.

The plan we created included:

- How to procure vaccines in partnership with the county;
- Getting equipment (special refrigerator) to store the vaccines;
- How to schedule people for initial and return vaccine appointments;
- How to use existing clinic staff and resources on Saturdays to provide "core staff";
- How to get and train additional staff as "volunteers";
- Creating a layout plan for workflow;
- How to bill for services; and
- Thinking through contingencies like how to not waste doses or how to politely decline to vaccinate people who did not meet eligibility requirements.

Phase 3: Expand Access Beyond Weekend Coverage and Address Vaccine Hesitancy (February–May 2021)

As the pandemic evolved and vaccines were developed, we turned our focus to vaccine-hesitant groups and worked to expand access by starting two weekday vaccine clinics, in coordination with the county health department and medical student volunteers. We also developed billboards in coordination with local public health experts (see Fig. 8.4), which were timed with the expansion of the Pfizer emergency use authorization to 12–17-year-olds. After we started looking at the numbers of patients (often 200+ people were signing up for vaccines), we realized we needed more volume. There was initial discussion of trying to do it at a large county site, but our academic health center institution had guidelines for logistics we needed to follow. We therefore set our sights on the satellite clinic across the parking lot; it was still officially a part of the campus, given it had the same physical address. This was important for staffing, especially for the union contracts for many of our staff, and for insurance. The county weekday clinic in the separate space took longer to operationalize because of the partnership with public health and the inherent red tape involved with creating a joint partnership between an academic health system and the county government.

During this phase, we created a weekly schedule of communications between key partners. For example, between the clinic and the county public health department to get vaccine doses and the list of people scheduled and between the clinic and the volunteer coordinator to determine how many vaccination teams would be needed based on how many people were scheduled. We conducted regular debriefings to refine the processes, workflows, and communication with clinic staff and volunteers. We held check-ins with clinic staff on well-being and burnout [9].

Phase 4: Address Burnout, Phase Out Events in Light of Decreased Demand, Transition to In-Clinic Vaccine Availability (May–June 2021)

By the end of June 2021, our teams were exhausted from the excessive workload (i.e., weekend and evening volunteers were also working full-time during the regular clinic hours). Additionally, demand dropped precipitously. We ultimately transitioned vaccine efforts to provide vaccines in clinic like our regular "influenza clinic" models. Teams shrunk back to the small core group at this point, reflecting a wave of involvement that started small and ended small, with the same people at the beginning and the end. Sadly, this difficult time coincided with the resignation of many of our RHC staff due to a state mandate that all health care workers be vaccinated.

We updated our initiative's primary objective to vaccinating patients of Scappoose clinic and community members during routine care. We began to plan to shut down the extended hours vaccination operations and moved to vaccinating in the clinic during normal clinic hours. The workflow had been developed and tested at another family medicine clinic, and an implementation toolkit was created, which we followed [10]. In this phase, we used routine care quality measures to assess success. We also prepared for anticipated "surges" in vaccine demand, e.g., when infants, children, and adolescents became eligible.

Sustainability and Evolution Through Phases

The outpouring of support in the first few weeks rapidly waned; after the first month, we became dependent on the same small group of volunteers, many of whom worked every weekend and many evenings for months. As a result, *many* people got really burned out. It is a false narrative to present this as a flash, because the real successes were in being able to sustain this in a way that we could eventually get everyone vaccinated.

The initial launch of the vaccination efforts in our clinic brought an inspiring burst of community support and volunteer engagement. In those early weeks, volunteers flooded in, eager to contribute to what felt like an historic public health effort. However, that excitement proved to be short-lived (weeks to a few months). As the excitement settled into the grueling reality of weekend after weekend spent administering vaccines, many volunteers understandably returned to their regular lives, and the once robust workforce dwindled into a small core of dedicated volunteers. These dedicated volunteers were the staff and providers of the Scappoose primary care clinic.

Sustaining these vaccine extension clinics, especially through the attrition of support, required innovative efforts to build resilience and community among those who carried the work forward long after the initial outpouring had faded. From a logistical standpoint, with volunteer numbers waning, it also became clear that the success of these clinics would depend on establishing a more dependable, streamlined operation that could carry on with fewer people and less external support. We primarily accomplished this in part by giving more responsibility and leadership opportunities to the individuals that frequently volunteered. Many became trainers who helped with improvement efforts aimed at finding efficiencies in our specific processes. For the frontline workers, vaccinators would also find ways to introduce elements of competition, tracking how many patients they could get through in a defined time, or how quickly they could turn over a room for the next patient. These friendly competitions made some of the mundane elements of the work more tolerable and also built camaraderie.

Zoom Out: Bigger Contextual Factors and How We Handled Them

Partnerships with County Public Health and Coordinated Care Organizations (CCO)

Our RHC's longstanding relationships with both the county health department and the CCO proved invaluable during the COVID-19 vaccine rollout. The former clinic medical director served as the county health officer, giving us a direct line to decision makers and allowing for a smooth collaboration. We were able to draw on these preexisting networks for critical support. The county health department was going through a major re-organization as the pandemic hit and was in the process of rapidly hiring and expanding under relatively new leadership. This was both helpful (more money, more interest in collaborating) and challenging (newer people with less experience, not a strong culture yet). Nevertheless, the county partnership was important to help us set up the vaccination site. The CCO, already a close partner of our RHC, provided substantial funding and some volunteers to sustain our vaccine efforts. The CCO's commitment was particularly driven by a shared focus on health equity, which aligned closely with our clinic's goals to reach underserved populations. Both of these established partnerships enabled us to mobilize resources quickly and leverage local expertise, helping us scale our vaccination efforts effectively despite the challenges of a rapidly changing environment.

Oregon's Approach to Vaccination

The US Centers for Disease Control and Prevention (CDC) provided a great deal of information about the COVID-19 vaccine. Based on this information and informed by state leaders, each state developed its own vaccine priorities, and counties developed plans to distribute vaccines to community members. The State of Oregon initially established three phases to prioritize vaccination of seven population groups. Oregon utilized a hub-and-spoke distribution model for vaccine distribution with thirteen Vaccine Redistribution Hubs for COVID-19 vaccines across the state, to widen vaccine access and prevent waste. Over about 5 months, from December 2020 to May 2021, vaccine supply shifted dramatically from scarcity and rationing to surplus.

In response to CDC guidelines and state directives, our RHC worked within Oregon's phased priority system, which aimed to allocate vaccines strategically across key population groups. As Oregon implemented the hub-and-spoke distribution model, our clinic served as one of the spokes, receiving vaccines from a regional hub and distributing them locally to ensure accessibility and minimize waste. For us, distribution was ultimately managed by the central pharmacy of our academic affiliate, which decreased the logistical burden many other clinics face.

Early on, vaccine scarcity required our team to focus on efficient allocation and careful outreach to priority groups, often scheduling doses meticulously to avoid any wasted supplies. This was challenging initially because our vaccine scheduling system was independent of our regular medical record, and so we ultimately relied on PCPs to review their own patient lists and pass along patient names they felt to be high risk. But as supply increased and moved toward surplus from May 2021 onward, our strategy shifted. We expanded outreach efforts, opening up vaccination to all eligible community members and increasing walk-in availability. Eventually, we pivoted our focus to try to encourage vaccine hesitant groups in our community to consider vaccination, primarily through our partnership with the county public health department. This adaptive approach allowed us to serve the broader population while managing fluctuating demand effectively.

Challenges of Equitable Access to Vaccination Sites

We worked with our local public health department to get our site listed on the state vaccination sign-up list. The RHC is physically located in a different county than the academic medical center and the vast majority of the other primary care clinics at our institution. The mass vaccination sites were too far away for our patients to go. There were all sorts of weather issues, and families could not bring multiple people (such as young children or elderly), travel, or wait several hours. The mass vaccination sites were heavily dependent upon personal vehicles putting those who used public transportation at a disadvantage. Those with disabilities had even more difficulty accessing the mass vaccination sites. We found that many people in our county and patients of our RHC tended to have more frontline jobs, so they had to be at work during the mass vaccination site hours.

What backfired about listing the vaccine site publicly was that people from Portland, at a time that vaccines were in very high demand, flooded our site the first few weekends. This was probably because the urban people were much savvier with online sign-up systems than our generally rural population. We ultimately never found a great solution for this. However, we mobilized our team-based care model to use PCPs and care teams to identify high-risk patients and get them scheduled before the online sign-ups went live, which helped prioritize people in our county.

Vaccination Was a Very Divisive Issue in the Community/County

After months of working together to vaccinate as many people in our rural county as possible, our clinic faced another huge challenge: Oregon implemented a COVID-19 vaccine mandate for all health care workers, and nearly one-third of our staff chose to resign rather than be vaccinated. The mandate hit particularly hard in our rural area, where vaccine hesitancy was widespread, and longstanding employees were deeply rooted in their personal beliefs. Furthermore, because the mandate was so well known, some staff feared that their ongoing employment at our clinic would effectively "out" them as having been vaccinated, which was a social liability in many community circles. To mitigate the impact, we engaged with leadership to consider potential exemptions and explored every option to retain our valued staff. Our medical director even sent a letter to the governor, outlining the repercussions that such a mandate could have in rural communities like ours, where institutional knowledge and trusted relationships are essential to care. However, the mandate stood firm, and in the end, we had to make the difficult decision to let many of these employees go.

Losing one-third of our team was an intense blow to morale, especially as several of those who left had been with us for decades and held irreplaceable knowledge about our clinic's operations, community connections, and patient care. There was no quick solution to rebuild what had been lost. To maintain morale and resilience among the remaining team members, we prioritized promoting junior staff where appropriate, offering additional mentorship to help them grow into their new roles. While these efforts helped us gradually regain stability, the full impact of the departures were felt for over a year, underscoring the long-term, complex ripple effects that rapid policy changes can create, especially in tight-knit, rural health care environments.

Lessons Learned

The relationship between the clinic and the community was improved when we were able to meet community needs regarding testing and vaccination. Many patients and community members voiced appreciation for our work to provide these services at primary care sites.

Staff and well-being were impacted both positively and negatively throughout the initiative. The shared mission and values enhanced staff well-being. However, the added workload, stress around health risks and changing practice guidelines, and the larger context of societal disruption and fraying of infrastructure continued to be stressful and harmed everyone's well-being, especially through the isolation of remote work. We are still seeing impacts today.

Looking back, there are some things we would approach differently if we were to stand up a vaccine clinic in our RHC today:

- We would focus on building a sustainable volunteer and staffing model from the start, recognizing the likelihood of initial enthusiasm waning and planning accordingly. This would involve creating staggered scheduling rotations and cross-training staff, so no one group bore the full burden of weekend and extended shifts over time.
- We would create a sustainable pace for our vaccination clinics, limiting the number of available slots to not overly burden the volunteers, and hopefully achieve better long-term sustainability.
- We would work more closely with community leaders and trusted local voices earlier in the process to help address vaccine hesitancy head-on, rather than waiting until demand slowed. Strengthening partnerships with local organizations could also allow us to better reach hesitant populations, providing education and outreach alongside vaccine delivery.
- We would prioritize streamlined workflows and simplified data systems to reduce administrative burden, allowing our team to focus more energy on patient interactions and maintaining morale during extended operations.

Summary Themes and Observations

Throughout this chapter, several themes emerged:

- **The dynamic balance between chaos and process**: The environment was chaotic, *and* there was a common framework among clinical leaders, that pre-dated the pandemic, for thinking about change and implementing new projects. This was because, as patient-centered medical homes (PCMHs) [11], the clinics already had a culture of process improvement and team-based care. Our clinics use a leadership core dyad of the medical director and clinic manager, with front- and back-office leads. Efforts to meet QI goals are led by a dyad of clinician and administrative QI leads. Together, these leadership teams manage priorities, typically focusing on performance metrics (e.g., preventive care and chronic disease management goals, meeting system or payer quality benchmarks). During the COVID-19 pandemic, we were monitoring data through both qualitative and quantitative means and adjusting processes, sometimes in real time, according to what we were finding. In that way, the QI work helped to organize the disruptions inherent to rapid deployment of new workflows into "managed chaos," which, with time, became efficient workflows.

- **Interdisciplinary nature of primary care teams and an "all-hands-on-deck" mentality**: Although the traditional health care hierarchy was still present, initiatives during the pandemic really became an all-hands-on-deck strategy where team members who are historically underrepresented in the leadership of the clinic (such as MAs and frontline staff) had their voices amplified.
- **Local autonomy and action balanced with and supported by centralized support**: Our FQHC and RHC are unique and based in community, and they are also linked with the larger public health and academic communities. The support with the EHR, central policies and guidelines, central supply chain access to testing supplies and PPE such as masks and gowns, our central laboratory, and the strong connection to the state lab were all critically important in our story. Having the central support for complicated logistics (like how to get PPE through the stressed supply chain) allowed local leaders to focus on the areas where they were truly experts, like how to structure a vaccine clinic in a way that was efficient in their unique community setting, acceptable to diverse stakeholders, and able to account for unique on-the-ground limitations and demands.
- **Values and benefits of community medicine**: Being an FQHC and RHC embedded within an academic health center influenced the mission, resources, and ability to implement these initiatives. The pre-existing culture really helped these two initiatives flourish in these settings with their teachings and learnings being applied more widely across the institution. We included teaching and learning in all efforts—not just in our mindset—but also in our commitment to our learners.
- **Authentic relationships and a focus on meeting unique needs**: There are so many different groups that are missed by "one-size-fits-all" approaches. The lesson for the future is we can do hard things in high-stakes situations with shared goals. The "how to" is about balancing the importance of strong and nimble professional relationships with constant negotiations and adjustments.
- **Health equity is part of the fabric of our work**: We knew inequities would be exacerbated in so many ways and that we needed to creatively respond to reduce the widening of health and health care disparities. We tried to simultaneously keep the patients and staff at the forefront of all the decisions to keep everyone safe and access to our clinical services open. It was a constant balance of managing science and emotion, given the perpetually changing guidelines and resources. This health equity focus eventually served as a model for our institution's wider testing and vaccine equity efforts.

- **Family medicine is a discipline of comprehensiveness, generalism, and leadership across boundaries**: Primary care, and specifically the specialty of family medicine, is well-positioned to bridge across clinical care and population health needs during a public health crisis like the COVID-19 pandemic. Our family medicine teams were capable of providing the perspective needed to translate the care at the individual and community level to the policies, procedures, and guidelines at the health systems level. Concepts and tenets of primary care were integrated into every aspect of our work. These were: person-and family-centered, continuous, comprehensive and equitable, team-based and collaborative, coordinated and integrated, accessible, high-value.

Final Reflections

What we knew in the beginning of the pandemic evolved. Our resources evolved. The emotions and fear dissipated over time. The prevalence of disease changed. All these pieces changed our recommendations and response. The fluidity of the situation was one of the most challenging pieces.

Chronic and preventive care backed up during the pandemic so things like preventable cancers were left unnoticed or unchecked which we are still trying to catch up on and manage today. Chronic diseases such as diabetes and hypertension became uncontrolled, which has had lasting effects.

Health care professionals across the board (e.g., PCPs, RNs, administrators, inpatient staff, specialists) either retired or left the field because of the moral injury leaving fewer people to do the same amount or more work than before.

> I am very proud of our work. When I see what we could accomplish quickly and successfully when the need was urgent and the values were shared, I take heart the health care system and the community at large has a much greater capacity to address our challenges than we may realize in the current polarized political context. (Medical Director)

Key Resources- Electronic Supplemental Materials

- Link to vaccination toolkit—https://www.ohsu.edu/sites/default/files/2021-11/Implementation_Toolkit_Final_November_2021.pdf
- Covid POC Testing workflow

References

1. Warren JB, Norton R, Nolt D, Khan FJ, Guzman-Cottrill JA. Medical facemasks are adequate for healthcare worker safety at outdoor coronavirus disease 2019 (COVID-19) drive-through testing centers. Infect Control Hosp Epidemiol. 2022;43(3):411–3. https://doi.org/10.1017/ice.2020.1430.
2. Freed SL, Thiele D, Gardner M, Myers E. COVID-19 evaluation and testing strategies in a federally qualified health center. Am J Public Health. 2022;112(S3):S284–7. https://doi.org/10.2105/ajph.2022.306827.
3. Coalition of Oregon Professional Associations for Counseling and Therapy. Telehealth Bill Passes House and Senate! Answers to FAQs Regarding HB 2508. https://www.copactoregon.com/news/telehealth-bill-passes-house-and-senate-faqs-answered
4. Fujimura SF. Purple Death: the Great Flu of 1918. https://www.paho.org/en/who-we-are/history-paho/purple-death-great-flu-1918. Accessed 2024.
5. Sara H. "OHSU opens centralized command center for statewide coordination of patient care." Published September 18, 2024. https://news.ohsu.edu/2024/09/18/ohsu-opens-centralized-command-center-for-statewide-coordination-of-patient-care
6. Oregon Health & Science University. Two mass vaccination sites tally more than 800,000 doses. https://news.ohsu.edu/2021/06/23/two-mass-vaccination-sites-tally-more-than-800-000-doses
7. United Census Bureau. QuickFacts. Columbia County, Oregon; Scappoose City, Oregon. 2024. https://www.census.gov/quickfacts/fact/table/columbiacountyoregon,scappoosecityoregon/POP010220
8. Matsumoto S. Think out loud. OHSU doctor on addressing vaccine hesitancy in Oregon. https://www.opb.org/article/2021/03/01/ohsu-doctor-on-addressing-vaccine-hesitancy-in-oregon/
9. Garvey B, Berger S, Garvin R, et al. COVID-19 Vaccination Clinic Implementation Toolkit. 2021. https://www.ohsu.edu/sites/default/files/2021-11/Implementation_Toolkit_Final_November_2021.pdf
10. Poarch H, Wideman K, Richardson J, DeVoe JE, Likumahuwa-Ackman S, Cohen DJ. Administration of COVID-19 vaccinations in primary care: an implementation toolkit. 2021. https://www.ohsu.edu/sites/defaul/files/2021-11/In-clinic_Vaccination_Toolkit_November_2021.pdf
11. Agency for Healthcare Research and Quality (AHRQ). Defining the PCMH. https://www.ahrq.gov/ncepcr/research/care-coordination/pcmh/define.html

Chapter 9
Implementation of Telephone and Video Visits in Primary Care: Informing the Future of Care Delivery

Tamar Wyte-Lake, Deborah J. Cohen, Steffani Bailey, Nathalie Huguet, and Kurt C. Stange

Introductory Quotes

> *My hope is that telehealth will continue to be a resource that we have, even with all of the limitations that I've talked about. I think the benefit of being able to have a visit with patients who can't make it physically to the clinic is incredibly valuable. I really hope that is something that insurances continue to reimburse for so that it can maintain its accessibility for patients.* —Licensed Clinical Social Worker

> *Telehealth is great for some issues, and not so great for others. It's certainly great for patients who live far away, or who have really busy schedules, or maybe just don't want to be out in public. It's good for mental health, to some extent. I think there's still something healing about being in the same room with an actual human being. Things that don't require a physical exam, or things that don't require a hands-on physical exam, so medication refills, blood pressure checks, talking about diabetes. Those sorts of visits, I think, are well-suited to the virtual realm. Things that require an in person visit: I need to listen to your heart, I need to move around one of your limbs, I need to look up close at a rash that you've got; those really need to be in person. Even some of the derm stuff that you can get a decent sense of, e.g., does that mole look dangerous, or what kind of rash is this virtually, or with the patient sending in a photo; but there's just some things that you really need to see as clear as possible, and even need to be able to put a magnifying glass on.* —Physician

T. Wyte-Lake (✉) · D. J. Cohen · S. Bailey · N. Huguet
Department of Family Medicine, Oregon Health & Science University, School of Medicine, Portland, OR, USA
e-mail: wytelake@ohsu.edu

K. C. Stange
The Larry A. Green Center, Richmond, VA, USA

Center for Community Health Integration, Case Western Reserve University, Cleveland, OH, USA

A. Cheng et al. (eds.), *Primary Care in a Public Health Emergency*,
https://doi.org/10.1007/978-3-032-12487-6_9

Introduction

Prior to March 2020, the term telehealth was not in the common discourse. Yet, like most new terms, people already had experience with it, even if that experience did not have a name. Most people could recall a time when they talked with their clinician, or someone in their clinician's office, about their health care by telephone. Much of this communication was ad hoc, used for triaging acute issues and questions, and often done when the traditional brick and mortar clinic site was closed. However, very few primary care clinics had formal mechanisms for scheduling, documenting, or paying for "visits" in this way. We use the term telehealth to include telephone and video communications to provide care when clinicians and patients are not in the same place. Our focus is on "real-time visits" that foster remote synchronous communication between a patient and clinician using audiovisual or audio-only technology.

In this chapter, we use numbers and narratives to make sense of telehealth implementation and use for preventive and chronic care in primary care clinics. We focus on telephone and video visits and do not consider other telehealth modalities such as remote patient monitoring, mobile health, or case-based teleconferencing. We describe how telehealth implementation varied across clinics and identify factors that influenced implementation. We examine how telehealth and hybrid care models (e.g., both telehealth and in-person options) are currently being used and discuss—with quotes and case examples from our research—some of the implications of hybrid care models for patients and clinical teams. Our examination of telehealth blends evidence from the literature and findings from studies that our team has conducted on this topic [1–6].

We use these lessons to make recommendations for sustaining and optimizing telehealth in the future and for considering what might be next regarding how to optimize hybrid models of care delivery.

Telehealth Implementation in the United States (US)

Early efforts toward telehealth use (pre-2000) were rare [7, 8]. Some health systems started rolling out the capacity for video-based ambulatory visits in the late 1990s and early 2000s. For many organizations, there was talk about video visits, but its implementation was not prioritized, nor was it in widespread use. Early adopters drove most of its volume, and patients and clinicians likely talked by telephone, as needed, with little documentation, enumeration, or recognition of this work. The Veterans Health Administration (VHA), an example of an early adopter, had begun exploring telehealth options to address access barriers, including perceived stigma for receiving health care, geographic and transportation challenges, and socioeconomic stressors. By 2017, there were over 700,000 Veterans receiving care via telehealth. And yet even in the VA, although there were initiatives to distribute iPads to patients' homes, much of this care was provided via in-clinic video, where patients had to come into local community-based outpatient sites to connect with clinicians at more distant facilities [9].

Telehealth use in primary care (and in many other health care settings) changed rapidly in late March 2020. Within weeks of the first US COVID-19 case, federal and state governments were issuing stay-at-home orders. Staying home included not visiting a health care facility unless it was an emergency. These regulations were aimed at reducing COVID-19 exposure [10]. In response, hospitals, health systems, and clinics across the US dramatically restricted in-person care and rapidly adopted and implemented telehealth visits. Video visits became more widespread [11–13], telephone discussions were recognized as visits and were reimbursable, even as data systems struggled to keep up with the new remote visit categories [14]. Early in the pandemic, more than three quarters of primary care clinics used telehealth [3, 15–18], with some reporting >500% increases in video and telephone visits in 2020 [3, 15–19]. And yet, even at a large academic medical center with a long history of information technology and telehealth innovation, there was variability in uptake, with telehealth use varying from 0% to 100% across clinicians for the same visit diagnosis for new patient visits [6].

While telehealth use declined within a few years after the peak of the pandemic, it remains an important modality for care among primary care clinicians [3, 20]. In 2022, more than half of primary care clinicians practiced in a setting that used videoconferencing for patient visits [21], and it was common by 2022 for primary care practices to have telehealth visits as an option. In community health centers, by 2022, telehealth visits had declined to less than a quarter of primary care visits—still a substantial change compared to the negligible number of telehealth visits in 2019 prior to the pandemic [22]. But in 2022, telehealth continued to account for the majority of behavioral health visits in community health centers, representing a sea change in how behavioral health services were being delivered [22].

Experiences with Telehealth Use

A systematic review found that over 60% of the studies that reported benefits of telehealth were from studies where this modality was used for chronic conditions and mental health/behavioral care, for medication management, and to care for existing patients [23, 24]. While fewer studies examine how patients and clinicians view and experience telehealth visits, those that do suggest that patients' and clinicians' experiences may be aligned [6]. Patients find telehealth visits suitable for medication management, discussions of lab results, and for following up with their clinician after a visit. Patients find the quality of these visits comparable in quality to an in-clinic visit. While both patients and clinicians tend to prefer in-clinic visits over telehealth, especially for initial appointments, appointments requiring a physical exam and for overall relationship building, they do see the value of telehealth and appreciate the option [6, 24, 25].

Evidence is emerging on how individual attributes, such as comfort level with technology, and demographic characteristics, such as age and race/ethnicity, may influence experience with and use of telehealth. For example, the lowest rates of telehealth use are observed among uninsured, young adults, and residents of Midwestern states [26]. Some of the highest rates are observed among Medicaid and Medicare beneficiaries. These attributes may also influence preference for modality (video or telephone). For example, Hispanic/Latino, Black, and Asian individuals are more likely than White individuals to use telehealth, specifically audio-only, but are less likely than White patients to use video telehealth [26]. In community health centers, already focused on caring for disadvantaged populations, disparities in preventive service delivery and chronic disease care persisted even with widespread use of telehealth [27, 28]. Yet, research in this area is quite limited, and more research is needed—post-pandemic—to understand how to optimize in-office and telehealth visits in today's emerging hybrid care models.

Implementation and Sustainability of Telehealth

Several studies identify the multilevel (e.g., policy, organization, care team, individual) barriers and facilitators of rapidly implementing telehealth modalities in response to the COVID-19 pandemic [29–36]. Figure 9.1 identifies the types of telehealth factors at each level and shows how these levels are interdependent.

Policy-related factors. Prior to the pandemic, to be reimbursed by the Centers for Medicare and Medicaid Services (CMS), telehealth visits could only be conducted by licensed providers, who had an established relationship with the patients and practiced in specific clinical sites. To be reimbursed, these needed to be video visits, using approved technology platforms. These video visits were reimbursed at a lower rate than an in-clinic visit, and payment policies contributed to the lack of adoption of telehealth in primary care prior to the pandemic.

During the pandemic, under the Coronavirus Preparedness and Response Supplemental Appropriations Act and the Coronavirus Aid, Relief, and Economic Security Act (2020) [37], CMS and private insurers implemented waivers that changed reimbursement for telehealth. These changes allowed for parity in reimbursement for telephone (audio only) and video (audio-video), which could be conducted by all providers using a wide range of technology platforms [38]. For rural health clinics (RHCs) and federally qualified health centers (FQHCs) who are reimbursed as an organization and not a specific provider, CMS allowed all providers to conduct telehealth visits without restricting where services were provided. This meant providers could conduct visits from their home. This change was important because clinical team members were contracting COVID-19 and needed to quarantine. Allowing clinicians who were feeling better but still quarantining to continue delivering care to patients facilitated patient access and kept some clinics in business.

Following the end of this public health emergency, states regulated their telehealth reimbursement for their Medicaid Program and CMS changed the

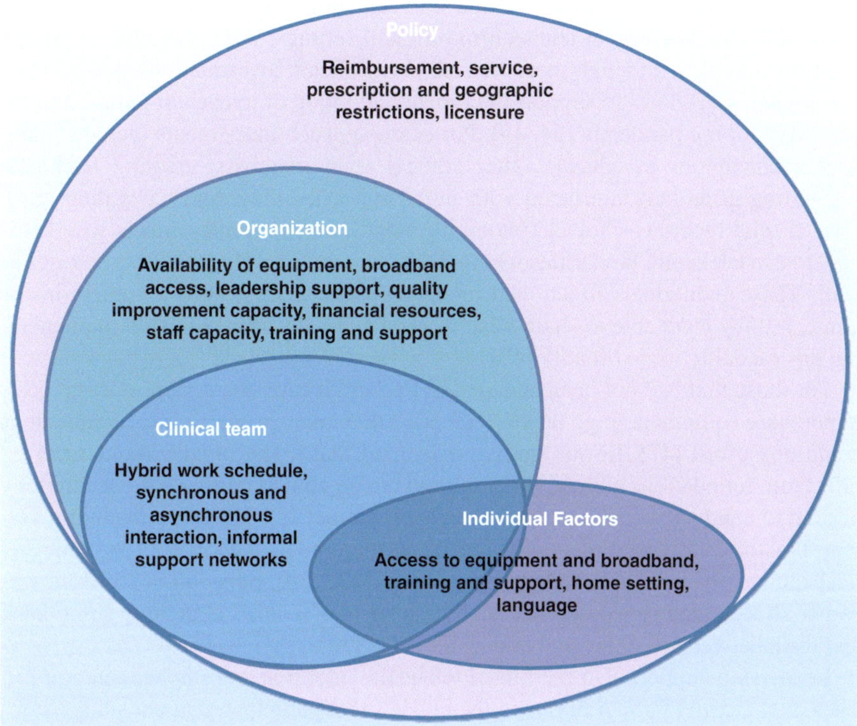

Fig. 9.1 Interdependent factors influencing telehealth implementation

comprehensiveness of reimbursement for Medicare [39]. Although at the time of this writing all state Medicaid programs continue to reimburse for certain video visits, states have flexibility in determining telehealth coverage [40]. Telehealth policies also can vary greatly, including by the types of services that can be delivered via video, reimbursement (or not) of telephone-only visits, where visits can be conducted (e.g., provider's home, patient is in the same state as the provider), and reimbursement for telehealth visits for certain patients (e.g., established patients only). The variability and complexity of telehealth reimbursement regulations are likely to have a differential impact on racial and ethnic minorities, rural populations, and socially and economically disadvantaged communities who engaged in telephone visits more frequently than video visits [4, 41–44], which can impact the clinics that serve these patients.

Organization-related factors. Implementation of telehealth during the COVID-19 pandemic was influenced by organizational leadership and support and resources, such as access to finances and technology infrastructure, as well as staff capacity, including quality improvement capacity. Primary care organizations varied in their access to computers, broadband, and technology to enable video visits. Organizations with experience with telehealth care prior to the pandemic, particularly video visits, had an advantage. These organizations had the equipment, knowledge, and scheduling capacity to rapidly expand this care modality. Organizations, such as VHA, that had invested in telehealth in limited settings, were also able to rapidly scale up activities, although there was still a significant investment needed to adapt the original workflows to support the broader adoption of telehealth required in the early days of the pandemic [34, 45]. For example, such investments included identifying champions to educate other clinical team members, creating telehealth scheduling grids that interfaced with in-person scheduling, and navigating questions around modality choices (phone vs. video). Having professionals who knew how to use telehealth modalities was an advantage in the VHA and other settings as well. These individuals functioned as champions and resources to others in the clinic, as they were able to share what worked and what to avoid when implementing this modality more broadly [46].

For those that had not been engaged in telehealth care, there were start-up costs to purchase equipment (e.g., tablets, cameras) that many primary care organizations could not afford [47]. In our study, we learned that a few organizations received gifts from foundations and applied for grants to be able to purchase the technology needed to conduct video visits [2]. Moreover, similar to VHA, the scheduling systems that these organizations used were not configured to support both in-clinic and telehealth visits, and this needed to be changed [32, 34]. Scheduling software was essential; it helped schedule visits in a manner that avoided clinicians going back and forth between in-clinic and telehealth visits [32].

Leadership support also facilitated telehealth adoption and implementation [3]. The Chief Quality Officer of one of the FQHCs that participated in our study examining telehealth use for cancer preventive care told us that the executive team in this clinic brought together an interdisciplinary team, with representation from across the organization, to plan and implement telehealth and a hybrid care model. This included developing and tasking several subcommittees to work on facilities and technology, to develop workflows and staff and clinician training. Leaders like this valued telehealth, and they viewed it as an integral part of primary care of the future. They saw its benefits for new billing revenues for services like follow-up calls, reductions in no-show rates, opportunity for improved access by reducing travel barriers, especially for follow-up visits, and behavioral and mental health visits, which may not require in-office visits [44]. They found ways to invest in the technology needed to facilitate work-from-home and telehealth visits, and they led and empowered others to make the operational changes needed to design new workflows and refine team roles to accommodate telehealth care (e.g., identifying staff to assist patients with their first video visit). These teams also led clinician and staff trainings [46].

Clinical team factors. As comfort around telehealth increases, and barriers begin to be addressed, there needs to be a consideration of the impact of hybrid work schedules on clinical teams. Beyond telehealth, which considers only how patient visits are conducted, hybrid care models must consider how the patient visit is conducted (i.e., telephone/video or in clinic) and where the clinician is conducting the visit (i.e., remotely vs. in clinic). The benefit of offering the hybrid care model is that it allows for the flexibility to meet the needs of individual patients it and allows clinicians flexibility in their personal schedules. Looking forward, organizations need to consider the impact of hybrid care models on clinical team work and patient care.

There are many facets to a primary care team's clinical success, and two critical components include the health of the individual clinic team members and the health of the clinical team [48, 49]. What we learned about the hybrid care delivery model is that it affects both the mental health of the individual team members, as well as team dynamics [5]. In our work we found that the hybrid work environment could result in fragmented schedules among team members and fewer in-clinic interactions. Similar to research that has shown that the layout of a physical workspace and the physical proximity and visibility among team members can impact both the individuals who work in a space, as well as their interprofessional interactions [50–52], clinical team members in our study contrasted their in-clinic, team interaction with asynchronous team interaction due to hybrid schedules, where the reduced ability to have in-person information sharing could adversely impact patient care.

> *Well, I think that having people in the building [again] has been a big positive, one for morale among staff, more camaraderie. People have relationships again. There's our whole team cohort that we have built up over years in these pod systems. People are sitting together again... that pod-based, team-based care is where the magic happens because you can just turn around and be like, "Hey, can you give this patient—" or, "Hey, this is—I have this question. What do you think about this?" Instead of sending an in-basket message that's 12 hours later they get back to you, and it just—it improves how quickly care can happen.... I mean [the on-line messaging application] works great, but it's not the same as just, you know, sitting next to somebody.*
>
> —*Primary Care Clinician* [5]

The hybrid schedules could also lead to a breakdown of informal support networks that clinicians described having when sitting together in the clinic. Unlike the culture working together in clinic fostered, where through informal check-ins, team members knew how others on the team were doing, clinicians described that the options for non-visual communication and virtual meetings did not foster this kind of knowing.

> *If we could just talk things out in person, like we used to, really affects the way that we work... this push to be virtual, the push to have an agenda that is very objective, and the absence of agenda to just say, "Hey, how are you doing? What's going on in your life? What did you do this weekend?" is gone, and we see each other as so transactional and not as human beings.*
>
> —*Primary Care Clinician* [5]

Recognizing both the advantages and the challenges of the hybrid work environment, many clinicians, although not all, noted that they preferred to have most of their clinical shifts occur in person and in clinic, with an ideal schedule of 1–2 sessions (e.g., 8 am–12 pm or 1 pm–5 pm) per week for in-home (remote) shifts. Although the impact of these hybrid models on the work of the individual or the social capital of the clinical team is not yet known, our findings suggest that clinical leaders need to think carefully about how to achieve the right mix of care delivery options because the incorporation of telehealth has the potential to have both positive and negative effects for the team and the individual clinician in terms of burnout, well-being, and meaningful collaboration, all of which in turn enrich patient care [49, 53].

Individual Factors. Individual attributes of patients and clinicians also influence telehealth use. Technology acceptance and literacy varied among clinicians regarding use of telehealth appointments software (e.g., Doximity, FaceTime, or other apps to facilitate video appointments).

Technology acceptance and literacy was also a challenge for some patients. Factors such as geographic location, access to broadband, access to equipment, and technology literacy were common challenges for patients engaging in video visits, although less so with telephone visits. There are clear barriers for elderly and rural patients, many of whom may prefer to use telephone visits over video visits [31, 34]. One behavioral health consultant we interviewed reported that many of her patients struggled to access MyChart, which was the portal application used to engage in a video visit:

> *I think I have been able to successfully have five video appointments [laughs] since COVID started...because of barriers. Some of that is education literacy, patients figuring out, "How do I even use MyChart?" [web-based patient portal]. I have a number of patients who still haven't been able to figure out how to access MyChart. That doesn't even include internet complications and all that stuff.*
> —*Behavioral Health Consultant* [4]

Telehealth visits could be particularly challenging for non-English speaking patients, if clinics did not have interpreter systems in place. For example, one of the clinic leaders in our study discussed the challenges with bringing an interpreter into a telehealth visit: "*With our tele-video visits...it becomes a bit more of a challenge because the interpreter services they're connected via telephone and it's one of those where it's putting the landline on speaker close to the computer. It's not ideal." (Primary Care Practice Leader)* [54]. Not only are the logistics of including an interpreter within a telehealth visit complex, getting patients to that visit is also challenging as pre-visit reminders, registration for, and patient portal entry at the time of the visit are not supported in all languages [54].

Early in the pandemic, a clinical team member might have been assigned to helping patients access and navigate telehealth appointments to avoid some of these challenges [55]. For example, medical assistants (MA) and front desk staff were sometimes trained to provide technical support to patients during either their virtual rooming or in advance, during scheduling [3]. At clinics with large Spanish-speaking populations, clinics developed educational materials in Spanish and brought in Spanish-speaking interpreters to help support successful telehealth visits [2, 3]. Family members could be an important asset in assisting patients with these barriers [54]. However, conducting a visit in the presence of family, in the home environment, could limit privacy and confidentiality and change visits in ways that are difficult to appreciate. Furthermore, many patients do not have family members to assist them and people who lack permanent housing experience serious barriers to telehealth care in general and video visits specifically [33].

Implications of Visit Modality on Care

Choices about which visit modality is used have not been well studied. It is likely that these decisions are either made by the patient or medical receptionist when the appointment is made, or they are made in the context of a clinician-patient relationship. This is an area where more research is needed. We did learn that patients' technology access, literacy, and social and economic situation influenced how clinicians see visit modality choices: "*How do we pick between phone or video? We typically leave it up to the patient. A lot of our patients are marginally housed or don't have a lot of privacy when they are housed. It's much easier to have a quiet phone conversation than have a video chat on their phone.*" *(Registered Nurse)* [6]. Decisions about the visit modality have implications for the visit and for patient care.

Telehealth visits can provide an opportunity for family members who live a distance from the patient to join a visit virtually. One of the clinicians who we interviewed cared for older adults, many of whom are living with dementia and struggling to care for themselves at home: "*Telemedicine's actually been wonderful. Twice now, at least, that out-of-town family member has been able to be part of the appointment on video...That's really enhanced that patient's care enormously.*" *(Medical Director)* [3].

Telehealth visits also promote scheduling flexibility and access for patients. Case Example 1 shows how access to care via telehealth was helpful to a patient with a substance use disorder.

Case 1: The Stable, Continuity Patient

Ms. S is a 34-year-old woman. She is the mother to two children who are six and nine and has a full-time job out of the home. She has been receiving care for her opioid use disorder for 6 years at this clinic. As a longstanding patient, she comes into the clinic once every 3 months for a check-in to receive a prescription renewal. Prior to 2020, Ms. S always had to take time off from work to come for her appointments and/or find childcare for her children. Since the option of a telehealth appointment became available, she can now schedule telehealth check-ins during her lunch break, where she conducts them by phone because her phone's Wi-Fi reception is spotty in the area where her office is located. Ms. S has continued her treatment and considers herself to be stable in her care.

Telehealth was effective for Ms. S as it allowed care to continue in an uninterrupted manner, and it reduced the burden the patient experienced trying to balance childcare, work, and travel for an in-clinic visit.

In cases such as these, clinicians emphasized that, for patients in recovery from an addiction, the option for a telehealth visit allowed stable patients to have more autonomy over their recovery process, and that this autonomy allowed patients to further distance themselves from their lives in addiction. However, this distance could also delay care delivery when a clinician learns of a patient's return to drug use as Case Study 2 shows. But this is complicated. On one hand the clinician might have learned of the patient's drug use sooner if appointments had been held in person; on the other hand, it was on the patient's terms and timeline that he talked with his doctor about this.

Case 2: Previously Stable Patient Returns to Opioid Use

Mr. G is a 32-year-old male. He lives with his sister and is finishing school and looking to get a job. Prior to the COVID-19 pandemic, Mr. G had not been using opiates for several years. When the pandemic hit, he continued his treatment program via telehealth. Although Mr. G and his clinician initially tried to conduct their visits via video, after a few sessions where the video did not connect, they switched to phone and from then on continued care via the phone visits. Throughout this time, although Mr. G continued filling his suboxone prescription, he slowly stopped taking it and returned to using opiates. After his sixth time trying to quit on his own, he decided to tell his physician what was going on. He went through a virtual induction [initiating medication for opioid use disorder] and then returned to consistently taking his suboxone. In describing his challenges in remaining stable, he included the lack of needing to provide a urine sample during his regular treatment sessions, that it was easier to lie to his clinician on the phone, in contrast to having to face him in person. He also reported missing the positive and supportive energy that he received during in-person visits. Yet, he continued to choose to conduct his visits by phone because he had moved out of town when he moved in with his sister, and getting to the office was difficult.

Clinicians who reflected on cases like Case 2 underscored that, in some situations, maintaining the relationship with the patient was the most important factor to successful treatment. Opioid use disorder treatment was seen as a long-term relationship that could have periods of high and low stability regardless of visit modality. For that reason, even though both the patient and the clinician recognized the limitations of telehealth care, the successful maintenance of the relationship was of prevailing value, as it allowed communication and relationship building, and an open path for the patient to re-engage in treatment when he was ready.

A key lesson learned regarding the modality of the visit (e.g., in person, phone, video) is being open with all options and choosing the visit modality best aligned with the medical care problem while balancing the patient's access preferences and needs. Case study 3 exemplified this flexibility and how that evolves overtime and in the context of a relationship between a patient and the clinical team.

Case 3: Person Stable in Their Recovery, Who Transfers Care to New Primary Care Clinic

Ms. T is 33-year-old female. She has been living in a sober living home for 2 years, works full time, and visits her child on the weekends. Ms. T was put on probation for a drug charge and through that was put into an outpatient opioid use disorder treatment program, which she continued for one and a half years. When she graduated and completed the course, she moved and established care at a new clinic. Ms. T's first appointment with her new primary care clinician was in person. Most of her subsequent visits with the opioid use disorder treatment team have been via video, although there has been a sprinkling of phone and in-person visits. Ms. T primarily sees the licensed clinical social worker (LCSW) for opioid use disorder-related care via video. When she has a need to see her primary care clinician for an issue that needs a physical exam, she comes in person and will often be asked to complete a urine analysis (UA) as part of that visit. On some occasions, she also has a virtual visit with the LCSW and then will come in separately, as requested by the LCSW, to complete a UA in the clinic. Ms. T describes all three visit types as being equal and generally uses video visits for the combination of flexibility (for her work schedule) and because it feels more personable to see her clinician's face.

For patients and clinicians who are developing a relationship, building rapport through initial in-person visits may foster greater confidence and comfort in conducting subsequent visits via a telehealth modality. As telehealth care evolves and improves, clinical teams and patients will need to continue to identify issues that require an in-clinic visit from those that do not, and sequence other medical data, such as the collection of blood, so that these test results efficiently inform clinician-patient communication and decision making, regardless of visit modality. These decisions will continue to shift, as the evidence base becomes more robust and reimbursement rules continue to evolve.

Thoughts on Implementation of Sustainable Telehealth in Primary Care

With the external factors that drove the spike in adoption of telehealth in primary care subsiding, there must be thoughtful consideration of the ways telehealth will continue to be incorporated into care delivery. Organizational and policy leaders, as well as those on the ground, must continue to learn from the early and evolving experience and review the positive and negative factors of telehealth to be able to implement sustainable practices moving forward. Tools and resources from leading

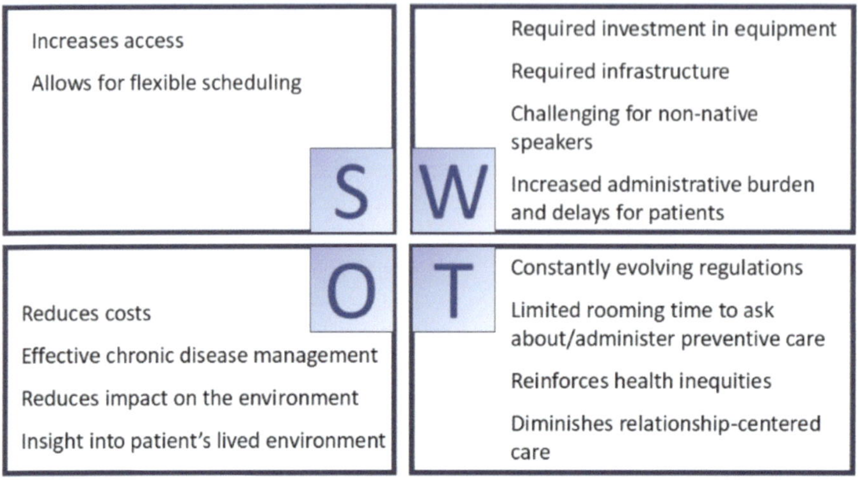

Fig. 9.2 Strengths, weaknesses, opportunities, and threats for continued telehealth implementation

organizations such as the Association of American Medical Colleges (AAMC) [56] and the American Medical Association (AMA) [57] have been developed to support effective strategies for the incorporation of telehealth into patient care, including leveraging the benefits of telehealth while maintaining a commitment to health care equity [58]. Figure 9.2 summarizes the strengths, opportunities, weaknesses, and threats that we see regarding telehealth technology implementation and use.

With in-person visits returning to the norm for most (primary) medical care, the question remains as to how telehealth can most helpfully remain as one option in the primary care armamentarium for providing access, quality medical care, and developing healing and health-promoting relationships [44, 59]. Incorporating telehealth into the primary care practice model while maintaining the core values of contextual care, continuity of care, access to care, comprehensive care, and care coordination for all individuals is possible, but requires adaptation [60].

Strengths and opportunities. One of the strengths of telehealth modalities is that time and travel barriers are reduced for those for whom the technical and social barriers are not prohibitive. For instance, patients who have to travel 2 hours for a visit to see their clinician, who do not own or operate a vehicle, who have limited sick leave, who have caregiving responsibilities, and other barriers to an in-person, in-office visit can use telehealth to access primary care. They can also use telehealth modalities to access services that are not available in their area. This can be a particular strength for medically underserved areas where few medical specialists may practice [44]. As reported above, telehealth modalities can be effective when clinicians and patients are following up to manage a chronic disease, including mental health and behavioral care, and accessing care in this way can prevent unnecessary emergency department visits [47]. Telehealth visits can also sometimes provide insight into the patient in their lived context, sometimes akin to a home visit. The opportunity for primary care today is to leverage these strengths and expand access to telehealth for visits where this modality is acceptable and effective. Also largely unexplored by research is the opportunity to meld a combination of in-person and telehealth visits to meet the circumstances of patients.

Weaknesses and threats. Telehealth requires equipment and equipment maintenance. This means that resources and capacity, including information technology expertise, are needed. Broadband access and speed are not equally distributed across the US. Broadband access impacts the rural clinics, rural patients, and patients and medical staff with lower income that may have lower-speed broadband. The ability to assist non-English speaking patients via telehealth modalities can be an asset but also a barrier, particularly if systems and workflow are not in place to facilitate use of the virtual platform and care interpretation. For those connected with a practice, telehealth could increase access. For those who are not connected, it could just be one more inaccessible way to (not) receive care. If these threats and weaknesses are not addressed, telehealth could end up reinforcing inequities, and/or creating new ones. In addition, telehealth visits represent another way that (primary) care can be commodified. For those who seek and receive isolated telehealth visits from different clinicians, rather than investing in developing a relationship with a single clinician or team, telehealth could result in a subtle reduction in access to quality of care, an important component of which is continuity of care [61–67], or at least relationship-centered care [59, 68–70].

Waiting room time is very different in telehealth visits. Research suggests that patients are less tolerant of waiting in a virtual environment relative to in-office visit [32, 46]. Perhaps more importantly, telehealth visits often do not include rooming activities such as screening. While some assessments such as height, weight, and blood pressure need to be done in person unless patients have at-home equipment, rooming activities that could be done virtually, such as assessing for tobacco use or reminding patients of overdue preventive services, are also not being completed [71, 72]. This could be due to MAs not being part of virtual visits. The impact of these changes, particularly the absence of rooming activities, on disease diagnosis due to delays in preventive care services, is unknown.

Mis-triaging care—scheduling patients for a telehealth visit that requires an in-clinic visit—can lead to administrative burden, increased workload, and an increase in patients' burden (e.g., extra visits, out-of-pocket cost). In addition, in-person visits can facilitate care that is unrelated to a patient's chief complaint, such as imaging and labs, immunizations, or preventive services. These opportunistic approaches to delivering preventive care, which often occur in primary care visits, may be less likely to happen and may require an additional visit, if not carefully planned.

Variations in telehealth regulations by payer and by state, which are continuing to change, are a challenge for clinics and health care organizations who need to stay on top of these regulations and who may need to offer care to patients differently if payers pay for care differently. These create uncertainty for clinicians and patients with regard to how they can access primary care. This variation and uncertainty are likely to increase, as the last vestiges of pandemic-induced payment changes expire or evolve.

In conclusion, telehealth now plays an important role in primary care delivery. We need to remain cognizant of and continue to address challenges related to telehealth and hybrid models of care to ensure quality care is delivered equitably. We make the following recommendations:

- Maintain the 5 Cs of primary care (contextual care, continuity, access to care, comprehensive, and care coordination) [60] at the center of patient care to ensure that telehealth adoption preserves the values of primary care.
- Upgrade clinical systems to integrate limited English proficiency access, such as automated interpreter links, multi-language platforms including text reminders, and longer visits to account for interpretation time to promote equity.
- "My telehealth visit should have been in person." Establish systems to triage visits and integrate rooming within virtual visits. To avoid repeated care, ensure timely diagnosis and detect needed behavioral counsel; developing smart triage systems is critical.
- Integrate systems to identify patients in need of vital monitoring (e.g., patients with history of high blood pressure) or that assist patients with obtaining monitoring devices to check vital metrics. These systems are paramount for the millions of people in need of chronic care management. These systems could also assist in promoting continuity of care by flagging patients in need of an in-person visit with a specific clinician. Such systems could be modelled after existing algorithms that identify at-risk patients for specific illnesses or preventive screening due dates.
- Bridge the digital divide. Infrastructure investments are needed to ensure access for all. While we wait, it is critical for federal and state rules and reimbursement to support telephone care as equal to video care to overcome discrimination against areas in internet deserts. The digital divide also includes disparities in digital literacy, which negatively impacts access to services, similar to language literacy.

Telehealth has been shown to be a formidable tool to facilitate access to care for many. Ensuring its continued use equitably and without overwhelming the primary care system is the next challenge to overcome.

References

1. Flocke SA, Huguet N, Bailey SR, Hodes T, O'malley JP. Impact of COVID-19 pandemic on assessing tobacco status in community health centers. Ann Fam Med. 2023;21(2):161–4.
2. Huguet N, Danna M, Baron A, et al. Delivery of cervical and colorectal cancer screenings during the pandemic in community health centers: practice changes and recovery strategies. Med Care. 2023;61(8):554–61. https://doi.org/10.1097/mlr.0000000000001879.
3. Holderness H, Baron A, Hodes T, et al. Community health centers rapid adoption of telemedicine during the COVID-19 pandemic: trends, barriers and successful strategies. J Prim Care Community Health. 2023;21(Suppl 3):4956.

4. Bailey SR, Wyte-Lake T, Lucas JA, et al. Use of telehealth for opioid use disorder treatment in safety net primary care settings: a mixed-methods study. Subst Use Misuse. 2023;58(9):1143–51.
5. Wyte-Lake T, Cohen DJ, Williams S, Bailey SR. Balancing access, well-being, and collaboration when considering hybrid care delivery models in primary care practices with team-based care. J Am Board Fam Med. 2023. https://doi.org/10.3122/jabfm.2024.240388R2.
6. Wyte-Lake T, Cohen DJ, Williams S, et al. Patients' and clinicians' experiences with in-person, video, and phone modalities for opioid use disorder treatment: a qualitative study. J Gen Intern Med. 2024;39:2179–86.
7. Brown FW. Rural telepsychiatry. Psychiatr Serv. 1998;49(7):963–4.
8. Parameswaran V, Koos H, Kalwani N, et al. Drivers of telemedicine in primary care clinics at a large academic medical centre. J Telemed Telecare. 2023:1357633X231219311. https://doi.org/10.1177/1357633X231219311.
9. Zulman DM, Wong EP, Slightam C, et al. Making connections: nationwide implementation of video telehealth tablets to address access barriers in veterans. JAMIA Open. 2019;2(3):323–9.
10. Severino R, Director OC. Notification of enforcement discretion for telehealth remote communications during the COVID-19 nationwide public health emergency. Washington: US Department of Health & Human Services; 2020. p. 22024–5.
11. Rockwell KL, Gilroy AS. Incorporating telemedicine as part of COVID-19 outbreak response systems. Am J Manag Care. 2020;26(4):147–8. https://doi.org/10.37765/ajmc.2020.42784.
12. Hong YR, Lawrence J, Williams D Jr, Mainous IA. Population-level interest and telehealth capacity of US Hospitals in response to COVID-19: cross-sectional analysis of google search and national hospital survey data. JMIR Public Health Surveill. 2020;6(2):e18961. https://doi.org/10.2196/18961.
13. Centers for Disease Control and Prevention (U.S.). Coronavirus disease 2019 (COVID-19): outpatient and ambulatory care settings: responding to community transmission of COVID-19 in the United States. https://www.hsdl.org/c/abstract/?docid=836457. Accessed 16 Aug 2024.
14. Larson AE, Stange KC, Heintzman J, et al. Identifying virtual care modality in electronic health record data. Learn Health Syst. 2024;8:e10411. https://doi.org/10.1002/lrh2.10411.
15. Shaver J. The state of telehealth before and after the COVID-19 pandemic. Prim Care. 2022;49(4):517–30. https://doi.org/10.1016/j.pop.2022.04.002.
16. Peden CJ, Mohan S, Pagán V. Telemedicine and COVID-19: an observational study of rapid scale up in a US academic medical system. J Gen Intern Med. 2020;35:2823–5.
17. Kane CK. Telehealth in 2020: survey data show widespread use across most physician specialties and for a variety of functions. Am Med Assoc. 2021;37:1915–2104. Policy research perspectives.
18. Keppel G, Cole AM, Ramsbottom M, et al. Early response of primary care practices to COVID-19 pandemic. J Prim Care Community Health. 2022;13:21501319221085374. https://doi.org/10.1177/21501319221085374.
19. Mann DM, Chen J, Chunara R, Testa PA, Nov O. COVID-19 transforms health care through telemedicine: evidence from the field. J Am Med Inform Assoc. 2020;27(7):1132–5. https://doi.org/10.1093/jamia/ocaa072.
20. Myrick K, Mahar M, DeFrances C. Telemedicine use among physicians by physician specialty. NCHS Data Brief. 2024;493:1–8.
21. Kane CK. Telehealth in 2022: availability remains strong but accounts for a small share of patient visits for most physicians. 2023. Policy research perspectives.
22. Cook N, McGrath BM, Navale SM, et al. Care delivery in community health centers before, during, and after the COVID-19 pandemic (2019–2022). J Am Board Fam Med. 2024;36(6):916–26. https://doi.org/10.3122/jabfm.2023.230081R1.
23. Ward K, Vagholkar S, Sakur F, Khatri NN, Lau AYS. Visit types in primary care with telehealth use during the covid-19 pandemic: systematic review. JMIR Med Inform. 2022;10(11):e40469. https://doi.org/10.2196/40469. PMID: 36265039. PMCID: 9745650.

24. Berry CA, Kwok L, Massar R, et al. Patients' perspectives on the shift to telemedicine in primary and behavioral health care during the COVID-19 pandemic. J Gen Intern Med. 2022;37(16):4248–56. https://doi.org/10.1007/s11606-022-07827-4.
25. Nguyen MT, Garcia F, Juarez J, et al. Satisfaction can co-exist with hesitation: qualitative analysis of acceptability of telemedicine among multi-lingual patients in a safety-net healthcare system during the COVID-19 pandemic. BMC Health Serv Res. 2022;22(1):195. https://doi.org/10.1186/s12913-022-07547-9.
26. Lee E, Grigorescu V, Enogieru I, et al. Updated national survey trends in telehealth utilization and modality: 2021–2022 (Issue Brief No. HP-2023-09). 2023. https://aspe.hhs.gov/sites/default/files/documents/7d6b4989431f4c70144f209622975116/household-pulse-survey-telehealth-covid-ib.pdf. Accessed 13 Aug 2024.
27. McGrath BM, Goueth R, Jones MWH, et al. Care quality and equity in health centers during and after the COVID-19 pandemic. Am J Prev Med. 2024. https://doi.org/10.1016/j.amepre.2024.05.011.
28. Gold R, Cook N, Dankovchik J, et al. Cardiovascular disease risk management during COVID-19: in-person vs virtual visits. Am J Manag Care. 2024;30(1):e11–8. https://doi.org/10.37765/ajmc.2024.8948.
29. De Vera K, Challa P, Liu RH, Fuller K, Feroz AS, Gamble A, Leung E, Seto E. Virtual primary care implementation during covid-19 in high-income countries: a scoping review. Telemed J E Health. 2022;28(7):920–931. https://doi.org/10.1089/tmj.2021.0377. Epub 2021 Nov 29. PMID: 34847758.
30. Hall TL, Connelly L, Staton EW, et al. Points of concordance, points of discordance: a qualitative examination of telemedicine implementation. J Am Board Fam Med. 2022;35(3):517–26. https://doi.org/10.3122/jabfm.2022.03.210325.
31. Sharma AE, Lisker S, Fields JD, et al. Language-specific challenges and solutions for equitable telemedicine implementation in the primary care safety net during COVID-19. J Gen Intern Med. 2023;38(14):3123–33. https://doi.org/10.1007/s11606-023-08304-2.
32. Rabinowitz G, Cho LD, Benda NC, et al. The telemedicine experience in primary care practices in the United States: insights from practice leaders. Ann Fam Med. 2023;21(3):207–12. https://doi.org/10.1370/afm.2967.
33. Rome D, Sales A, Cornelius T, et al. Impact of telemedicine modality on quality metrics in diverse settings: implementation science-informed retrospective cohort study. J Med Internet Res. 2023;25:e47670. https://doi.org/10.2196/47670.
34. Der-Martirosian C, Wyte-Lake T, Balut M, et al. Implementation of telehealth services at the US Department of Veterans Affairs during the COVID-19 pandemic: mixed methods study. JMIR Form Res. 2021;5(9):e29429. https://doi.org/10.2196/29429.
35. Rangachari P, Mushiana SS, Herbert K. A scoping review of applications of the Consolidated Framework for Implementation Research (CFIR) to telehealth service implementation initiatives. BMC Health Serv Res. 2022;22(1):1450. https://doi.org/10.1186/s12913-022-08871-w.
36. Godfrey EM, Fiastro AE, Jacob-Files EA, et al. Factors associated with successful implementation of telehealth abortion in 4 United States clinical practice settings. Contraception. 2021;104(1):82–91. https://doi.org/10.1016/j.contraception.2021.04.021.
37. Coronavirus Preparedness and Response Supplemental Appropriations Act, 2020, 116–123, 116th congress (Representative Lowey NM 2020).
38. American Medical Association. CARES Act: AMA COVID-19 pandemic telehealth fact sheet. https://www.ama-assn.org/delivering-care/public-health/cares-act-ama-covid-19-pandemic-telehealth-fact-sheet. Accessed 13 Aug 2024.
39. Center for Connected Health Policy. Summary report: the highlights & findings of a comprehensive scan of 50 states, D.C., Puerto Rico and the Virgin Islands. State Telehealth Laws and Medicaid Program Policies. https://www.cchpca.org/2023/10/Fall2023_ExecutiveSummaryfinal.pdf. Accessed 13 Aug 2024.

40. Medicaid.gov. Reimbursement for telehealth and provider and facility guidelines. Centers for Medicare & Medicaid Services. https://www.medicaid.gov/medicaid/benefits/telehealth/reimbursement-for-telehealth-and-provider-and-facility-guidelines.
41. Weber E, Miller SJ, Shroff N, Beyrouty M, Calman N. Recent telehealth utilization at a large federally qualified health center system: evidence of disparities even within telehealth modalities. Telemed J E Health. 2023;29(11):1601–12. https://doi.org/10.1089/tmj.2022.0511.
42. Chang JE, Lindenfeld Z, Thomas T, Waldman J, Griffin J. Patient characteristics associated with phone versus video telemedicine visits for substance use treatment during COVID-19. J Addict Med. 2022;16(6):659–65. https://doi.org/10.1097/adm.0000000000000985.
43. Rodriguez JA, Betancourt JR, Sequist TD, Ganguli I. Differences in the use of telephone and video telemedicine visits during the COVID-19 pandemic. Am J Manag Care. 2021;27(1):21–6. https://doi.org/10.37765/ajmc.2021.88573.
44. Nkodo AF, Gonzalez MM, Reves S, Etz RS. Telemedicine adoption during COVID-19 pandemic: perspectives from primary care clinicians in safety-net settings. J Am Board Fam Med. 2024;37(3):409–17. https://doi.org/10.3122/jabfm.2023.230339R1.
45. Der-Martirosian C, Chu K, Steers WN, et al. Examining telehealth use among primary care patients, providers, and clinics during the COVID-19 pandemic. BMC Prim Care. 2022;23(1):155. https://doi.org/10.1186/s12875-022-01738-3.
46. DePuccio MJ, Gaughan AA, McAlearney AS. Making it work: physicians' perspectives on the rapid transition to telemedicine. Telemed Rep. 2021;2(1):135–42. https://doi.org/10.1089/tmr.2020.0038.
47. Fraze TK, Beidler LB, De Marchis EH, Gottlieb LM, Potter MB. "Beyond just a supplement": administrators' visions for the future of virtual primary care services. J Am Board Fam Med. 2022;35(3):527–36. https://doi.org/10.3122/jabfm.2022.03.210479.
48. Lanham HJ, McDaniel JRR, Crabtree BF, et al. How improving practice relationships among clinicians and nonclinicians can improve quality in primary care. Jt Comm J Qual Patient Saf. 2009;35(9):457–AP2.
49. Miller WL, Crabtree BF, Nutting PA, Stange KC, Jaén CR. Primary care practice development: a relationship-centered approach. Ann Fam Med. 2010;8(Suppl 1):S68–79.
50. Halawa F, Madathil SC, Gittler A, Khasawneh MT. Advancing evidence-based healthcare facility design: a systematic literature review. Health Care Manag Sci. 2020;23:453–80.
51. Gunn R, Davis MM, Hall J, et al. Designing clinical space for the delivery of integrated behavioral health and primary care. J Am Board Fam Med. 2015;28(Supplement 1):S52–62.
52. Nguyen MH, Armoogum J. Perception and preference for home-based telework in the COVID-19 era: a gender-based analysis in Hanoi, Vietnam. Sustainability. 2021;13(6):3179.
53. Edwards ST, Marino M, Solberg LI, et al. Cultural and structural features of zero-burnout primary care practices: study examines features of primary care practices where physician burnout was reported to be zero. Health Aff. 2021;40(6):928–36.
54. Payán DD, Frehn JL, Garcia L, Tierney AA, Rodriguez HP. Telemedicine implementation and use in community health centers during COVID-19: clinic personnel and patient perspectives. SSM Qual Res Health. 2022;2:100054. https://doi.org/10.1016/j.ssmqr.2022.100054.
55. Balut MD, Wyte-Lake T, Steers WN, et al. Expansion of telemedicine during COVID-19 at a VA specialty clinic. Healthcare. 2022;10(1):100599. https://doi.org/10.1016/j.hjdsi.2021.100599.
56. Association of American Medical Colleges, Vizient. Effective strategies for sustaining and optimizing telehealth in primary care. 2023. https://store.aamc.org/downloadable/download/sample/sample_id/584/.
57. American Medical Association. Telehealth integration and optimization: improve patient care through virtual health care delivery. https://edhub.ama-assn.org/steps-forward/module/2813038. Accessed 3 Dec 2024.
58. Association of American Medical Colleges. Digital health equity current practices and approaches of academic medical centers. 2023. https://store.aamc.org/digital-health-equity-current-practices-and-approaches-of-academic-medical-centers.html. Accessed 3 Dec 2024.

59. Bergman D, Bethell C, Gombojav N, Hassink S, Stange KC. Physical distancing with social connectedness. Ann Fam Med. 2020;18(3):272–7. https://doi.org/10.1370/afm.2538.
60. Cheng A, Guzman CEV, Duffield TC, Hofkamp H. Advancing telemedicine within family medicine's core values. Telemed E-Health. 2021;27(2):121–3. https://doi.org/10.1089/tmj.2020.0282.
61. Stange K, Burge F, Haggerty J. RCGP continuity of care toolkit: promoting relational continuity. Br J Gen Pract. 2014;64:274–5.
62. Haggerty JL, Roberge D, Freeman GK, Beaulieu C. Experienced continuity of care when patients see multiple clinicians: a qualitative metasummary. Ann Fam Med. 2013;11(3):262–71.
63. Loxterkamp D. Benefits of continuity of care. Fam Med. 2009;41(5):312.
64. Guthrie B, Saultz JW, Freeman GK, Haggerty JL. Continuity of care matters. BMJ. 2008;337:a867. https://doi.org/10.1136/bmj.a867.
65. Saultz JW, Lochner J. Interpersonal continuity of care and care outcomes: a critical review. Ann Fam Med. 2005;3(2):159–66.
66. Saultz JW, Albedaiwi W. Interpersonal continuity of care and patient satisfaction: a critical review. Ann Fam Med. 2004;2(5):445–51. https://doi.org/10.1370/afm.91.
67. Mainous AG 3rd, Goodwin MA, Stange KC. Patient-physician shared experiences and value patients place on continuity of care. Ann Fam Med. 2004;2(5):452–4. https://doi.org/10.1370/afm.84.
68. Frankel RM. Relationship-centered care and the patient-physician relationship. J Gen Intern Med. 2004;19(11):1163–5.
69. Beach MC, Inui T, Network R-CCR. Relationship-centered care: a constructive reframing. J Gen Intern Med. 2006;21:3–8.
70. Epstein RM, Fiscella K, Lesser CS, Stange KC. Why the nation needs a policy push on patient-centered health care. Health Aff. 2010;29(8):1489–95.
71. Flocke SA, Huguet N, Bailey SR, Hodes T, O'Malley JP. Impact of COVID-19 pandemic on assessing tobacco status in community health centers. Ann Fam Med. 2023;21(2):161–4. https://doi.org/10.1370/afm.2948.
72. Bailey SR, Lucas JA, Holderness H, et al. Smoking assessment by visit modality among community-based primary care clinics. Am J Prev Med. 2025;68(3):607–10. https://doi.org/10.1016/j.amepre.2024.11.020.

Chapter 10
Lessons on Employee Health and Caring for the Team from the COVID-19 Pandemic

Te-Yu Ruth Chang and Brian Park

Introduction—A Rapid Shift in Leadership Thinking

> *It's Friday night, February 28, 2020, near midnight on the East Coast, and I am sitting on a bed in a chilly dorm room. I am here to attend a leadership training program in my role as the Chief People Officer for Kaiser Permanente Northwest and missing my family back in Portland, Oregon. My family and my team back home suddenly feel so much farther away as I hunch over my computer, conferring with our organization's Director of Benefits and HR Operations as we quickly edit a policy. A couple of minutes earlier, the Medical Director of Hospital and Post-Acute Care notified me that we needed an Employee Health Exposure to Infectious Disease policy—and we needed it now. Our hospital had the first presumptive case in Oregon of a patient infected with the novel COVID-19 virus. We needed to know what to do for the staff and clinicians who had been caring for this patient.*
>
> *Serving as a family physician and a people leader for a medical group of over 1400 clinicians that cares for over 600,000 members, that evening required a shift in thinking from how to solve complicated yet predictable problems, towards tackling complex issues with many unknowns.* —Dr. Ruth Chang, physician leader at Kaiser Permanente Northwest

While the issues we tackled in human resources, people, and culture were complex, this chapter outlines lessons learned and practical considerations in managing and caring for the health care workforce during the early years of the COVID-19 pandemic. The demands on health care during the pandemic introduced many

T.-Y. R. Chang (✉)
Family Medicine, Kaiser Permanente Northwest, Portland, OR, USA
e-mail: Ruth.Chang@kp.org

B. Park
Department of Family Medicine, Oregon Health & Science University School of Medicine, Portland, OR, USA

A. Cheng et al. (eds.), *Primary Care in a Public Health Emergency*,
https://doi.org/10.1007/978-3-032-12487-6_10

challenges for personnel management. These include reducing the risks of infectious diseases, managing exposures, workplace accommodations, and caring for the health care team. This chapter offers a guide and a summary of lessons learned; it is not intended to replace the expert advice of HR professionals and employment lawyers. The federal, state, and local laws governing employment and benefits are numerous and complex.

The first half will focus on guidelines about necessary policies and protocols that focus on employee health, and the second half of the chapter details proactive strategies deployed to support retention and well-being of the workforce.

Policies and Procedures that Focus on Employee Health

Written documents are a critical management tool generally and especially during a crisis. Policies and procedures documents provide consistent guidance, expectations, and accountability in how an organization operates. They help improve efficiency, and in times of crisis, they can help provide certainty. Here, we will describe our approach to policies and procedures focusing on employee health, including quarantine, symptom self-check and self-report, personal protective equipment (PPE), vaccinations, and medical accommodation, as well as how these functions were challenged during the pandemic and lessons learned. In addition to policies to help prevent the spread of COVID-19, we approached employee health from a broad perspective of caring for the psychological and mental health of the team (see later section on well-being of the workforce).

Employee health offices are governed by their organizational policies, as well as national guidelines defined by the Occupational Safety and Health Administration (OSHA), which is tasked with ensuring a safe working environment for American workers. OSHA mandates encompass a wide range of regulations designed to protect workers from hazards such as exposure to harmful substances, physical dangers, and ergonomic risks. Employers are obligated to assess workplace hazards, implement appropriate controls, provide necessary training, and maintain records of incidents and corrective actions. Compliance with OSHA requirements not only minimizes the risk of workplace injuries and illnesses but also fosters a culture of safety and well-being among employees. By prioritizing employee health in alignment with OSHA standards, organizations demonstrate their commitment to providing a safe and healthy work environment for all [1].

Employee health is a critical aspect of any organization, encompassing various functions and principles aimed at ensuring the physical, emotional, and psychological well-being of workers. Basic principles of employee health include promoting a safe work environment, providing access to health care services, and implementing preventive measures. These principles guided our response to the COVID-19 pandemic.

Quarantine Policy

In the process of admitting and caring for the first patient diagnosed with COVID-19 in Oregon, over 80 staff members were exposed to the patient. At the time, the US did not have any PPE requirements in place at the federal, state, or local levels. The staff who cared for the patient did not wear PPE. Once we knew they had been exposed to patient zero, we had to instruct the staff to quarantine either at home if they had a private room or in a hotel if they did not have access to a private room in their homes. The policy was created to define who would need to go into quarantine, for what length of time, and how the organization would support workers during this time—in other words, this was paid administrative time in quarantine, and hotel rooms were paid for if the employee did not have a private room at home. This policy was written to decrease the risk of disease spread in the workplace, protect the employees' families and the community, and outline the responsibilities of the impacted employees and the employer.

Symptom Self-Checking and Reporting Policy

As COVID-19 spread in the community, it was imperative for employees to stay home when feeling sick. A policy that outlined a checklist for employees to self-check each morning reinforced the expectation to not come to work if any symptom typical of COVID-19 was present. By coming to work, the employee was attesting that they were symptom-free. If employees were experiencing any symptoms associated with COVID-19 such as fever, sore throat, cough, or runny nose, then they were to immediately report the symptoms to employee health. The employee then needed to test negative for COVID-19 before returning to work. Again, this policy aimed to decrease the risk of transmission in the workplace—between colleagues and between staff and patients.

Personal Protective Equipment (PPE)

In the COVID-19 pandemic, the primary mode of virus transmission was via respiratory droplets, which resulted in a focus on masks and respirators, but it was not entirely clear in the early days of the pandemic whether there were other modes of transmission. One might expect future pandemics to follow a similar evolution with full PPE required while research clarifies transmissibility of the pathogen.

Once the Centers for Disease Control and Prevention (CDC) issued clear guidelines for masking, health care organizations worked as quickly as possible to acquire and deliver PPE to staff and ensure staff complied. Early in the pandemic there was a shortage of PPE, and health care systems had to prioritize how this resource was allocated before consistent supplies were secured. Clinical staff at the highest risk of exposure—those performing aerosol-generating procedures, e.g., intubation, noninvasive positive pressure ventilation, tracheotomies, cardiopulmonary resuscitation, bronchoscopies, and sputum induction—were prioritized for N-95 and respirator use. Clear communication about why certain teams were prioritized over others was essential to ensure staff felt they were being fairly treated.

In addition to prioritization and allocation of resources, religious and medical exceptions were needed in the fitting of protective equipment. A proper fit of an N-95 mask requires close adherence of the mask against the face. This meant that those with facial hair needed to remove it to ensure a proper fit. To accommodate religious observances that require growth of facial hair, people were offered the use of powered air-purifying respirators (PAPRs). In addition, people with a medical contraindication to wearing masks, such as severe contact dermatitis, or severe claustrophobia, were also offered PAPRs.

Over time as staff tired of wearing masks for their entire shifts, policies around strict masking needed to be reinforced through communication, reminders, and corrective conversations. Once masks became optional in the workplace per CDC and state health authority recommendations, their use became highly variable, even during times of high prevalence of COVID-19 in the community. The arc of mask wearing preferences throughout the pandemic demonstrated the full spectrum of human behavior in relation to PPE. Early in the pandemic, health care teams wanted masks that were in short supply; later, when the PPE supply was more plentiful, some team members did not want to comply with mask mandates. Over time, as more information became known about the virus and vaccines became widely available, individuals were eager to make their own decisions about mask wearing based on their individual and family risks.

Vaccination Mandates

Fortunately, vaccinations were developed to protect against the COVID-19 virus, which marked a turning point in the pandemic. With a backdrop of general unrest and civil discord, vaccines became politicized, and employers faced difficult challenges with vaccine mandates. In contrast to seasonal influenza vaccinations, which have historically been a requirement with little resistance from health care workers, the COVID-19 vaccine mandates were met with significant concerns. Recall that the COVID-19 vaccines were the first mRNA ones to receive full Food and Drug Administration approval and in record time from development to market. The speed of development raised safety and efficacy concerns. In addition, false information and conspiracy theories were widely disseminated through the internet and social media regarding the government using the vaccines to track people or to alter their DNA. Furthermore, in a society that values individual choice, any mandate faces skepticism and opposition simply because people do not want to be told what to do.

Employers learned several valuable lessons about vaccination mandates during the COVID-19 pandemic. First, of utmost importance, is clear communication and consistent messaging to employees regarding the rationale behind vaccination mandates, emphasizing workplace safety and public health concerns. Two recommendations based on our experiences include:

- **Be nuanced with exemptions**: Develop a process to accommodate exemptions based on medical or religious reasons, while working towards balancing individual rights with collective well-being. Implementation of a vaccination mandate requires careful consideration of legal implications, including compliance with federal, state, and local regulations, local community practice, as well as potential risks of litigation.
- **Consider the role of incentives**: Consider offering an incentive to employees for completing vaccinations. The Bureau of Labor Statistics reported that nearly half of establishments that required COVID-19 vaccinations offered incentives, including financial, paid time off, and remaining on the clock to obtain a vaccine [2]. Overall, the pandemic highlighted the significance of vaccination mandates as a proactive measure to protect employees, patients, and the broader community against infectious disease.

Workplace Accommodation

In addition to employee health policies, we implemented workplace accommodations to help protect the health of employees. A workplace accommodation is an adjustment to a job or work environment that enables an individual with a disability to perform their job functions. Title I of The Americans with Disabilities Act defines a reasonable accommodation as a modification or adjustment to a job, the work environment, or the way a hiring process usually proceeds. These changes enable an individual with a disability to have an equal opportunity to obtain a job and successfully perform their job duties to the same extent as persons without disabilities [3].

Making reasonable accommodations in the workplace involves balancing operational needs and the needs of the employee seeking the accommodation, all the while adhering to federal regulations. "Reasonable" accommodation means that it is feasible for the employer. HR principles emphasize the importance of clear communication, confidentiality, and respect for employee privacy throughout the accommodation process.

Accommodations during the pandemic evolved as our understanding of risk of transmission increased along with the availability of PPE and vaccines. Initially we took a conservative approach to make reasonable accommodations to protect staff who may be at higher risk of severe illness due to conditions such as immunocompromise, immunosuppression, chronic lung disease, or cancer treatment. Whenever possible, as requested by persons at higher risk, accommodation was given to perform work remotely via telehealth platforms. Any granted accommodation was reviewed after a specific time interval. As the supply of PPE increased and vaccines became widely available, some of the initial requests for accommodation were no longer needed.

Recommendations based on our experiences include:

- Open communication is essential. Meet with the employee seeking accommodation to discuss their specific needs and limitations resulting from their medical condition. Listen and seek to understand their challenges and how they impact their ability to perform their job.
- Work collaboratively to explore potential accommodations that meet both the employee's needs and the operational requirements of the job. This may involve adjusting work hours, modifying tasks, providing assistive technology or ergonomic accommodations, or allowing for telecommuting if feasible.
- Maintain confidentiality and sensitivity to the employee's privacy.
- Revisit accommodations after a specific time interval.
- By integrating federal laws with HR best practices, organizations can effectively accommodate employees' medical needs while upholding legal requirements and fostering a supportive work environment that values diversity and inclusion. Again, given the complexity of regulations governing accommodations, balance inquiry of employee needs through open communication channels alongside consulting with HR professionals when making medical accommodations.

Caring for the Team

During a public health and/or medical crisis, the health care team is expected to perform exceptionally when they are also under stress. Leaders can implement practices of mutual care and compassion to bolster the resiliency of their teams. In addition, leaders also must take care of themselves through stressful times. Follow the adage of "put your own oxygen mask on first." For example, some leaders prioritized exercise every morning to center themselves to tackle the rest of the day.

Caring for the health care team remained a central focus during the pandemic. The Northwest Permanente Medical Director of Mental Health Services astutely referenced Abraham Maslow's hierarchy of needs to prioritize how we organized support for the teams. Maslow's 1943 paper [4] (on the "Theory of Human Motivation," originally published in Psychology Review) used the terms "physiological," "safety," "belonging and love," "social needs" or "esteem," "self-actualization," and "transcendence" to describe the basic needs that humans experience in a hierarchical fashion. This means that, according to the theory, for motivation to arise at the next stage, each prior stage must be satisfied.

For example, our initial priority during the earliest stages of the pandemic was often not to help our teams "make meaning" of the crisis, but rather to provide supplemental nutritional support for our hospital staff. Due to staffing shortages, the hospital cafeteria had reduced its nighttime hours. The overnight staff had limited hours and options to access hot food. In addition to providing a wider array of foods that could be distributed by vending machines, and working to increase hours of the cafeteria, the facilities team started inviting food trucks, from a wide variety of cultures, to come onto the hospital campuses on a rotating basis to offer a wider selection of food. The facilities team also arranged food trucks to visit urgent care locations and as budget allowed, meals were hosted by the local management teams. While this seems like a small gesture, staff gave very positive feedback on having access to food trucks—they felt cared for by their leaders who took the time to make these arrangements.

In the early days of the pandemic, prior to the availability of vaccines, Kaiser Permanente offered to pay for hotel stays for health care workers who had been exposed to COVID-19 and needed to quarantine but did not have a private room at home. There was also a large-scale effort to distribute additional access to scrubs for hospital workers, so that staff did not have to launder contaminated clothing themselves. Providing food, clothing, and shelter fulfilled the most basic "physiologic" need on the Maslow hierarchy of needs.

With ongoing attention to physiologic needs, safety and security, we were able to also develop programs focused on love and belonging. These included a peer support program, caring calls program, and COVID-19 debriefs.

Peer Support

Clinicians face stressors and challenges that are unique to the profession and having a peer to turn to is invaluable. Peer support offers an important layer of support for physicians and clinicians, who are negatively impacted when their patients experience an unanticipated adverse outcome, known as second victims. A definition, by international consensus, of the second victim is "any health care worker, directly or indirectly involved in an unanticipated adverse patient event, unintentional health care error, or patient injury and who becomes victimized in the sense that they are also negatively impacted" [5]. The negative impact is significant and can lead to attrition.

In a 2010 survey of 898 health care professionals at University of Missouri Health Care (MUHC), 30% reported second victim symptoms because of a patient safety event. Psychological symptoms could include depression, fear, self-doubt, and anger, and physical symptoms could include sleep disturbances, difficulty concentrating, and eating disturbances, among others. Of those experiencing these symptoms, nearly 15% reported seriously contemplating leaving their profession [6].

Another framework relevant to peer support is the MUHC Scott model of tiered support (see Fig. 10.1). The base of support, tier 1, comes from local colleagues and leaders who offer reassurance to the second victim. The second level of support, tier 2, consists of peer supporters or patient safety managers. This serves a subset of employees who need a higher level of support. The third level of support, tier 3, consists of an expedited referral network to an employee assistance program,

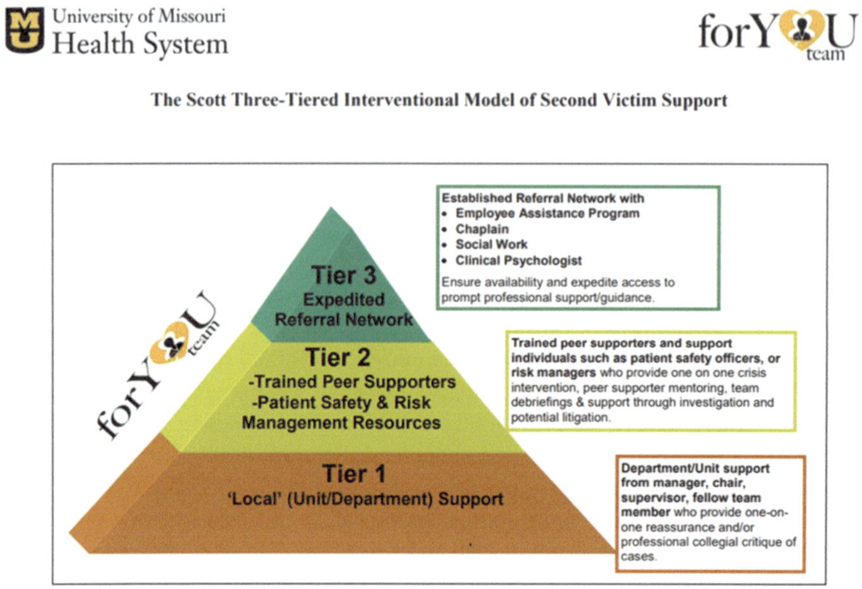

Fig. 10.1 The Scott Three-Tiered Interventional Model of Second Victim Support. (Reprinted with permission from Scott, et al. [6])

chaplain, social work support, and/or clinical psychologists. The third tier serves second victims with severe or persistent symptoms [7].

While the planning for a peer support program was underway before the COVID-19 pandemic, the start of the pandemic fast-tracked the creation of this program at Northwest Permanente. Over three dozen physicians and clinicians volunteered to serve as peer supporters. These volunteers were ones that colleagues tended to gravitate toward to talk about stressors. The identified peer supporters completed education on the second victim phenomenon and training on how to best offer support and identify those with mental health concerns who would require referral to the employee assistance program for professional assessment. The wellness team which leads this program also offered broad education to departmental leaders on the concept of peer support and how to self-refer or refer colleagues to the program. The peer support program continues to provide confidential one-on-one sessions to our clinicians for emotional processing of unintended adverse patient outcomes or for any concern that the clinician seeking support wants to discuss. There are unique pressures and challenges that clinicians face because of their profession and having access to peer support is key to caring for mental health.

Caring Calls

A year and a half into the pandemic, the isolation and strain of the pandemic was palpable. While clinicians came to work every day and continued to provide care for patients, the lack of connection with colleagues generated feelings of loneliness. With this lack of connection, the core clinicians were wondering if the work they did mattered and if they themselves mattered. One of the Northwest Permanente physicians offered the idea of caring calls. Each clinician would receive a personal outreach and invitation to check in over the phone with a colleague. Over three dozen of our administrators volunteered to individually outreach to all 1400+ clinicians. This one-time outreach to all the clinicians occurred over a period of 4 months. The response from clinicians varied. Some people responded to a text stating they were fine and appreciated the outreach. Others welcomed a call that lasted anywhere from a few minutes to an hour. Overall, the response from the caring calls was very positive and those who chose to talk with a colleague felt cared for, valued, seen, and heard. The administrative team provided an invaluable service and those who participated felt they were contributing to the mission by caring for those who provide direct care to patients.

COVID Debriefs

Commemorating the anniversaries of major tragic events, such as the start of the COVID-19 pandemic, holds significant importance for several reasons. The commemorations serve as a means of honoring and remembering the lives lost and the profound impact the event had on individuals, teams, communities, and societies worldwide. Additionally, commemorations provide an opportunity for reflection and introspection, allowing us to assess lessons learned, evaluate our responses, and identify areas for improvement in crisis management within our health care systems.

On the first anniversary of caring for the first patient in the state of Oregon diagnosed with COVID-19, Kaiser Permanente leaders acknowledged our clinicians, administrators, and staff with a special town hall broadcast. Recall that in the first year, health care workers were celebrated as heroes and then as the pandemic continued, the tone and tenor shifted. Due to numerous factors, including distrust and conspiracy theories about the available vaccines, fatigue over COVID-19 precautions, social isolation, and lack of everyday social interactions, clinicians began to experience increasing instances of difficult interactions with patients over the course of the second year. While checking in with clinicians, the question of "How are we going to collectively process our trauma?" was posed. In response to this need for collective processing and commemoration of the second anniversary of the pandemic, Northwest Permanente leaders facilitated discussions called the COVID Debriefs. Using three simple questions, team members shared as little or as much as they wanted to in their team meetings. The debriefs were optional, and the degree of participation in the debriefs was up to each individual.

The questions posed during the debriefs were:

1. What was the hardest thing for you since the pandemic started?
2. What is one thing you lost?
3. What is one thing you learned?

Starting with the senior leadership team, each member shared their personal stories and then led the same discussion with the teams that reported to them. As each cadre of leaders experienced the debriefs, they were then asked to facilitate a discussion using the same questions for their teams. This cascade structure relied on the framework of "see one, do one, teach one." Some teams devoted an entire departmental meeting to the debrief while others conducted them with a lighter touch. Departmental chiefs and medical office medical directors decided how much time they would dedicate to the COVID Debriefs based on the needs of their teams. The feedback was positive from core clinicians. Being able to share their personal experiences, losses, and learnings, clinicians reported they felt less lonely, more connected, and a bit lighter. Using this broad-based approach to discussing the pandemic and its impact on all of us also helped to normalize conversations about mental health.

In addition to these large, company-wide initiatives, many work teams held daily or weekly check-ins. These were unstructured meetings for team members to call into a video conference and connect with each other, share learnings, tips around patient care, or to vent. The employee assistance program and wellness team also set up topic-focused facilitated discussions around managing anxiety and parenting during COVID-19 (and when online learning was the norm), among other topics. These topical sessions were also well received and repeated due to interest.

During the second winter of the COVID-19 pandemic, hospital censuses across the country were at record high levels and resources were running low compared to demand. Hospital leaders made plans to ration resources if communities experienced more disease burden than resources available. Part of this resource allocation required the creation of a bioethics triage team who would serve as consultants to care teams and run the process of resource allocation through evaluation of survivability of patients, as well as random number generation to assign ventilators, in the event the community ran out of this resource. The bioethics triage team members were all volunteer physicians who received training and education on the process. This team set up a call schedule and a debrief meeting following each scheduled shift. Luckily, we did not activate our bioethics triage teams in Oregon, but had we needed to, we had trained coaches, and mental health therapists on standby to support the team.

Mental Health

Even with optimal support in place, chronic stress can cause many employees to experience burnout and psychological distress. The HR teams of organizations have an important role to play in supporting the mental health and well-being of physicians and staff. The prevalence of stress, burnout, and psychological distress among physicians has been an increasing concern and worsened during the pandemic [8]. The increased levels of burnout have significant implications for the health of patients and populations. HR can offer multilayered strategies to help mitigate burnout by running mental health awareness campaigns, offering employee assistance programs, and promoting stress management [9].

Everyone Has Mental Health

To increase awareness of and to promote mental health, it needs to be discussed openly. The Mental Health Coalition, a not-for-profit organization, was "formed with the understanding that the mental health crisis is fueled by a pervasive and devastating stigma, preventing millions of individuals from being able to seek the critical treatment they need" [10]. Just as physical health can fluctuate for individuals during times of health or times of illness, mental health also fluctuates. Mental well-being or mental fitness (analogous to physical fitness) is on a continuum that is always in flux. This framework acknowledges and normalizes conversations about mental health (see Fig. 10.2 for an example of how this continuum is visually represented by The Mental Health Coalition).

Organizations can adopt cultures and build programs to support mental health. One powerful way to normalize it is for leaders to talk about how they care for their own mental health, as they see fit. Northwest Permanente's President and CEO, Dr.

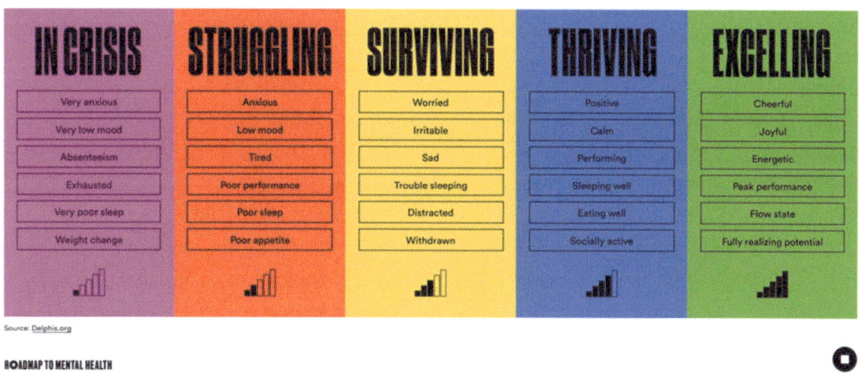

Fig. 10.2 Original Mental Health Roadmap. (Source: thementalhealthcoalition.org. Used with permission [11])

Leong Koh, openly shares at new hire orientation about the company's employee assistance program, Permanente Advocate Resource, and his own access to the program for himself and his family members. The author, Dr. Ruth Chang, also welcomes the new hires and reinforces the president's message by sharing her own families' use of counseling over the years. Everyone benefits from recognizing what their mental health state is and accessing resources to meet their needs. It is imperative that organizations offer support and development, no matter where a person is on their mental health roadmap. In support of this continuum of mental health, ideally workplaces offer resources to support those in crisis or who are struggling in the form of employee assistance programs that include professional counseling. Peer support can help provide a boost to those in the surviving state. For people who are thriving or excelling, professional development and coaching helps them continue to flourish.

In the spirit of everyone having mental health, Northwest Permanente undertook a series of actions to create programs, provide support, and advocate for improved mental health. The HR team built a new peer support program, made outreach calls to every clinician, designed and facilitated structured debriefs, and advocated for statewide changes to remove barriers that prevent physicians from accessing mental health services.

A Call to Action

Our employees' health is affected by factors throughout society and while leaders cannot influence all domains of their employees' lives, they may have more influence than they would think. An example for health care workers is state-level accrediting boards. Here, we share an example of how organizational advocacy has reduced stigmatizing language from physician credentialing processes, a change that will have impact on thousands of physicians for years to come.

On April 26, 2020, Dr. Lorna Breen, an emergency medicine physician, daughter, sister, and friend died by suicide. Seventeen days prior to her death, she had called her sister to tell her that she could not move. She had been working around the clock to care for patients dying of COVID-19 in a busy New York hospital, contracted COVID-19 herself, and was not getting any sleep. She was worried that she would lose her medical license if she sought help for her mental health. Dr. Breen had no known prior history of anxiety or depression. Her only known risk factor was that she was a physician [12]. Well before the pandemic, in a 2005 article published in the New England Journal of Medicine, it was noted that physicians have a higher risk of suicide than the general population. Male doctors have suicide rates 40% higher than the general population, and female doctors up to 130% higher [13].

The Dr. Lorna Breen Heroes' Foundation was founded in her honor and seeks to reduce the stigma that prevented Dr. Breen from seeking the care that she desperately needed. One area of focus of the foundation advocates for the removal of stigmatizing language and intrusive mental health questions from state medical licensing applications and the hospital credentialing forms whose language often follows state forms. These questions serve as a barrier to care. Four in 10 physicians said that they did not seek help for burnout or depression because they worried that their employer or state medical board would find out, according to the Medscape 'I Cry but No One Cares': Physician Burnout & Depression Report 2023 [14]. In a 2023 cross-sectional review of medical licensing forms (from 2022) from 50 states, Washington, DC, and 4 territories, the authors note that only 3 states/territories met the 2018 recommendations from the Federation of State Medical Boards regarding questions on mental health to (1) ask only if impaired, (2) ask only if current, (3) allow for safe haven non-reporting, and (4) include supportive language normalizing physician wellness [15].

Inspired by the Dr. Lorna Breen Heroes' Foundation call to action, Northwest Permanente physician wellness director, Dr. Laura Ryan, served on The Oregon Health Authority's Advisory Committee on Physician Credentialing Information (ACPCI) [16] to help change the language on the Oregon hospital credentialing forms [17]. The ACPCI develops the content and format of the uniform applications used by credentialing organizations to credential and recredential health care practitioners in the State of Oregon: the Oregon Practitioner Credentialing Application (OPCA) and the Oregon Practitioner Recredentialing Application (OPRA). The Committee meets at least once every calendar year to review and confirm that the applications comply with current credentialing standards and regulations. The Committee solicits application change suggestions from the public on a regular basis. Those suggestions are reviewed and evaluated by the ACPCI at its annual meeting. Any approved Committee recommendations are brought to the Director of the Oregon Health Authority for approval.

The language in a prior version:

L.	Do you currently have any physical condition, mental health condition, or chemical dependency condition (alcohol or other substance) that currently affects your ability to practice, with or without reasonable accommodation, the privileges requested?
	If reasonable accommodation is required, please specify the accommodation(s) required on a separate sheet.

The updated language, approved by the ACPCI in the summer of 2024:

We recognize that providers encounter health conditions, including those involving physical and mental health and substance use disorders, just as their patients do. It is imperative that providers address their health concerns for their own well-being as well as for patient safety.
I attest to no current physical, mental health, or chemical dependency conditions (alcohol or other substances) that currently affect my ability to practice, with or without reasonable accommodation.
Please disclose any current conditions requiring employer-provided accommodation(s) on a separate sheet.

In Dr. Ryan's words: This was an invaluable learning experience as it allowed me to recognize and appreciate the many lines of sight that must be addressed when implementing a change of this magnitude. The work group within the ACPCI considering this change consisted of myself, an Oregon Health & Science University internal medicine physician, and

> a credentialing specialist, and learning the perspectives of stakeholders on both sides of the issue was crucial. We were thus prepared to address one another's concerns, effectively preempting objections from our larger committee. Additionally, our chair, Mark Bonanno, General Counsel and Director of Health Policy for the Oregon Medical Association, assisted us with legal wording and also facilitated a listening session prior to our committee meeting, in order to introduce the proposed change and get any feedback. Mark invited two national advocates for this change to this listening session (Corey Feist, along with another health care lawyer, from the Dr. Lorna Breen Heroes' Foundation) in order to discuss the importance of removing intrusive mental health questioning and answer any questions about this change. This added expert perspectives to the proposal and certainly galvanized the initiative's importance. I credit a multi-disciplinary work group, representing both sides of the argument, and an experienced health care lawyer advocating for effective lobbying of the issue, with our success. The proposed change was rapidly and unanimously recommended at our annual meeting.

For too long, licensed health care professionals were hesitant to care for themselves as it would mean needing to disclose this information to regulatory agencies. If your state medical licensing forms still contain intrusive language about mental health, now is the time to advocate for change. By removing this barrier, more physicians will seek the care they need, without worrying that they will lose their jobs.

Conclusion

The realm of HR, like other parts of health care, required agility and creative problem solving as we navigated the COVID-19 pandemic. Lessons learned included the importance of caring for the whole person, not just limiting the spread of disease in the workplace. Attention to basic needs such as food and physical safety is paramount. In addition, hosting structured debriefs, encouraging check-ins, and supporting mental health helped address burnout and emotional exhaustion during this stressful period.

In addition to long hours, worrying about staying healthy, and not bringing home disease to loved ones, health care workers faced a heavy mental and emotional toll from the death of patients, and possibly colleagues and loved ones. Promoting mental health by normalizing its existence with "everyone has mental health" and decreasing barriers to care such as eliminating intrusive language in licensing and credentialing forms, are ways that organizations can act.

Health care organizations promote the health and wellness of our patients and must simultaneously care for our employees. This caring can take the form of comprehensive and compassionate policies, internally focused well-being programs, a humanistic leadership culture, and advocacy to improve the external environment.

References

1. U.S Department of Labor. About OSHA. Accessed 18 Mar 2024. https://www.osha.gov/aboutosha.
2. U.S. Bureau of Labor Statistics. TED: The Economics Daily. United States Department of Labor. Accessed 19 Mar 2024. https://www.bls.gov/opub/ted/2022/nearly-half-of-establishments-that-required-covid-19-vaccinations-offered-incentives.htm.
3. U.S Department of Labor Office of Disability Employment Policy. Accomodations. Accessed 17 Mar 24. https://www.dol.gov/agencies/odep/program-areas/employers/accommodations.
4. Green CD. A.H. Maslow. Theory of Human Motivation (1943). Accessed 7 Mar 2024. https://psychclassics.yorku.ca/Maslow/motivation.htm.
5. Vanhaecht K, Seys D, Russotto S, et al. An evidence and consensus-based definition of second victim: a strategic topic in healthcare quality, patient safety, person-centeredness and human resource management. Int J Environ Res Public Health. 2022;19(24). https://doi.org/10.3390/ijerph192416869.
6. Scott SD, Hirschinger LE, Cox KR, et al. Caring for our own: deploying a systemwide second victim rapid response team. Jt Comm J Qual Patient Saf. 2010;36(5):233–40. https://doi.org/10.1016/s1553-7250(10)36038-7.
7. University of Missouri Health Care Office of Clinical Effectiveness. forYOU Team. Accessed 16 Mar 2024. https://www.muhealth.org/sites/default/files/Scotts_Three_Tier_Support.pdf.
8. Alkhamees AA, Aljohani MS, Kalani S, et al. Physician's burnout during the COVID-19 pandemic: a systematic review and meta-analysis. Int J Environ Res Public Health. 2023;20(5). https://doi.org/10.3390/ijerph20054598.
9. Mhlongo N, Elufioye O, Asuzu OF, Ndubuisi N, Olatoye F, Ajayi-Nifise A. The role of HR in promoting mental health and well-being in healthcare settings: a comprehensive review. Int J Manag Entrep Res. 2024;6:380–91. https://doi.org/10.51594/ijmer.v6i2.777.
10. The Mental Health Coalition. About Us. Accessed 17 Mar 2024. https://www.thementalhealthcoalition.org/about-us/mission/.
11. The Mental Health Coalition. Roadmap to Mental Health. Accessed 17 July 2024. https://www.thementalhealthcoalition.org/wp-content/uploads/2020/12/MHC_Roadmap_16-9_R2-1.pdf.
12. Foundation DLBH. About Lorna. Accessed 17 Mar 2024. https://drlornabreen.org/about-lorna/.
13. Schernhammer E. Taking their own lives – the high rate of physician suicide. N Engl J Med. 2005;352(24):2473–6. https://doi.org/10.1056/NEJMp058014.
14. Kane L. I cry but no one cares': physician burnout and depression report 2023. 2023. https://www.medscape.com/slideshow/2023-lifestyle-burnout-6016058.
15. Douglas RN, Sharpe EE, Kraus M, Saddawi-Konefka D, Hanson AC, Pulos B. Mental health questions on state medical license applications and evaluation of updates. JAMA Netw Open. 2023;6(9):e2333360. https://doi.org/10.1001/jamanetworkopen.2023.33360.
16. Oregon Health Authority. Advisory Committee on Physician Credentialing Information. https://www.oregon.gov/oha/hpa/ohit-acpci/pages/index.aspx.
17. Garvey G. Fighting for physicians' right to access mental health care. American Medical Association; 2025. https://www.ama-assn.org/practice-management/physician-health/fighting-physicians-right-access-mental-health-care.

Chapter 11
Lessons on Workforce Management During the Pandemic

Te-Yu Ruth Chang and Brian Park

In early December 2020, I received a welcome call from the Medical Director of Hospital and Post-Acute Care. "Good news, we should start receiving large shipments of vaccines by late January and we need a lot of people to deliver hundreds of thousands of doses." As the Chief People Officer of Northwest Permanente, the medical group that partners with Kaiser Foundation Health Plan and Hospitals to serve over 600,000 members in Oregon and Southwest Washington, I knew it was time to get creative. —Ruth Chang, MD, MPH

The COVID-19 pandemic introduced pressures on staffing decisions. With the rapidly increasing demands on hospitals and clinics, there was also a need for additional non-licensed staff to manage the volume of patients and help direct workflow. Once vaccines became available, we needed as many qualified people as possible to administer vaccines and monitor for allergic reactions. While the demand for qualified health care workers was high, the US system also saw an increase in involuntary and voluntary turnover. In the early years of the pandemic, health care systems faced an abrupt drop in revenues due to deferred care leading to necessary cost reductions. Simultaneously, many health care workers voluntarily left the workforce due to isolation, disengagement, and burnout. Depleted reserves and a diminished workforce have set enduring challenges for health care organizations, even as the volume of services returns to pre-pandemic levels. For leaders, understanding how these challenges impact the teams, and how to best address them, are a critical part of the pandemic response.

T.-Y. R. Chang (✉)
Family Medicine, Kaiser Permanente Northwest, Portland, OR, USA
e-mail: Ruth.Chang@kp.org

B. Park
Department of Family Medicine, Oregon Health & Science University School of Medicine, Portland, OR, USA

A. Cheng et al. (eds.), *Primary Care in a Public Health Emergency*,
https://doi.org/10.1007/978-3-032-12487-6_11

The SCARF (Status, Certainty, Autonomy, Relatedness, Fairness) psychological theory helped leaders at Northwest Permanente frame and address issues by centering on the social needs of individuals. This model, developed by neuroscientist David Rock in 2008, helps explain that people perceive situations as threat or reward [1]. Based on neuroscience research, the theory states that each individual has the need for five social domains, the first being status, defined by how important someone feels in relation to others. People also have a need for certainty which is the ability to predict the future. Humans want autonomy or sense of control over events. As social beings, relatedness, or a sense of safety and friendship with others is crucial. Lastly, fairness, a sense of just and impartial exchanges, rounds out the SCARF model. Each person may have varying degrees of how important each social domain is to them. The ability to problem solve and collaborate with others is reduced when one is feeling threatened and, conversely, increased when one feels rewarded. Threat responses tend to be more intense and more common and need to be mitigated in social interactions. This model can help leaders anticipate communications or actions that might provoke an emotional response in others.

The SCARF model helps frame the great upheaval that health care providers, clinicians, and physicians experienced at the start of the pandemic. Medical experts' status was challenged and questioned by patients as the knowledge about COVID-19 was ever evolving. No one had any certainty about how the pandemic was going to impact us globally or locally. Health care workers lost a sense of control as it was imperative to follow the orders from the local and national health authorities. People became socially isolated given the restrictions on group gatherings. As essential workers, it also felt unfair that we were risking our lives every day coming to work when some people worked from home 100% of the time. Understanding and applying the SCARF model throughout decisions and communications about the workforce helped address the social needs of workers during the pandemic.

The demand for non-licensed staff increased at the very beginning of the pandemic and one way to solve this workforce need was through redeployment of staff. Clinics and hospitals needed "greeters" at entrances to scan people's temperatures and help enforce masking as they entered the buildings. Keeping in mind the SCARF model, we asked administrative staff to volunteer to fill these roles so that clinical staff could continue to provide care to patients. If staff volunteered, their teammates helped cover the administrative work. We tried to avoid mandates for redeployment of staff because it would have threatened their autonomy at a time when it was already low. For each type of job, we created a clear job description, contact information, dress code, parking instructions, breakroom locations, etc. We provided as much detail as possible because people needed certainty during these uncertain times. The volunteer staff were also stepping out of their comfort zone and interacting with the public, which was a risk to them. While the administrative staff volunteered to work in the clinical sites, they continued to receive their usual salaries, which acknowledged their status and felt fair. The organization also publicly celebrated the staff who voluntarily redeployed to elevate their status.

When faced with the prospect of an effective vaccine by the end of the calendar year 2020, we immediately strategized on how to increase the workforce in anticipation of delivering vaccines at large scale. Being part of a large medical group with engaged retirees, we developed a creative solution to scale up the workforce. We created a new job description of a "vaccinator" role and recruited retired and community physicians who wanted to help. This approach addressed a few regulatory requirements and financial constraints. As a for-profit medical group, we could not have volunteers. To cover medical liability, the clinicians giving vaccines needed to be employed within our system. The vaccinator role also had a pay rate that was de minimis compared to the usual pay scale of physicians. Not-for-profit groups can have volunteers, but they were not staffed to onboard large numbers of physicians which required background, license, and reference checks. During just a couple of months, we recruited and onboarded over 250 physicians as vaccinators who became an integral part of the staff for the All 4 Oregon mass vaccination site when it opened in January 2021. Since we were hiring the retirees and community physicians as locums, they were eligible for vaccines when staff were first eligible. This served as an incentive to sign up as a vaccinator and ensured our retirees and staff were immunized before they started work in the mass vaccination site.

Signing up as a vaccinator served the retirees' status, certainty, autonomy, relatedness, and fairness needs. The retirees who signed up to be vaccinators shared with me that they felt well cared for, that they mattered, and were delighted to help make a difference in the community. Since they were receiving their vaccines before starting as vaccinators, they also had certainty about the timing of their vaccines. Some had expressed worry about how soon they were going to be able to get the vaccine if they had to wait along with the general public. They chose to sign up as a vaccinator and exercised their autonomy in that decision making. Many also told me that this was their first time leaving the house, other than grocery shopping, since the start of the pandemic. They were delighted to see their friends and former colleagues during the onboarding for the vaccinators program. Lastly, they felt they were being treated fairly as they had equal access to vaccines, along with all other active health care staff.

As the pandemic unfolded and demand for health care decreased in some specialties, medical groups and health systems conducted layoffs. While the demand for primary care remained high, this specialty still experienced high turnover. Reported Oct 4, 2021, 18% of health care workers quit their jobs during the COVID-19 pandemic, while another 12% were laid off [2]. For practices that faced negative economic impact during the pandemic, difficult decisions had to be made to balance the budget.

When strategizing cost structure reductions, organizations must thoughtfully consider whether to implement temporary or permanent measures. Temporary reductions may involve furlough days, decreased full-time equivalent (FTE) positions or fewer workdays, and adjustments to base pay. These measures provide short-term relief during economic downturns while allowing companies to retain talent for future growth. Conversely, permanent reductions in force, necessitated by economic factors, require thorough consideration of employees' skills, performance records, and seniority. When planning for any reduction in force, either voluntary or involuntary, it is crucial to navigate national and local labor laws and regulations to ensure compliance, especially regarding protected classes and age-related considerations.

Consulting with HR experts or employment lawyers can provide invaluable guidance, particularly concerning special considerations for demographics impacted by layoffs, such as women and individuals identifying as non-binary, individuals holding racially/ethnically minoritized identities, or individuals over the age of 40. For instance, the Older Workers Benefit Protection Act mandates extended periods for considering separation packages for employees over 40 years old, highlighting the importance of legal expertise in navigating such complex detailed processes [3].

When considering employee separations, it is important to be generous and compassionate [4]. One approach is to offer a separation package to support individuals during the transition, which may include financial assistance equivalent to several months' salary. However, if providing such a package, it would be beneficial to the employer to present a separation agreement to protect the practice from potential legal disputes, ensuring that the departing employee cannot file lawsuits related to their dismissal or layoff. Depending on the circumstances, different incentives or benefits may be offered, such as retirement benefits for those nearing the end of their careers, incentives for voluntary separations, or support for those being involuntarily separated. To ensure incentives are distributed fairly, entire departments or classes of workers should be offered the same incentive. Additionally, including outplacement services in the package can assist employees in finding new employment opportunities.

Viewed through the SCARF model, layoffs strip the status of the impacted employee and cause a lot of uncertainty for their future. In involuntary layoffs, the impacted employees have no say, and people lose friendships and relationships they have cultivated at work. Fairness also comes into question as people wonder why their jobs were eliminated and others were not. It is important for organizations to document the rationale for why certain roles were eliminated and to communicate these reasons. Recognizing the full breadth of impact on employees and teams helps leaders communicate the reduction in force plans and acknowledge the depth of loss people experience. Applying the SCARF model to anticipate the needs of the employees who are not laid off also helps leaders move their team forward.

Expect decreased morale for employees who remain in a workforce after a layoff, known as the "survivors." The survivors may have a decreased sense of job security, for they may fear that their job is next in the future round of layoffs. The surviving staff may also face an increase in workload as work that their former colleagues performed may need to be redistributed. People can also experience a strong sense of survivor guilt, causing them to ask why not me and why the person who sat next to me? As with any major loss, expect staff to go through different stages of grief: shock/disbelief, anger, bargaining, depression/disengagement, and at some point, acceptance. As staff grieve, there will likely be a loss of productivity of about 20% [5].

After a layoff, there are key approaches that leaders can make to support the grieving process of surviving staff. Layoffs disrupt many work relationships and friendships. A fundamental approach is to help people feel reconnected to the mission of the organization and the day-to-day work. Leaders speaking to why their work is important for the patient, for the team, and for the organization help the staff connect to the mission. Making these connections demonstrates that the leader values the work and sees the employee and their efforts. Recognize staff for a job well done by sharing acknowledgements from patients, colleagues, and managers. Research shows that recognition results in increased employee morale, motivation, and sense of ownership, and helps foster a supportive and conducive work environment, thereby improving retention [6]. Recognition serves as a key element in building trust between managers and staff [7, 8]. Rebuilding trust is foundational to retention, especially after a reduction in force.

It would be important also to show individuals that the organization wants to develop and retain them. Managers can invest in co-creating an individual development plan for each staff member. Spending time discussing and encouraging staff's professional development plans demonstrates that the manager values the staff as individuals. This sense of value serves the need for status. Another facet managers need to carefully consider is the reallocation of work and to intentionally discuss what work to prioritize. This rebuilds a sense of autonomy of team members and ensures a sustainable workload. With a smaller team, it would be unreasonable to think the surviving team can continue all the work that was performed prior to the layoff. Overworking the surviving team risks increased turnover, which is already high after a layoff.

It is also imperative that leaders speak well of those who have separated from the organization. It is critical in maintaining the morale of the surviving staff by speaking positively of those who left. For the health of the team dynamics, layoffs should not be construed as a workaround to performance management. Because people have uncertainty that they may be next, the last thing they want to hear is negative talk about those who are no longer with the organization. Furthermore, employees who have been laid off may have enduring friendships with those who remain. It is also important to uphold the status of the employees who were laid off as a show of respect.

Effective communication is key throughout this process, involving clear messaging to the impacted teams and holding meetings with leaders to address any concerns or questions that may arise. Effective communication reduces uncertainty and serves the status and relatedness needs of staff. Leaders taking the time to communicate, convey to employees that they are important, and the interaction builds relationships. If the organization has a larger team and layers of leadership, be sure to support the frontline managers. They may not always be directly involved in making the tough decision to lay off staff, and they need to continue to lead the surviving teams. The managers may need debriefing and training from their leaders on how to lead the teams through a layoff, especially if they have not managed one in the past. Layoffs are traumatic to everyone impacted–those who are laid off, the survivors, and the leaders. By following a thoughtful and comprehensive approach to employee separations, organizations can mitigate potential challenges and maintain positive relationships with both departing and remaining staff members.

Conclusion

Given the volatility of the demand for health care during the pandemic, we had to employ creative solutions such as the "vaccinator" program and then respond to the negative impact on the finances. Many practices had to exercise cost reduction measures such as unpaid furloughs, reduction in FTE, reduction in pay, or reduction in force, either voluntary or involuntary. All cost reduction tactics impact the morale of a team, especially the reduction in force, and we shared what one might expect if facing such a difficult situation. Transparency in communication, being generous with separation packages and outplacement services decrease the negative impact of layoffs. For remaining employees, it is important for managers to reprioritize work and continue to focus on career development.

During a pandemic, when everything is uncertain and volatile, serving the social needs of status, certainty, autonomy, relatedness, and fairness, helps teams stay cohesive. The application of the SCARF psychological model can help leaders better anticipate reactions, and proactively communicate and address them upfront, especially through something as disruptive as a layoff during a pandemic. Recognizing when teams or individuals are in a threat response state and helping them move to a reward response state creates a more productive work environment. This practical framework for leaders helps them navigate changes and stay human centered during the most challenging times.

References

1. NeuroLeadership Institute. SCARF®: a brain-based model for collaborating with and influencing others, vol. 1. Accessed 12 Dec 2024. https://membership.neuroleadership.com/material/scarf-a-brain-based-model-for-collaborating-with-and-influencing-others-vol-1/?utm_term=&utm_campaign=Solutions+-+NA&utm_source=adwords&utm_medium=ppc&hsa_acc=6445333425&hsa_cam=15017298938&hsa_grp=135603230083&hsa_ad=594742821016&hsa_src=g&hsa_tgt=dsa-19959388920&hsa_kw=&hsa_mt=&hsa_net=adwords&hsa_ver=3&gad_source=1&gclid=Cj0KCQjwzYLABhD4ARIsALySuCTQ9qKWWSe0b7BN1aFe1q5ssaUiF6o5C1UUOaZ7q45n9qQFrHlhOZwaAnpBEALw_wcB.
2. Galvin G. Nearly 1 in 5 health care workers have quit their jobs during the pandemic medical workers cited COVID-19, poor pay and burnout as reasons for layoffs, resignations. Accessed 5 Mar 2024. https://thepcc.org/2022/01/07/nearly-1-5-health-care-workers-have-quit-their-jobs-during-pandemic.
3. US Equal Employment Opportunity Commission. Older Workers Benefit Protection Act of 1990. US Equal Employment Opportunity Commission website. Accessed 5 Mar 2024. https://www.eeoc.gov/history/older-workers-benefit-protection-act-1990.
4. Sucher S, Gupta S. A better, fairer approach to layoffs. Harvard Business Review. Accessed 5 Mar 2024. https://hbr.org/2018/05/a-better-fairer-approach-to-layoffs.
5. Philip R. The paradox of layoffs: engagement drops when you need it most. Accessed 5 Mar 2024. https://www.forbes.com/sites/radhikaphilip/2020/07/23/the-paradox-of-layoffs-engagement-drops-when-you-need-it-most/?sh=7c6cd8d93fd2.
6. Sverke M, Hellgren J, Näswall K. No security: a meta-analysis and review of job insecurity and its consequences. J Occup Health Psychol. 2002;7(3):242–64.

7. Mngomezulu N, Challenor M, Munapo E, Mashau P, Chikandiwa C. The impact of recognition on retention of good talent in the workforce. J Gov Regul. 2015;4. https://doi.org/10.22495/jgr_v4_i4_c3_p2.
8. Bingham S. How HR leaders can adapt to uncertain times. Accessed 7 Mar 2024. https://hbr.org/2020/08/how-hr-leaders-can-adapt-to-uncertain-times.

Chapter 12
Long COVID and Primary Care

Aluko A. Hope, Louise Vaz, and Nathalie Huguet

Yes, I am seeing [Long COVID]. [Its] presentation is quite variable but the most consistent feature I am seeing is fatigue. It is frustrating for patients, and [for] us, because we have few answers to their questions such as what can I do and how long this will last. —Primary Care Clinician

History and Definitions

History With the onset of the coronavirus disease 2019 (COVID-19) pandemic, early reports emerged from patients in online forums and mainstream media about lingering symptoms for months after SARS-CoV-2 infection [1]. In March 2020, Body Politic started a COVID-19 support group using the Slack app for patients who were struggling to find resources after lingering symptoms from what was considered "mild" COVID-19 infection. Patients shared their experiences on these and other social media platforms and referred to themselves as COVID long haulers. Elisa Perego, from Lombardy, Italy, first used #LongCOVID to summarize her protracted illness experience; over time, this term was taken up by the medical and scientific community [1]. Since these early accounts from individual experiences, patient-scientists have been crucial for advocacy as well as forging scientific advancements in understanding Long COVID. For example, Hannah Davis with

A. A. Hope (✉)
Department of Medicine, Division of Pulmonary, Allergy, and Critical Care Medicine, Oregon Health & Science University, Portland, OR, USA
e-mail: hopeal@ohsu.edu

L. Vaz
Department of Pediatrics, Division of Infectious Diseases, Oregon Health & Science University/Doernbecher Children's Hospital, Portland, OR, USA

N. Huguet
Department of Family Medicine, Oregon Health & Science University School of Medicine, Portland, OR, USA

A. Cheng et al. (eds.), *Primary Care in a Public Health Emergency*,
https://doi.org/10.1007/978-3-032-12487-6_12

other Long COVID patients started the Patient Led Research Collaborative which has published seminal articles on Long COVID, funded grants to biomedical researchers, and advocated for more funding for Long COVID research [2–5].

Terminology and Definitions Numerous other terms have been in use to describe the long-term health effects of SARS-CoV-2, often with differing definitions. The broad clinical condition that we are calling Long COVID in this chapter has also been called post-acute sequelae of SARS-CoV-2 (PASC), post-covid syndrome, and post-covid condition(s) among other terms [6–9]. For the purposes of this chapter, we have chosen to use the patient-developed term Long COVID for its clarity and resonance across patient and scientific communities. The term post-acute sequalae of SARS-CoV-2 (PASC), coined by the National Institutes of Health, encompasses both acute and chronic health effects that may emerge four or more weeks after a SARS-CoV-2 infection [6]. The World Health Organization (WHO) developed a consensus definition of a post–COVID-19 condition as a chronic condition which occurs in individuals with a history of probably or confirmed SARS-CoV-2 infection, usually within 3 months of onset with symptoms lasting at least 2 months and not explained by an alternative diagnosis [9]. The National Academies of Sciences, Engineering, and Medicine (NASEM) has defined Long COVID as an infection-associated chronic health condition that occurs after SARS-CoV-2 infection that is characterized by at least 3 months of symptoms that are either continuous, relapsing or remitting, or progressive disease state that affects one or more organ systems [10].

Epidemiology

Prevalence and Incidence Long COVID has affected a striking number of people. A lack of awareness of the condition may result in under identification and under-treatment in day-to-day medical practice. Data from the National Health Interview Survey (NHIS) conducted by the U.S. Centers for Disease Control and Prevention (CDC) show that in 2022, 6.9% of U.S. adults and 1.3% of children have had Long COVID (defined in the survey as persistent symptoms for more than 3 months after a SARS-CoV-2 infection) at some point; notably, 3.4% of adults and 0.5% of children had Long COVID at the time of the NHIS interview [11, 12]. Data on the evolving prevalence of Long COVID shows that the prevalence of Long COVID decreased from 7.5% in June 2022 to 5.3% in January 2023 [7].

Risk factors Long COVID can occur across all age groups, genders, races/ethnicities, and among all socioeconomic groups. Predisposing factors are those factors that increase risk of developing acute SARS-CoV-2 or that increase risk of an acute COVID-19 infection developing into Long COVID. Data from 2022 suggest that women (vs. men), middle-aged adults (vs. $\geq$ 65 years), people of Hispanic ethnicity (vs. non-Hispanic ethnicity), and those residing in rural areas (vs. metropolitan areas) have higher prevalence of Long COVID. Among children, girls (vs. boys), those aged 12–17 years (vs. younger age groups), those of Hispanic ethnicity (vs. non-Hispanic) have higher prevalence of ever having Long COVID [7, 11, 12]. In a large retrospective matched cohort study using data from primary care medical records across the UK, researchers found that adults with certain pre-existing health conditions such as chronic obstructive pulmonary disease (COPD), benign prostatic hyperplasia, fibromyalgia, or migraine disorders were associated with higher odds of developing Long COVID [13]. In a similar US-based study using the Behavioral Risk Factor Surveillance System, adults with obesity, pulmonary disease, depression, and arthritis were found to have higher odds of developing Long COVID [14].

Precipitating factors for Long COVID include the many factors related to the nature, severity, and approach to treatment of the acute SARS-CoV-2 infection. Across multiple studies, the individual risk of developing Long COVID has been shown to be proportional to the severity of the acute COVID-19 infection with patients who were hospitalized for severe acute COVID-19 at higher risk of Long COVID than those patients who were not hospitalized [15–17]. However, from a population perspective, the fact that most patients who get a SARS-CoV-2 infection have not been hospitalized means that the vast majority of Long COVID patients that will be seen by primary care clinicians will have had mild or asymptomatic SARS-CoV-2 infections. Some studies have found that receipt of a COVID-19 vaccination was associated with a lowered risk of developing Long COVID [18, 19]. Some studies have found treatment with antivirals during acute COVID-19 to be associated with a lowered risk of Long COVID [20, 21], while there are other studies that have not found this association [22, 23].

Protective or perpetuating factors include those that may affect the risk of protracted Long COVID symptoms. So far, few studies have explored protective or perpetuating factors that decrease or increase risk of prolonged symptoms after being diagnosed with Long COVID. For example, an observational study, using the UK COVID Symptom Study Biobank, found that features of hypermobile spectrum disorders (e.g., Ehlers Danlos Syndrome) were associated with 30% higher odds of developing Long COVID and refractory fatigue symptoms after COVID-19 infection [24, 25].

Conceptual Framework and Pathophysiology

Systems Biology Framework The best approach to understanding Long COVID is through a "systems biology" approach, which acknowledges that the condition is occurring within complex biological systems that strive to maintain function despite internal or external disruptions [26]. Health and disease are seen as emergent phenomena, where biological systems self-organize in ways that cannot be predicted by examining the individual components alone [26]. This approach to understanding disease helps us better understand why multiple factors across many different levels (e.g., genes, cells, organs, and the environment) can work together to collectively trigger a chronic condition [27]. In turn, an overlapping set of biopsychosocial factors can sustain the impact of the condition on a patient's quality of life [28].

This approach may also help identify distinct stages of illness over time, based on shifts in the adaptability of the biological systems involved. A key concept here is "allostasis"—the process by which organisms maintain stability through adaptation [29]. This helps explain how biologic systems change and adapt to stressors [29, 30]. In response to a threat like SARS-CoV-2 infection, the human organism can adjust regulated variables to different set points through complex, dynamic communication between the autonomic nervous system, neuroendocrine, cardiovascular, metabolic, and immune systems [30]. Typically, these allostatic processes are temporary, allowing systems to return to baseline functioning after a stressor. However, persistent dysregulation can lead systems to adopt a new rhythm or to be reset to a suboptimal level. Such shifts in system regulation come at the cost of accelerated wear and tear and increased energy utilization thereby creating the milieu for multiple chronic symptoms [31–33] (See Fig. 12.1).

Pathophysiology Several biological mechanisms are being investigated to elucidate how SARS-CoV-2 infection can contribute to the initiation of Long COVID including viral persistence, reactivation of endogenous viral or microbial reservoirs, infection triggered autoimmunity or other immunologic dysfunction [5, 34–36]. Possible biologic factors that have been postulated to be involved in the clinical presentation and course of Long COVID include cerebral hypoperfusion, gastrointestinal dysbiosis, autonomic dysregulation, mitochondrial dysfunction, hyperinflammation, increases in oxidative stress, endothelial dysfunction, immunologic abnormalities, and autoimmunity [5, 35–37]. In terms of potential upstream biologic mechanisms that can be used to understand the complexity of Long COVID, we would posit three: (1) neuroglial dysfunction with or without dysregulation in neurovascular coupling [32]; (2) autonomic nervous system signaling [30, 31, 38, 39]; and (3) mitochondrial dysfunction [32, 40–43]. Neuroglial cells are the non-neuronal cells of varying types across the central, peripheral, and enteric nervous systems that serve multiple homeostatic roles, including nutritional support, blood flow regulation, and immunologic defense [44, 45]. The extended autonomic nervous system which includes the central autonomic network, the autonomic nervous system, the neuroendocrine systems, and the immune and inflammatory systems provide much of the regulatory foundation for homeostatic regulation [30]. Importantly, the extended autonomic nervous systems can regulate variables using negative and positive feedback processes, as well as by anticipatory feedforward processes which can clarify the role of anticipatory cues in system regulation [30, 31]. Mitochondrial dysfunction—whether characterized by increases in reactive oxygen species or decreases in antioxidant defenses, altered mitochondrial membrane permeability, disrupted calcium homeostasis, or impaired adenosine triphosphate (ATP) production—may underlie many of the physical and cognitive fatigue symptoms in Long COVID [41–43].

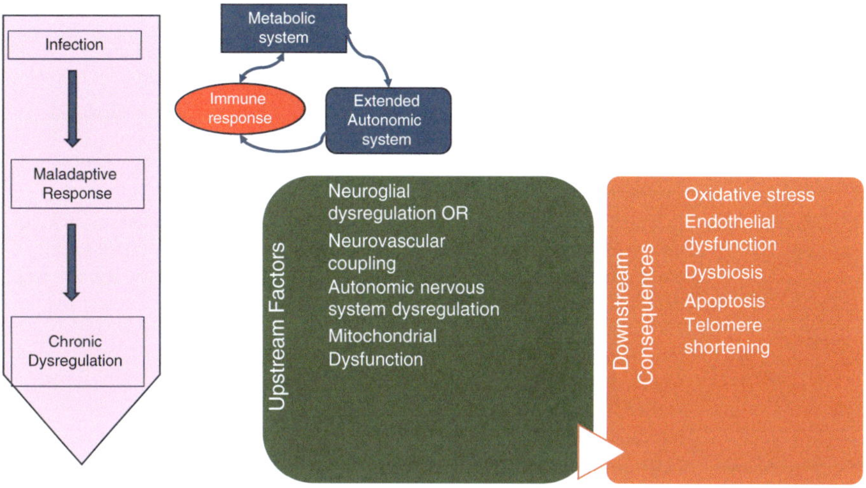

Fig. 12.1 Framework for understanding Long COVID with possible upstream and downstream biologic factors that can contribute to chronic symptoms

Clinical Presentation and Diagnosis

Signs and Symptoms Long COVID has been associated with over 200 signs or symptoms [4]. Most commonly, Long COVID patients present with signs or symptoms across multiple organ systems. The most common signs or symptoms include chronic fatigue; post-exertional malaise or post-exertional symptom exacerbation; sleep changes; cognitive impairment or subjective cognitive changes often termed "brain fog"; orthostatic intolerance symptoms such as dizziness, lightheadedness, headache, and pre-syncope; gastrointestinal disturbances such as constipation or diarrhea; altered sensory perception including increased pain, changes in hearing, smell, or visuospatial impairment (see Table 12.1 for a list of the most common signs or symptoms) [37, 46–64]. These signs or symptoms may be a continuation of those present during an acute SARS-CoV-2 infection, or they may develop in the weeks or even months after the SARS-CoV-2 infection. The symptoms can range from mild to severe and can either improve steadily over the period of weeks to months, be persistent, or follow a relapsing/remitting pattern. Long COVID signs and symptoms, whether through changes in patients' physiological structures and/or function or through restrictions in their ability to do their usual activities (e.g., work, school, social activities) can be associated with functional decline and/or decreased quality of life.

Diagnosing Long COVID As of this writing, there is no biomarker or diagnostic test with high specificity or sensitivity for Long COVID. Long COVID is diagnosed based on the proximity to presumed history of acute SARS-CoV-2 infection, the presence of Long COVID signs or symptoms, and careful consideration of other conditions that could be contributing to these signs or symptoms. Primary care providers should not assume that confirming acute SARS-CoV-2 infection is necessary

Table 12.1 The most common signs and symptoms of Long COVID

Signs or Symptoms	Detailed Descriptions	Identification or Screening Approaches
Chronic fatigue and exercise intolerance	Physical, cognitive, social, and emotional fatigue is out of proportion to activity and not alleviated by rest; shortness of breath	By self-report; can use validated surveys [46–48]
Post-exertional malaise	Increase in symptom severity and/or new symptoms after physical, emotional, sensory, or cognitive exertion often manifesting after a 12–72-hour delay; heavy "leaden" legs; sensitivity to light, sound, smells, or temperature; palpitations, nausea, vertigo, dizziness, brain fog, increased pain	By self-report; validated surveys can be modified for the clinical setting; 2-day cardiopulmonary exercise test [46, 47, 49]
Sleep problems	Difficulty falling asleep; awakening; increased restless symptoms at night; daytime sleepiness	By self-report; screen for obstructive sleep apnea [50]; modify validated sleep or insomnia symptom surveys [51]; formal sleep study
Cognitive problems	Impairments in attention, executive functioning, expressive or receptive language, memory or processing; visuospatial impairment	By self-report; can use validated surveys for subjective cognitive dysfunction; formal cognitive screening tools such as MoCA, SLUMS, or MMSE [52]; more detailed neuropsychological batteries may be needed in some patients [53]
Orthostatic intolerance symptoms	Headache; dizziness; weakness; difficulty with prolonged standing or upright posture; palpitations; mental confusion with prolonged standing; nausea or vomiting; postural orthostatic tachycardia syndrome	By self-report; can use validated surveys such as COMPASS-31 [54]; active standing test; 10-min NASA Lean Test; tilt table testing where available [55]
Gastrointestinal symptoms	Diarrhea; constipation; retrosternal chest pain or burning; heartburn; lump in throat feeling; postprandial fullness	By self-report [56]; validated surveys such as the Gastrointestinal Symptom Rating Scale or the Rome IV Diagnostic Questionnaire for disorders of gut-brain interaction [57, 58]
Olfactory and gustatory dysfunction	Complete loss of smell (anosmia); reduced sense of smell (hyposmia); distorted smells (parosmia); unpleasant smell (cacosmia); smelling an odor that is not present (phantosmia); ageusia; abnormal or altered taste sensations; phantogeusia	By self-report [59–61]

(continued)

Table 12.1 (continued)

Signs or Symptoms	Detailed Descriptions	Identification or Screening Approaches
Chronic pain syndromes	Increased chronic pain intensity; neuropathic pain; chronic headache; central sensitivity features, including allodynia; complex regional pain syndromes; paresthesia, dysesthesia [62, 63]	Validated surveys such as central sensitization inventory [64]; ask about co-morbid illnesses such as bladder pain syndromes or interstitial cystitis; ask about previous nerve injuries or traumatic brain injury

Abbreviations: *MoCA* Montreal Cognitive Assessment, *SLUMS* Saint Louis University Mental Status, *MMSE* Mini-Mental State Examination, *COMPASS-31* Composite Autonomic Symptom Score-31, *NASA* National Aeronautics and Space Administration

to diagnose Long COVID since many people with signs and/or symptoms of SARS-CoV-2 infection may not have undergone testing to confirm the infection, may not report their home test results to their primary care providers, or may not have been symptomatic enough to even recognize their SARS-CoV-2 infection [65]. Most of the current definitions of Long COVID are meant to be inclusive and may include: chronic conditions due to new or worsening organ damage after SARS-CoV-2 infection (e.g., interstitial lung disease); new or worsening chronic conditions with well characterized objective biomarkers that can occur after SARS-CoV-2 such as type 1 or type 2 diabetes mellitus or chronic kidney disease, and, new multisystem, immune-related conditions that have been reported after SARS-CoV-2 such as lupus, rheumatoid arthritis, Sjogren's syndrome, and other rheumatologic disorders with highly specific classification criteria [66–68]. Given the inclusivity of the current Long COVID definitions, primary care clinicians need to diagnose Long COVID as well as understand when the diagnosis is likely to provide value in improving their patients' health, function, or quality of life [69].

A Practical Approach to Long COVID Identification in Primary Care As most cases of Long COVID involve multiple organ systems and rely on clinical judgment, primary care teams have often been the ones managing and diagnosing patients. A comprehensive symptom inventory can be used to document the relevant symptoms that are new or worsening since the SARS-CoV-2 infection. Table 12.2 summarizes the common symptom complexes along with diagnostic considerations for these symptoms [38, 66, 70–84]. We would suggest that primary care clinicians assume an empathic posture, one that seeks to interpret the patient's lived experience collaboratively while acknowledging both the scientific uncertainty as well as the complexity of the patient's symptoms [85–88]. Screening for post-exertional malaise (PEM) or post-exertional symptom exacerbation early in the evaluation process is crucial since patients with severe PEM may need to have the diagnostic process modified to prevent symptom exacerbation. PEM refers to an increase in the severity of symptoms and/or the appearance of new symptoms after physical, emotional, or cognitive exertion ("triggers"), often with the worst manifestations occurring 12–72 hours after the specific trigger [46, 47]. PEM can also include worsening in pain, fever, sore throat, or more difficulty with cognitive processing [89–93].

Table 12.2 Common overlapping conditions and diagnostic considerations for symptoms commonly seen in patients with Long COVID

Symptom Complex	Differential Diagnoses	Distinguishing Features
Cardiopulmonary symptoms such as shortness of breath, cough, palpitations	Reactive airway disease; GERD; upper airway cough syndrome; dysautonomia; generalized anxiety disorder	Ask about positioning during symptoms to identify orthostatic intolerance; check for hypoxemia; assess for dysfunctional breathing patterns [70, 71]
PEM or post-exertional symptom exacerbation [48]	Other infection-associated chronic conditions such as: myalgic encephalomyelitis/ chronic fatigue syndrome [48]; fibromyalgia; primary biliary cholangitis [72]; other rheumatologic conditions [66, 73, 74]	PEM is more likely to be associated with *both* physical and cognitive exertion; laboratory testing can identify primary biliary cholangitis and other rheumatologic conditions; physical exam can identify multiple pain sites associated with fibromyalgia
Orthostatic intolerance which includes symptoms or signs that get worse in an upright position such as dizziness, lightheadedness, fatigue, or even fainting [38, 70, 75]	Postural orthostatic tachycardia syndrome; supraventricular tachycardia; myocardial ischemia; inappropriate sinus tachycardia; hypertension; diabetes; Sjogren's syndrome; GBS; CHF; PTSD	History and symptom survey can help identify PTSD; ambulatory cardiac monitoring can identify supraventricular tachycardia or other cardiac rhythm abnormalities; electrocardiogram can be used to identify myocardial ischemia; laboratory testing can identify chronic conditions like type 2 diabetes mellitus or Sjogren's syndrome; neurologic examination can increase identification of GBS
Cognitive changes such as changes in attention, executive functioning, communication, memory or processing, visuospatial impairment [51, 76–78]	Post-concussion syndrome [79]; ADHD; major depressive disorder or general anxiety disorder; dementia	Age or developmental stage or developmental history can help disentangle dementia or ADHD
Sleep changes [51, 80]	Obstructive sleep apnea; restless leg syndrome; periodic limb movement disorder; narcolepsy; circadian rhythm sleep disorder	Home polysomnography; sleep laboratory polysomnography; asking about cataplexy, hallucinations, excessive daytime sleepiness, sleep paralysis, and sleep disruption can help with early identification of high risk for narcolepsy [81]

(continued)

Table 12.2 (continued)

Symptom Complex	Differential Diagnoses	Distinguishing Features
Gastrointestinal symptoms [11]	DGBI such as IBS; dyspepsia, gastroparesis; dysphagia; GERD; inflammatory bowel disease; dysautonomia; esophageal disorders	Trial of low FODMAP diet to see if there is improvement; pharmacologic co-management with chronic pain, depression, or insomnia can be considered; referral to gastroenterologist to consider the utility of more invasive diagnostic testing
Changes in mood, anxiety; emotional dysregulation [82]	Major depressive disorder; generalized anxiety disorder; bereavement disorder; PTSD; dysautonomia; cognitive impairment	History can help disentangle MDD and GAD from bereavement; screen for adverse childhood events; neuropsychological assessment can help identify cognitive impairment
Multiple medical allergies; chemical sensitivities; increased frequency or severity of respiratory, skin, or other allergic-type symptoms [83, 84]	Allergic rhinitis; exercise-induced reactive airway disease; asthma; MCAS	Avoiding triggers; tryptase level has low sensitivity but can be reordered during crisis; urine testing for MCAS also with low sensitivity; treatment trial with antihistamine; IgE level; pulmonary function testing for asthma
Visual or auditory processing impairment	Cognitive impairment; unmasking of learning disabilities in the context of fatigue; ADHD; autism; PTSD; dementia syndrome	Age or neurodevelopmental stage; neuropsychological testing; visual processing can be evaluated ideally after acuity is tested and corrected

Abbreviations: *PEM* post-exertional malaise, *ADHD* attention deficit hyperactivity disorder, *MDD* major depressive disorder, *GAD* general anxiety disorder, *MCAS* mast cell activation syndrome, *PTSD* post-traumatic stress disorder, *DGBI* disorders of gut-brain interaction, *GERD* gastroesophageal reflux disease, *IBS* irritable bowel syndrome, *FODMAP* fermentable oligosaccharides, disaccharides, monosaccharides, and polyols, *GBS* Guillain-Barré syndrome, *CHF* congestive heart failure

Clinicians may need to operationalize approaches to identify common Long COVID phenotypes that may be relevant to clinical management: cognitive or neuropsychiatric symptoms such as brain fog, executive dysfunction, anxiety, depression, post-traumatic stress; exercise intolerance manifested by muscle weakness, exertional shortness of breath, physical fatigue, post-exertional symptom exacerbations; chronic pain manifested by such symptoms as small fiber neuropathy, paresthesia, chronic headache; complex regional pain syndromes, or dysautonomia manifested by orthostatic intolerance, palpitations, low blood pressure, subjective fever, or changes in heat tolerance [94]. Clinicians should assess how the Long COVID symptoms have impacted the patient's function and quality of life, including their activities of daily living, instrumental activities of daily living, work, or school life. Clinicians should be aware that patients will often accommodate milder symptoms by reducing their activities in one life domain to preserve function in another domain [92, 95, 96].

Clinicians should be mindful to avoid premature misattribution of patients' symptoms to psychological comorbid conditions which can be deeply stigmatizing to patients, delay the diagnosis, and be associated with inappropriate management decisions [97–100]. We think for clinicians to form a collaborative and trusting relationship, it is essential that they are able to articulate clearly that Long COVID is not solely due to psychological factors, even as they are willing to acknowledge that the mental and physical aspects of health are deeply intertwined, often influencing and amplifying one another. Adopting an integrative perspective helps clinicians appreciate the full context of a patient's condition, validating all their lived experience of the illness as potentially important. This approach not only enhances trust and rapport but also supports a more comprehensive understanding of the patient, leading to more personalized and effective care in Long COVID [101, 102].

Chronic Conditions like Long COVID Long COVID shares similarities with other multisystem chronic conditions such as myalgic encephalomyelitis/chronic fatigue syndrome (ME/CFS) and fibromyalgia (see Table 12.2) [38, 66, 70–84]. Regarding the overlap between ME/CFS and Long COVID, several studies when taken together would suggest that a significant proportion of Long COVID patients may meet criteria for ME/CFS [91, 103–105]. There are several studies that suggest that about 30% of Long COVID patients may also meet criteria for fibromyalgia [73]. There are also some observational studies to suggest that in patients with a pre-COVID fibromyalgia diagnosis, Long COVID prevalence is comparable to the prevalence of Long COVID in other rheumatologic diagnoses [106]. Understanding the overlap between Long COVID and these other complex conditions may help clinicians in recognizing the broader impacts of Long COVID. For example, in a patient with a known history of fibromyalgia who presents with fatigue and post-exertional malaise, the clinician can spend less time ruling out other comorbid illness, start strict energy management earlier in the diagnosis course, and ramp up both pharmacologic and non-pharmacologic options for chronic pain early in the illness. On the other hand, a patient without a prior past medical history who presents with several months of fatigue, post-exertional malaise, and mild orthostatic intolerance may start off with a Long COVID diagnosis mixed with other diagnoses based on their chronic symptoms such as orthostatic intolerance, post-viral fatigue, and psychophysiologic insomnia. By 12 months, if all of these chronic symptoms remain and a patient remains at risk for PEM, it may help to label the patient as having myalgic encephalomyelitis/chronic fatigue syndrome.

Differential Diagnosis and Comorbid Conditions Patients with severe Long COVID symptoms may be more likely to have other comorbid conditions, many of which are summarized in Table 12.2. Broadly speaking, dysautonomia, disorders of the enteric nervous system such as irritable bowel syndrome [107], connective tissue disorders [25], and immune dysregulation disorders such as mast cell activation syndrome [83, 84], are quite common in Long COVID patients. In patients with severe cognitive and/or emotional symptoms, comorbid diagnoses of anxiety, depression, or post-traumatic stress disorder may be important to identify [108, 109]. Similarly, the neurocognitive symptoms in Long COVID may appear like post-concussion syndrome [110] or neurodevelopmental disorders such as attention deficit hyperactivity disorder [111, 112].

Role of Laboratory testing or Imaging studies in Diagnosis Table 12.3 summarizes the common laboratory or diagnostic testing recommendations for Long COVID symptoms. Since there is no one specific laboratory abnormality that will be diagnostic for Long COVID, clinicians should rely on their medical history and physical examination [113]. Most laboratory testing is used to evaluate other co-morbid conditions that can be associated with the symptoms or be important for perpetuating the chronic symptoms. Similarly, there are no definitive radiologic or imaging studies that need to be ordered to diagnose Long COVID. Additional testing may be needed to evaluate the extent of the impairment from a specific symptom. For example, a formal sleep study may be needed to evaluate sleep symptoms given the high prevalence of obstructive sleep apnea or restless leg syndrome in Long COVID patients. Both Tables 12.2 and 12.3 provide some important complementary details on this topic.

Patients with orthostatic intolerance symptoms may need an office evaluation such as the active stand test or the 10-min NASA Lean Test to help determine how their blood pressure or heart rates respond to changes in body position. Before the NASA Lean Test, the patient should be instructed to limit fluid intake to 1–2 liters 24 hours before the test, limit sodium intake within 24–48 hours before testing, and withhold medications that may raise blood pressure or heart rate. To conduct the NASA Lean Test, the patient is first placed supine for a period of 2 minutes followed by 10 minutes standing straight leaning against a wall with shoulder blades contacting the wall and heels 6 inches from the wall. During the testing, serial measurement of their pulse and blood pressure at some reasonable interval (e.g., 1 or 2 minutes based on symptom severity) is recorded along with any symptoms or challenges [114].

Patients with Long COVID cognitive changes (e.g., brain fog, concentration problems, word finding difficulties, reduced verbal fluency, blurred vision, or worse cognitive fatigue) may need some basic laboratory testing such as vitamin B12 level or thyroid studies and may benefit from brief cognitive screening tests such as the MoCA or SLUMS examination [52, 115]. In some patients, a comprehensive neuropsychological evaluation may be helpful in documenting the degree of impairments and to disentangle undiagnosed depression or anxiety [77–79]. Table 12.3 summarizes some of the common diagnostic or laboratory tests that are commonly considered as part of the diagnosis and management of Long COVID symptoms.

Table 12.3 Laboratory or diagnostic testing recommendations for Long COVID symptoms

Symptom Complex	Parsimonious Approach to Laboratory or Diagnostic Testing
Cardiopulmonary symptoms	Pulmonary function testing; chest x-ray; 12-lead electrocardiogram where appropriate
Chronic fatigue and post-exertional malaise	CBC with differential; iron studies including ferritin; comprehensive metabolic panel; urinalysis; vitamin B12 levels; ESR; CRP; ANA; TSH with free T4 if abnormal
Orthostatic intolerance	10-min NASA Lean Test or active stand test; tilt table testing (where appropriate or available)
Cognitive changes	Vitamin B12; homocysteine; methylmalonic acid; comprehensive metabolic panel; MRI brain where appropriate
Sleep changes	CBC with differential; ferritin; home or laboratory polysomnogram; home sleep apnea testing
Gastrointestinal symptoms	Liver function tests; gluten antibodies
Changes in mood, anxiety; emotional dysregulation	TSH with free T4; ANA; gluten antibodies if consistent with the history
Multiple medical allergies; chemical sensitivities; increased frequency or severity of respiratory, skin, or other allergic-type symptoms	Baseline tryptase; repeat tryptase within hours of symptom crisis; IgE levels; skin examination

Abbreviations: *CBC* complete blood count, *ESR* erythrocyte sedimentation rate, *CRP* C-reactive protein, *ANA* antinuclear antibodies, *TSH* thyroid stimulating hormone, *NASA* National Aeronautics and Space Administration, *IgE* immunoglobulin E, *MRI* magnetic resonance imaging

Prognosis The prognosis for recovery from Long COVID is complex and varies widely, with epidemiologic research still in its initial stages. Long COVID often follows a fluctuating course, with cycles of symptom exacerbation and temporary relief. While some patients gradually improve over months, others remain in a prolonged state of fluctuating or worsening symptoms. Chronic symptoms frequently impact daily functioning, leading patients to adapt or compensate in ways that can mask the illness' true impact. Regularly assessing these adaptations can help clinicians better understand and address the patient's evolving needs. Given that Long COVID may share pathophysiological features with other chronic conditions like ME/CFS and fibromyalgia, similar patterns of prolonged recovery, episodic relapses, and susceptibility to PEM may be anticipated. In the absence of definitive biomarkers for recovery, a patient-centered, adaptable approach is essential, allowing for the possibility of long-term symptoms while prioritizing quality of life.

Long COVID Management

An overall approach Since there are no disease modifying treatments, most guidelines recommend an individualized, multimodal approach to management. Primary care clinicians can focus on developing an empathic connection with their patient using trauma-informed communication strategies that empower patients and their caregivers to be more engaged in their health care while having reasonable expectations of the health system. Depending on where a particular patient may be in their recovery trajectory, we conceptualize Long COVID primary care management as having multiple overlapping domains: (1) harm reduction or symptom stabilization; (2) symptom and impairment management; and (3) enhancing performance or capacity (Fig. 12.2). Tables 12.4 and 12.5 give general and more specific management recommendations for Long COVID symptoms, respectively [116].

Harm Reduction and Symptom Stabilization This domain focuses on understanding the multiple factors contributing to the Long COVID symptoms or conditions, ruling out relevant diagnoses that could be an explanation for the specific symptom or discussing the role of other comorbid diagnoses in contributing to the symptom

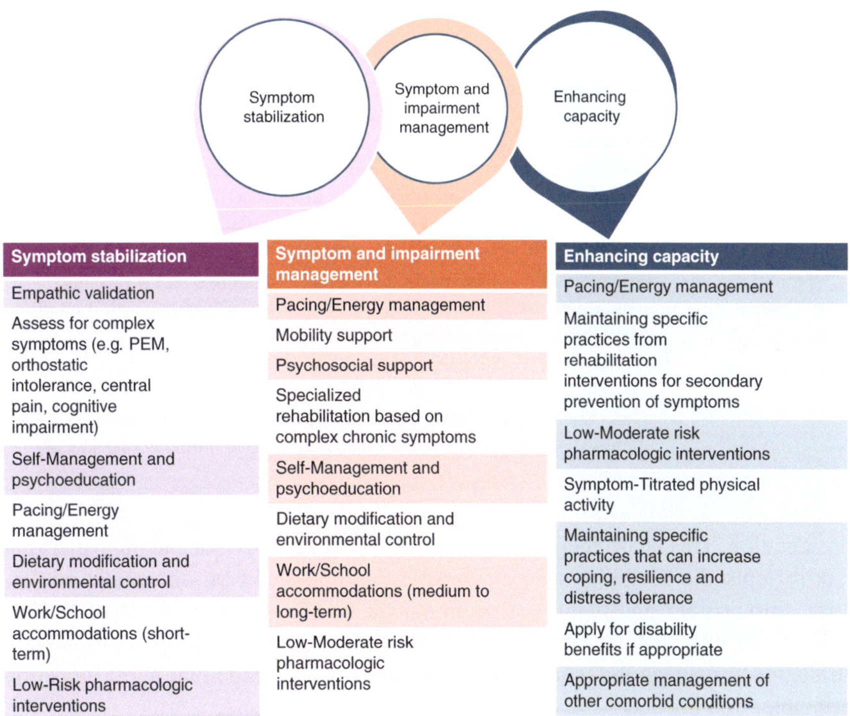

Fig. 12.2 Overall approach to managing Long COVID

Table 12.4 General management principles and considerations in Long COVID

Domains	Rationale and Details
Pacing/energy management	Most important strategy for patients with chronic fatigue and post-exertional malaise, focused on dividing activities into small chunks interspersed by proactive rest; provides an approach to reduce burden of fatigue and post-exertional symptoms.
Specialized rehabilitation interventions	Based on specific symptom complex, specialized rehabilitation approaches can be utilized including autonomic rehabilitation for patients with orthostatic intolerance or dysautonomia; visual processing rehabilitation for patients with visuospatial impairment; vestibular rehabilitation for vestibular symptoms.
Mobility support	These can include (1) disability parking permits; (2) wheelchairs or motorized scooters and/or appropriate home modifications; and (3) shower chairs and handrails.
Multidisciplinary care and care coordination	Primary care services along with rehabilitation; mental health care needs mixed with care coordination services.
Self-management and psychoeducation	Formal or informal patient education and empowerment approaches aimed at providing knowledge, skills, and confidence in chronic disease management both during crises and during day-to-day ups and downs. Helps to individualize the care plan and allows patients to match their care plans to their symptoms, which is particularly important because chronic symptoms can be associated with structural, functional, or chemical neurologic changes that may lead to lowered sensitivity to pain or other sensory stimuli [116].
Psychosocial support	Psychological support is often crucial not only because of the psychological co-morbidities that can co-occur but also because there is no specific biomarker or FDA-approved treatments as of yet, so leveraging the neuroplasticity of the brain requires avoiding some maladaptive psychological coping strategies; support groups and forums may be helpful for patients to learn about the illness and to feel validated; housing, employment, and financial support may be important in those patients whose social factors are worsened by their chronic conditions.
Dietary modifications	For autonomic gastrointestinal symptoms: small frequent meals and avoiding big meals; for orthostatic intolerance: liberalizing salt if no other contraindication; increasing hydration.
Environmental control	Patients with sensitivities to light, noise, or odors may benefit from removing perfume and chemicals from their environment; using eye masks and ear plugs where appropriate. For patients with specific allergies, including dietary allergies, may need to eliminate the specific triggers.

presentation. This phase focuses on assessing key symptoms that can put patients at risk for episodic disability such as exercise intolerance, PEM, orthostatic intolerance, chronic pain, and cognitive or communication challenges. When PEM is identified, educating patients on the importance of pacing or energy management strategies to manage the worst of their symptoms is an important harm reduction principle.

Table 12.5 More specific management considerations for Long COVID based on symptoms

Symptom Complex	Specific Management Consideration
Cardiopulmonary symptoms	Personalized cardiopulmonary rehabilitation; strengthening and flexibility; mindfulness training.
Chronic fatigue and/or post-exertional malaise	Pacing and energy management; low-dose naltrexone; low-dose aripiprazole; anti-inflammatory diet; disability accommodations such as proactive rest breaks may be needed for patients to continue working.
Orthostatic intolerance	Fluids/electrolytes/compression; propranolol or other beta-blockers can be used as needed or standing; midodrine or fludrocortisone for low blood pressure symptoms; ivabradine; pyridostigmine; physical activity in semi-recumbent position; leg strengthening exercises; disability accommodations such as permission to change to semi-recumbent position may be needed for patients to continue working.
Cognitive changes	Cognitive rehabilitation interventions; cognitive behavioral therapy; careful use of stimulants such as amantadine, methylphenidate, or suvorexant where appropriate; avoiding polypharmacy.
Sleep changes	Sleep hygiene; melatonin; light therapy; formal sleep evaluation; dietary changes; trazodone; gabapentin/pregabalin; sleep restriction therapy; avoiding polypharmacy.
Gastrointestinal symptoms	Dietary changes; small meals; antidiarrheals; antihistamines; fiber or motility agents for constipation.
Changes in mood, anxiety; emotional dysregulation	Antidepressants; consider cognitive behavioral therapy and its derivatives such as acceptance and commitment therapy or dialectical behavioral therapy to help with distress tolerance; neuropsychological testing where appropriate.
Changes in visual or auditory processing impairment	Specialized rehabilitation; tinted glasses; noise cancelling headphones; low-dose aripiprazole; fall prevention with mobility aids where appropriate.
Multiple medical allergies; chemical sensitivities; increased frequency or severity of respiratory, skin, or other allergic-type symptoms	H1 blockers such as cetirizine, fexofenadine, or levocetirizine may be needed at higher doses or more frequently than normally prescribed; H2 blockers may be needed up to twice per day; leukotriene modifiers such as montelukast can be tried; assess for hypermobile spectrum disorders; central-acting antihistamines with more sedation can be used at night.
Support for disability application	Document patient's symptoms and functional impact in clinical notes; use validated symptom surveys where available; no single performance test will be able to ascertain eligibility for disability benefits; consider whether returning to work is likely to exacerbate or aggravate symptoms.

Patients with orthostatic intolerance symptoms may need psychoeducation about the importance of lifestyle modifications such as liberalizing hydration and salt, light physical activity with attention to body posture and use of compression garments. Patients with orthostatic intolerance symptoms may need to have explicit plans for crisis symptoms that help to minimize their use of the emergency department for their symptoms.

Patients with chronic pain symptoms may need a thorough evaluation to categorize the type of post-COVID pain: nociceptive pain is attributable to the activation of peripheral receptive terminals of the afferent neurons in response to noxious stimuli; neuropathic pain is associated with a lesion or disease within the somatosensory nervous system and limited to an anatomically plausible distribution; nociplastic pain (often termed central sensitization) is pain primarily due to an increased responsiveness of the central nervous system nociceptive neurons [62]. Often a multimodal approach to chronic pain that can address both the peripheral (nociceptive and neuropathic) and central (nociplastic) pathways will be crucial to start early in Long COVID patients since often pain crises can further exacerbate dysautonomia and fatigue symptoms [62–64]. Crisis planning for severe pain crises can be helpful as well as personalized psychoeducation that matches the specific pain phenotype [117].

The harm reduction phase may also include ensuring that patients take appropriate steps to reduce the effects of chronic stress on their physiologic systems. This might include: (1) psychoeducation on deep breathing; (2) work accommodations or short-term disability to minimize the impact of work overexertion on their symptoms, and (3) accurate information sources about their Long COVID symptoms, including how their symptoms are related to their other comorbid medical or social conditions.

Symptom and Impairment Management This domain focuses on the non-pharmacologic and pharmacologic approaches to decrease symptoms and impairments. This may include helping patients to better understand how to modify their environment to avoid external triggers for their symptoms. Managing internal sources of distress (e.g., pain, emotional dysregulation, elevated heart rate, difficulty sleeping) may be important during this phase. Managing comorbid illnesses using new coping approaches consistent with Long COVID symptoms may become urgent as well during this phase. For example, patients with chronic fatigue and PEM who were using vigorous physical activity to help cope with depression or anxiety symptoms, may need to develop new coping strategies for these comorbid conditions.

Managing impairment may include any interventions meant to optimize function, which may include providing information, education, peer support, and rehabilitation interventions such as physical, occupational, or speech therapy. Depending on the nature of the symptoms, other specific rehabilitation approaches may be needed either in isolation or in combination. Autonomic rehabilitation can help Long COVID patients with orthostatic intolerance, while vestibular rehabilitation helps patients with balance impairment. Visual processing rehabilitation can help people with visual processing disorders which can make it difficult for these patients to interpret and understand visual information. When primary care clinicians refer patients to rehabilitation interventions, it is important that they be willing to assess whether these programs are safe and appropriate for the patient. If patients' symptoms get worse during rehabilitation intervention, it may mean that the specific intervention or the nature of how the intervention is being integrated into their disease management is not appropriate for this patient at this time. For example, some patients may need to be intentional about decreasing work or school obligations to ensure that they can participate fully in the rehabilitation intervention. Often the rehabilitation intervention uncovers strengths and deficits in the patient's behaviors, attitudes, and skills, which will need to be addressed alongside the rehabilitation intervention to sustain symptom improvement.

Effective symptom and impairment management will also benefit from a collaborative approach that values the insights and preferences of both the patient as well as the clinician. Patients may wish to explore various approaches to symptom management that may be unfamiliar to the clinician or for which evidence is still emerging. For instance, complementary and integrative medicine options—such as acupuncture, acupressure, chiropractic care, medical massage, and traditional Chinese medicine—show promising potential for improving certain Long COVID symptoms [118–122]. Clinicians can work together with patients to thoughtfully consider how to incorporate these approaches into the treatment plan, expanding the options available within symptom management. Open communication is essential, especially when discussing potential concerns about any specific treatment approaches, including practical considerations such as financial cost if a treatment is not covered by insurance. For patients who have experienced chronic symptoms resistant to traditional treatment, clinicians and patients can partner in exploring new therapeutic trials. By working together to develop a mutually agreeable treatment course, both clinician and patient can establish clear, patient-centered goals—such as identifying meaningful patient-reported outcomes and setting intervals for monitoring symptoms—thereby creating a treatment plan that is both innovative and responsive to the patient's needs.

Enhancing Performance or Capacity This domain focuses on helping patients improve their performance of their social and occupational roles and obligations, including physical or leisure activities as tolerated. The goal during this phase is to leverage neuroplasticity principles—strategies that harness the brain's natural capacity to adapt and reorganize—with targeted, purposeful training [123]. By choosing activities or specific practices that are aligned with patient's individual goals and values that can be done at the right intensity and frequency level, we can enhance brain function in ways that optimize physical, cognitive, or emotional recovery. These approaches are highly individualized and may change over time, and yet meaningful engagement in the right mix of these activities ensures that there is a tailored foundation for sustained improvement in capacity. This phase may also include the use of chronic medications (see Table 12.5 for examples) to help patients manage impairments that have plateaued so that patients can continue to work or engage in their important social roles. For patients whose impairments are chronic, this phase may also include support for accommodation at work or school or help applying for long-term disability.

Special Section on Pediatrics

Terminology and Scope While children and adolescents who have been infected with SARS-CoV-2 are more likely to experience asymptomatic or mild disease compared to adults, they can develop ongoing, relapsing, or new health effects after the acute phase of infection [124–126]. In fact, researchers have attempted to develop research definitions for Long COVID using modified Delphi consensus approaches with similar definitions as have been proposed for adults [127]. Particularly relevant in pediatrics is for primary care clinicians to recognize and disentangle de novo acute or chronic conditions such as type 1 diabetes mellitus, chronic kidney disease, or thromboembolic events that can emerge in the weeks after a SARS-CoV-2 infection [128, 129]. For the purposes of this chapter, we do not include Multisystem Inflammatory Syndrome in Children (MIS-C), a rare hyperinflammatory condition characterized by high fevers and multisystem signs of inflammation across multiple organs, as part of the Long COVID spectrum of conditions since it most often occurs within a few weeks of a SARS-CoV-2 infection and is managed in the hospital setting [130, 131].

Epidemiology The estimated rates of pediatric Long COVID are lower than in adults (1.3% prevalence in pediatrics compared with 6.9% in adults) although epidemiologic studies have similar methodological limitations as in the adult population such as small cohorts, lack of control groups, and selection and recall biases. In addition, studies use various definitions of Long COVID. Risk factors associated with increased risk for developing Long COVID in the pediatric population overlap with that of adults and include such factors as the severity of the initial SARS-CoV-2 infection, hospitalization, number of symptoms at initial SARS-CoV-2 infection [127, 132–134], vaccination status [135], older age, or atopic chronic conditions [132].

Differences in Clinical Diagnosis in Pediatrics In the pediatrics and adolescent population, distinguishing symptoms related to Long COVID from those related to psychosocial stressors such as social isolation, loss of family members, school closures, increased stress, and worsening social determinants of health can be more challenging than in adults [136]. Pediatric Long COVID is therefore more likely to be a diagnosis of exclusion and may require co-management with other pediatric conditions such as depression and anxiety. Additionally, symptoms, such as chronic cough, may reflect exacerbation of underlying conditions (e.g., asthma) [126]. As in adults, the initial evaluation includes obtaining a thorough history of symptoms and physical exam [137–139]. As is true in pediatrics generally, symptoms may need to be gathered from caregivers such as parents and teachers as well as from the child. Young children or those with developmental disabilities may express their symptoms differently than those children without these challenges.

Pediatric Management Differences Consensus guidelines for the management of pediatric Long COVID have been published to help in the diagnosis and management of this condition [129]. In pediatrics, comprehensive, holistic care is much more likely to continue through the primary care setting that can help address access to care, psychosocial support, and other social drivers of health outcomes [140]. The dearth of pediatric Long COVID centers [134, 137, 141] also likely contributes to why pediatric Long COVID is more likely to remain at the primary care setting [138, 139]. However, specialized interdisciplinary Long COVID consultation may be needed in complex cases.

Importantly, lifestyle management interventions include normalizing routines and optimization of sleep hygiene; adequate hydration and proper nutrition; and cognitive symptoms and fatigue should be managed with a gradual return to activity. School 504 plans can provide accommodations related to test taking, assignments, and rest for energy conservation [137, 141]. Addressing limited social participation and school absenteeism is helpful [140]. Personalized physical activity plans may be an important aspect of Long COVID symptom management along with energy management strategies and principles [142]. Working with trained physical or occupational therapists familiar with Long COVID can help patients who need specific modifications to allow for sports and extracurricular activities and to facilitate exercise progression while understanding symptom limitations [143].

Children with Long COVID may experience increased anxiety and depression symptoms, which can either be exacerbations of underlying chronic mental health conditions or a maladaptive response to their Long COVID symptoms [144]. In children, signs of depression include altered eating or sleeping habits, behavioral changes, and lack of interest in day-to-day activities; anxiety in children can manifest as fear of being away from a parent, physical symptoms of panic, and absenteeism at school [137, 143]. Management of mood disorders in pediatric Long COVID patients is the same as management for those without Long COVID; however, other Long COVID symptoms may complicate how these mood disorders present in pediatric patients [137]. For example, PEM may mean a decrease in school-related activities, leading to social isolation and depression. In children, brain fog or cognitive impairment may present as behavioral changes or declining school performance. There are a few studies that suggest there may be an increased risk of symptoms of attention deficit in children with intact executive function and processing speed along with changes in mood [77, 145]. For example, a recent cross-sectional survey of 510 children between the ages of 8 and 13 years found that a high proportion reported difficulty concentrating, memory concerns, difficulty completing everyday tasks, and difficulty processing information [138].

Health System Challenges and Opportunities

Health care systems continue to be ill-equipped to care for the considerable proportion of patients with Long COVID. The lack of knowledge about the types and duration of symptoms and treatment options led to significant variations in how health care systems responded to this new condition. Some health care systems engaged with their patients to try to find solutions and understand the condition [146–148], while others dismissed their patients saying that they could not do anything [146–149], or, even worse, some systems disbelieved patients that their symptoms could be a sequelae of a SARS-CoV-2 infection.

Across many health systems in the US, Long COVID clinics were created to address the clinical challenge of providing care for this chronic condition using various models of care [150]. Long COVID Alliance publishes an online list of Long COVID clinics across the US [151]. Most of the Long COVID clinics were newly created within tertiary care medical centers, with some evolving from pre-existing clinics with various referral processes, intake methods, and management infrastructure. A recent systematic review of the models of care for Long COVID synthesized five key principles that were essential in these specialty clinics: (1) a core lead team with expertise in Long COVID and other chronic complex conditions; (2) access to broad multidisciplinary expertise; (3) broad access to diagnostic and therapeutic services; (4) the ability to provide personalized and equitable care, and (5) the capacity to meet the local demand for Long COVID care [150].

With the emergence of these Long COVID clinics, primary care clinicians face new challenges of deciding when to refer patients to these clinics, particularly in the context of known barriers in access to these Long COVID clinics including long wait times and travel distance from these clinics for patients who live outside of metropolitan areas. Social determinants of health such as socioeconomic status, geographic location, health literacy, and race and ethnicity are all variables that affect access to health care broadly, but particularly these factors impact access to these specialty approaches to managing Long COVID. No specific model of care for Long COVID has been shown to be effective. Integrating primary care into these subspecialty approaches to managing Long COVID is a research gap that needs future innovation. One recent community-based primary care approach to managing Long COVID suggests that high-value, community-based Long COVID primary care approaches need to focus on three pillars: (1) validating and attending to patients' subjective experience of this condition while developing the clinical expertise about what is known and unknown about Long COVID; (2) enhancing clinical services that can be provided in the community primary care setting which can include diagnostic equipment not usually present in the primary care setting or integrated services such as behavioral health, and (3) ensuring sustainability by integrating population health metrics and measuring impact and outcomes of the program [152].

Research Gaps

Broadly speaking, the biggest research gap is in the understanding of the biologic pathways for the most common symptom complexes in Long COVID including exercise intolerance and PEM, orthostatic intolerance, cognitive and neuropsychiatric impairment, and chronic pain. Insights into cellular, molecular, and genetic factors that may contribute to Long COVID symptoms may be helpful in improving diagnosis, risk stratification, and unfolding new treatments. For both orthostatic intolerance and PEM, there is a need for more valid diagnostic approaches that are responsive to interventions. In adults, clinical trials on best approaches to manage the most prevalent chronic symptom complexes are needed with a focus on repurposing already approved medications as well as testing novel therapies. As more patients with Long COVID recover, qualitative exploration of the lived experience of recovery may provide insights on how to personalize recovery management. At the health system level, studying various models of care will be important, as well as strategies for enhancing patient engagement throughout the research pipeline.

Regarding research gaps in pediatric Long COVID, much work still needs to be done to better define the incidence, prevalence, and risk factors for Long COVID. For those with pediatric Long COVID, long term follow-up is desperately needed to ensure we can fully elucidate the potential long-term consequences as these patients transition to adulthood [126, 153]. Although some studies indicate that pediatric Long COVID symptoms resolved in most patients over several months, few studies have examined outcomes after 1 year [154, 155]. Some children may develop symptoms that can have a major impact on family life [156]. While the trajectory for children affected by Long COVID is more favorable compared to adults, additional studies are needed to better understand and characterize the diversity of presentations and clinical course in children, the impact of reinfection, and long-term implications related to quality of life and function.

Conclusion

Long COVID represents a complex health condition that has emerged since the COVID-19 pandemic and has required primary care teams to rapidly equip themselves with new knowledge and innovative approaches to providing care to patients with Long COVID. As more research emerges about the epidemiology, pathophysiology, diagnosis, and management of Long COVID, primary care clinicians and leaders will be called upon to continue developing approaches to diagnose and longitudinally manage patients with this condition. Continued research and innovation in Long COVID care may help improve patients' quality of life and has the potential to improve the ability of the primary care system to better address other infection-associated chronic conditions (Boxes 12.1, 12.2, and 12.3).

Boxes 12.1, 12.2, and 12.3: Each Present a Clinical Case and Summarize Key Strategies Used During the Long COVID Recovery Process

16-year-old female who presented 2 months after SARS-CoV-2 infection with palpitations, dizziness, headaches, lightheadedness, and poor exercise tolerance; multiple absences from school with depressed mood; Past medical history: ADHD diagnosed during elementary school and managed with occupational therapy interventions; Social and family history: three siblings, mother with hypermobile spectrum disorder and chronic pain.

Harm Reduction Phase (~4 months)	Symptom and Impairment Management (~8 months)	Enhancing Capacity (continues currently)
Physician validated symptoms; decided to see patient for a complex follow up visit monthly for 4 months with caregivers present to provide more time for psychoeducation.	Continued liberalizing salt, hydration, daily bouts of diaphragmatic deep breathing, compression stockings and abdominal binders, small frequent meals	Strict energy management continued
Visit 1 was a complex follow-up visit during which PEM, orthostatic intolerance, anxiety, and depression were assessed and a physical exam was performed	Occupational therapist suggested a wheelchair to allow for movement around school without PEM crashes	Continued liberalizing salt, hydration, daily bouts of diaphragmatic deep breathing, compression stockings and abdominal binders, small frequent meals
At visit 1, a 3-month disability accommodation was instituted for school	Disability accommodations continued indefinitely at school to allow more help with note taking, frequent proactive breaks, and more time to complete homework	Symptom-titrated physical activity for 30–60 minutes up to 4–5 times/week was initially supervised by a personal trainer and then sustained by patient
During visit 2, a referral to occupational therapy was instituted to provide more psychoeducation and to decide on utility of mobility devices	With the help of a psychopharmacologist, a trial of stimulants was started to help with cognitive endurance given the ADHD diagnosis	Continued a stable dose of a stimulant for her ADHD
Behavioral strategies such as strict energy management, liberalizing salt, recumbent physical activity, deep breathing, and hydration were all discussed during visit 1 and challenges were discussed during visit 2	Recumbent physical activity was started and encouraged for up to 4 times/week	Continued to have propranolol available, but this was only rarely needed
Low-risk medications started during this phase included propranolol 10 mg PO TID PRN	Low-risk medications continued during this phase: propranolol 10 mg PO TID PRN	

(continued)

Boxes 12.1, 12.2, and 12.3 (continued)

46-year-old woman with a history of fibromyalgia who now presents 4 months after SARS-CoV-2 infection with worsening diffuse pain, fatigue, and exercise intolerance. Severe depressed mood and suicidal thoughts. Past medical history: fibromyalgia; major depression; Social and family history: multiple drug sensitivities, including to morphine and Singulair.

Harm Reduction Phase (~6 months)	Symptom and Impairment Management (~18 months and ongoing)
Physician validated symptoms; saw patient monthly	Continued liberalizing salt, hydration, daily bouts of diaphragmatic deep breathing, compression stockings and abdominal binders, small frequent meals
Used validated surveys to assess PEM, orthostatic intolerance, depression, PTSD, anxiety; patient was found to have PEM, depression, and complex PTSD features	Care coordination with a psychiatric provider led to the continuation of the SSRI, the addition of low-dose ariprazole as an adjunct for depressive symptoms; psychotherapy focused on improving distress tolerance using dialectical behavioral therapy approaches
A referral to a physical therapist with expertise in Long COVID was done during visit 1	Continued low-dose naltrexone daily at 3mg PO daily since patient endorsed benefit
CBC with differential was within normal limits; B12 was 220 pg/mL which is considered borderline; and so B12 injections were provided monthly	Patient participated in a breath by breath mindfulness support group for 6 weeks which was helpful in providing mindfulness strategies for improving parasypmpathetic tone
Behavioral strategies such as strict energy management, liberalizing salt, recumbent physical activity, deep breathing, hydration, and strict sleep hygiene were all discussed during visit 1 and challenges were discussed during visit 2	Patient initiated a change in her diet towards a more anti-inflammatory approach
Low-risk medications started during this phase: a trial of an SSRI was started for depression symptoms; propranolol 10 mg PO TID PRN; insomnia was managed with melatonin slow release at 2 mg before bedtime and Neurontin 100–300 mg PO QHS; for chronic pain sensitivity: low-dose naltrexone started at 1mg and titrated up to 3 mg PO daily	Chronic pain psychoeducation was reinforced by physical therapist and physician during this period

(continued)

Boxes 12.1, 12.2, and 12.3 (continued)

55-year-old man with morbid obesity, class III congestive heart failure (diastolic and systolic) who now presents with worsening fatigue and exercise intolerance and a chronic cough 3 months after being hospitalized for severe COVID-19 pneumonia that required high-flow nasal cannula for 5 days in the hospital. Past medical history: systolic and diastolic CHF; type 2 diabetes mellitus on insulin; morbid obesity; severe obstructive sleep apnea; Social and family history: lives alone, is socially isolated; already on SSI disability.

Harm Reduction Phase (~3 months)	Symptom and Impairment Management (but the Long COVID diagnosis is no longer providing value to this patient's health or function during this phase)
Physician validated symptoms; saw patient every 6 weeks during this phase	Once cough and sleep symptoms were stabilized, PEM improved
Used validated surveys to assess PEM, orthostatic intolerance, depression, OSA; patient was found to have mild PEM and fatigue; physical exam focused on lung and heart examination; gait, balance, and lower extremity strength	It made more sense to leverage his CHF diagnosis and the prolonged admission to the hospital to focus his cardiopulmonary rehabilitation plan
Basic laboratory and diagnostic testing were ordered during visit 1 which included CBC with differential, comprehensive metabolic panel, spirometry, and PA/lateral chest x-ray	Patient was referred to the heart failure cardiology team
A referral for a laboratory-based polysomnogram found a mix of both obstructive sleep apnea and central sleep apnea; bi-level positive airway pressure therapy was started at night	
Chronic cough management started for upper airway cough syndrome using PPI BID before breakfast and dinner; behavioral interventions to address reflux symptoms were started such as sleeping with head elevated, avoiding eating within 2 hours of bedtime, and avoiding certain trigger foods; discontinuing ACE inhibitors was also associated with improvement in cough	
Medication reconciliation led to a discontinuation of some other sedating medications that were started during the hospitalization	

References

1. Callard F, Perego E. How and why patients made Long COVID. Soc Sci Med. 2021;268:113426. https://doi.org/10.1016/j.socscimed.2020.113426.
2. Stelson EA, Dash D, McCorkell L, et al. Return-to-work with Long COVID: an Episodic Disability and Total Worker Health(R) analysis. Soc Sci Med. 2023;338:116336. https://doi.org/10.1016/j.socscimed.2023.116336.
3. Fitzgerald ML, Cohen AK, Jaudon TW, et al. A call from patient-researchers to advance research on Long COVID. Cell. 2024;187(20):5490–6. https://doi.org/10.1016/j.cell.2024.09.011.
4. Davis HE, Assaf GS, McCorkell L, et al. Characterizing Long COVID in an international cohort: 7 months of symptoms and their impact. EClinicalMedicine. 2021;38:101019. https://doi.org/10.1016/j.eclinm.2021.101019.
5. Davis HE, McCorkell L, Vogel JM, Topol EJ. Long COVID: major findings, mechanisms and recommendations. Nat Rev Microbiol. 2023;21(3):133–46. https://doi.org/10.1038/s41579-022-00846-2.
6. RECOVER. FAQs. RECOVER: researching COVID to enhance recovery. Updated 2024. Accessed 2024.
7. US Centers for Disease Control and Prevention. Long COVID. Centers for Disease Control and Prevention. Updated 6 Feb 2024. Accessed 2024.
8. Munblit D, O'Hara ME, Akrami A, Perego E, Olliaro P, Needham DM. Long COVID: aiming for a consensus. Lancet Respir Med. 2022;10(7):632–4. https://doi.org/10.1016/S2213-2600(22)00135-7.
9. Soriano JB, Murthy S, Marshall JC, Relan P, Diaz JV. A clinical case definition of post-COVID-19 condition by a Delphi consensus. Lancet Infect Dis. 2021. https://doi.org/10.1016/S1473-3099(21)00703-9.
10. National Academies of Sciences, Engineering, and Medicine. A Long COVID definition: a chronic, systemic disease state with profound consequences. Washington, DC: The National Academies Press; 2024.
11. Adjaye-Gbewonyo D, Vahratian A, Perrine CG, Bertolli J. Long COVID in adults: United States, 2022. NCHS Data Brief. 2023;(480):1–8.
12. Vahratian A, Adjaye-Gbewonyo D, Lin JS, Saydah S. Long COVID in children: United States, 2022. NCHS Data Brief. 2023;(479):1–6.
13. Subramanian A, Nirantharakumar K, Hughes S, et al. Symptoms and risk factors for Long COVID in non-hospitalized adults. Nat Med. 2022;28(8):1706–14. https://doi.org/10.1038/s41591-022-01909-w.
14. Hejazian SS, Sadr AV, Shahjouei S, Vemuri A, Abedi V, Zand R. Prevalence and determinants of long-term post-COVID conditions in the United States: 2022 behavioral risk factor surveillance system. Am J Med. 2024. https://doi.org/10.1016/j.amjmed.2024.02.010.
15. O'Mahoney LL, Routen A, Gillies C, et al. The prevalence and long-term health effects of Long COVID among hospitalised and non-hospitalised populations: a systematic review and meta-analysis. EClinicalMedicine. 2023;55:101762. https://doi.org/10.1016/j.eclinm.2022.101762.
16. Ma Y, Deng J, Liu Q, Du M, Liu M, Liu J. Long-term consequences of asymptomatic SARS-CoV-2 infection: a systematic review and meta-analysis. Int J Environ Res Public Health. 2023;20(2). https://doi.org/10.3390/ijerph20021613.
17. Tsampasian V, Elghazaly H, Chattopadhyay R, et al. Risk factors associated with post-COVID-19 condition: a systematic review and meta-analysis. JAMA Intern Med. 2023;183(6):566–80. https://doi.org/10.1001/jamainternmed.2023.0750.
18. Byambasuren O, Stehlik P, Clark J, Alcorn K, Glasziou P. Effect of covid-19 vaccination on Long COVID: systematic review. BMJ Med. 2023;2(1):e000385. https://doi.org/10.1136/bmjmed-2022-000385.

19. Notarte KI, Catahay JA, Velasco JV, et al. Impact of COVID-19 vaccination on the risk of developing long-COVID and on existing long-COVID symptoms: a systematic review. EClinicalMedicine. 2022;53:101624. https://doi.org/10.1016/j.eclinm.2022.101624.
20. Fung KW, Baye F, Baik SH, McDonald CJ. Nirmatrelvir and molnupiravir and post-COVID-19 condition in older patients. JAMA Intern Med. 2023;183(12):1404–6. https://doi.org/10.1001/jamainternmed.2023.5099.
21. Xie Y, Choi T, Al-Aly Z. Association of treatment with nirmatrelvir and the risk of post-COVID-19 condition. JAMA Intern Med. 2023;183(6):554–64. https://doi.org/10.1001/jamainternmed.2023.0743.
22. Congdon S, Narrowe Z, Yone N, et al. Nirmatrelvir/ritonavir and risk of Long COVID symptoms: a retrospective cohort study. Sci Rep. 2023;13(1):19688. https://doi.org/10.1038/s41598-023-46912-4.
23. Durstenfeld MS, Peluso MJ, Lin F, et al. Association of nirmatrelvir for acute SARS-CoV-2 infection with subsequent Long COVID symptoms in an observational cohort study. J Med Virol. 2024;96(1):e29333. https://doi.org/10.1002/jmv.29333.
24. Eccles JA, Cadar D, Quadt L, Hakim AJ, Gall N, Bowyer V, Cheetham N, Steves CJ, Critchley HJ, Davies KA. Is joint hypermobility linked to self-reported non-recovery from COVID-19? Case–control evidence from the British COVID Symptom Study Biobank. BMJ Public Health. 2024;2(1):e000478.
25. Wilson GN. A clinical qualification protocol highlights overlapping genomic influences and neuro-autonomic mechanisms in Ehlers-Danlos and Long COVID-19 syndromes. Curr Issues Mol Biol. 2023;45(7):6003–23. https://doi.org/10.3390/cimb45070379.
26. Noell G, Faner R, Agusti A. From systems biology to P4 medicine: applications in respiratory medicine. Eur Respir Rev. 2018;27(147). https://doi.org/10.1183/16000617.0110-2017.
27. Rothman KJ. Causes. 1976. Am J Epidemiol. 1995;141(2):90–5; discussion 89. https://doi.org/10.1093/oxfordjournals.aje.a117417.
28. Juszko K, Szary P, Mazurek J, et al. Long-term consequences of COVID-19 disease specific to women: exploratory research. Int J Environ Res Public Health. 2022;20(1). https://doi.org/10.3390/ijerph20010150.
29. Sandifer PA, Juster RP, Seeman TE, Lichtveld MY, Singer BH. Allostatic load in the context of disasters. Psychoneuroendocrinology. 2022;140:105725. https://doi.org/10.1016/j.psyneuen.2022.105725.
30. Goldstein DS. The extended autonomic system, dyshomeostasis, and COVID-19. Clin Auton Res. 2020;30(4):299–315. https://doi.org/10.1007/s10286-020-00714-0.
31. Goldstein DS. Post-COVID dysautonomias: what we know and (mainly) what we don't know. Nat Rev Neurol. 2024;20(2):99–113. https://doi.org/10.1038/s41582-023-00917-9.
32. Renz-Polster H, Tremblay ME, Bienzle D, Fischer JE. The pathobiology of myalgic encephalomyelitis/chronic fatigue syndrome: the case for neuroglial failure. Front Cell Neurosci. 2022;16:888232. https://doi.org/10.3389/fncel.2022.888232.
33. Leng A, Shah M, Ahmad SA, et al. Pathogenesis underlying neurological manifestations of Long COVID syndrome and potential therapeutics. Cells. 2023;12(5). https://doi.org/10.3390/cells12050816.
34. Serviente C, Decker ST, Layec G. From heart to muscle: pathophysiological mechanisms underlying long-term physical sequelae from SARS-CoV-2 infection. J Appl Physiol (1985). 2022. https://doi.org/10.1152/japplphysiol.00734.2021.
35. Hope AA, Evering TH. Postacute sequelae of severe acute respiratory syndrome coronavirus 2 infection. Infect Dis Clin N Am. 2022;36(2):379–95. (In eng). https://doi.org/10.1016/j.idc.2022.02.004.
36. Tsilingiris D, Vallianou NG, Karampela I, et al. Laboratory findings and biomarkers in Long COVID: what do we know so far? Insights into epidemiology, pathogenesis, therapeutic perspectives and challenges. Int J Mol Sci. 2023;24(13). https://doi.org/10.3390/ijms241310458.

37. Chang K, Zaikos T, Kilner-Pontone N, Ho CY. Mechanisms of COVID-19-associated olfactory dysfunction. Neuropathol Appl Neurobiol. 2024;50(2):e12960. https://doi.org/10.1111/nan.12960.
38. Dani M, Dirksen A, Taraborrelli P, et al. Autonomic dysfunction in 'Long COVID': rationale, physiology and management strategies. Clin Med (Lond). 2021;21(1):e63–7. https://doi.org/10.7861/clinmed.2020-0896.
39. Bisaccia G, Ricci F, Recce V, et al. Post-acute sequelae of COVID-19 and cardiovascular autonomic dysfunction: what do we know? J Cardiovasc Dev Dis. 2021;8(11). https://doi.org/10.3390/jcdd8110156.
40. Lopez-Otin C, Blasco MA, Partridge L, Serrano M, Kroemer G. The hallmarks of aging. Cell. 2013;153(6):1194–217. https://doi.org/10.1016/j.cell.2013.05.039.
41. Molnar T, Lehoczki A, Fekete M, et al. Mitochondrial dysfunction in Long COVID: mechanisms, consequences, and potential therapeutic approaches. Geroscience. 2024. https://doi.org/10.1007/s11357-024-01165-5.
42. Jamieson A, Al Saikhan L, Alghamdi L, et al. Mechanisms underlying exercise intolerance in Long COVID: an accumulation of multisystem dysfunction. Physiol Rep. 2024;12(3):e15940. https://doi.org/10.14814/phy2.15940.
43. Dirajlal-Fargo S, Maison DP, Durieux JC, et al. Altered mitochondrial respiration in peripheral blood mononuclear cells of post-acute sequelae of SARS-CoV-2 infection. Mitochondrion. 2024;75:101849. https://doi.org/10.1016/j.mito.2024.101849.
44. Chagas LDS, Serfaty CA. The influence of microglia on neuroplasticity and Long-term cognitive sequelae in Long COVID: impacts on brain development and beyond. Int J Mol Sci. 2024;25(7). https://doi.org/10.3390/ijms25073819.
45. Chaves-Filho AM, Braniff O, Angelova A, Deng Y, Tremblay ME. Chronic inflammation, neuroglial dysfunction, and plasmalogen deficiency as a new pathobiological hypothesis addressing the overlap between post-COVID-19 symptoms and myalgic encephalomyelitis/chronic fatigue syndrome. Brain Res Bull. 2023;201:110702. https://doi.org/10.1016/j.brainresbull.2023.110702.
46. Bedree H, Sunnquist M, Jason LA. The DePaul Symptom Questionnaire-2: a validation study. Fatigue. 2019;7(3):166–79. https://doi.org/10.1080/21641846.2019.1653471.
47. Cotler J, Holtzman C, Dudun C, Jason LA. A brief questionnaire to assess post-exertional malaise. Diagnostics (Basel). 2018;8(3). https://doi.org/10.3390/diagnostics8030066.
48. Grach SL, Seltzer J, Chon TY, Ganesh R. Diagnosis and management of myalgic encephalomyelitis/chronic fatigue syndrome. Mayo Clin Proc. 2023;98(10):1544–51. https://doi.org/10.1016/j.mayocp.2023.07.032.
49. Davenport TE, Stevens SR, Stevens J, Snell CR, Van Ness JM. Development and measurement properties of the PEM/PESE activity questionnaire (PAQ). Work. 2023;74(4):1187–97. https://doi.org/10.3233/WOR-220553.
50. Chung F, Abdullah HR, Liao P. STOP-bang questionnaire: a practical approach to screen for obstructive sleep apnea. Chest. 2016;149(3):631–8. https://doi.org/10.1378/chest.15-0903.
51. Orru G, Bertelloni D, Diolaiuti F, et al. Long-COVID syndrome? A study on the persistence of neurological, psychological and physiological symptoms. Healthcare (Basel). 2021;9(5). https://doi.org/10.3390/healthcare9050575.
52. Valdes E, Fuchs B, Morrison C, et al. Demographic and social determinants of cognitive dysfunction following hospitalization for COVID-19. J Neurol Sci. 2022;438:120146. https://doi.org/10.1016/j.jns.2022.120146.
53. Jennings G, Monaghan A, Xue F, Duggan E, Romero-Ortuno R. Comprehensive clinical characterisation of brain fog in adults reporting Long COVID symptoms. J Clin Med. 2022;11(12). https://doi.org/10.3390/jcm11123440.
54. Larsen NW, Stiles LE, Shaik R, et al. Characterization of autonomic symptom burden in Long COVID: a global survey of 2,314 adults. Front Neurol. 2022;13:1012668. https://doi.org/10.3389/fneur.2022.1012668.

55. Blitshteyn S, Whiteson JH, Abramoff B, et al. Multi-disciplinary collaborative consensus guidance statement on the assessment and treatment of autonomic dysfunction in patients with post-acute sequelae of SARS-CoV-2 infection (PASC). PM R. 2022;14(10):1270–91. https://doi.org/10.1002/pmrj.12894.
56. Ghoshal UC, Ghoshal U. Gastrointestinal involvement in post-acute Coronavirus disease (COVID)-19 syndrome. Curr Opin Infect Dis. 2023;36(5):366–70. https://doi.org/10.1097/QCO.0000000000000959.
57. Elmunzer BJ, Palsson OS, Forbes N, et al. Prolonged gastrointestinal manifestations after recovery from COVID-19. Clin Gastroenterol Hepatol. 2024;22(5):1098–1107.e3. https://doi.org/10.1016/j.cgh.2023.11.009.
58. Ashktorab H, Challa SR, Singh G, et al. Gastrointestinal manifestations and their association with neurologic and sleep problems in Long COVID-19 minority patients: a prospective follow-up study. Dig Dis Sci. 2024;69(2):562–9. https://doi.org/10.1007/s10620-023-08176-w.
59. Liebell D. Part two: perspectives on olfactory and gustatory dysfunction pathophysiology, management, and relevance to COVID-19: current approaches. Altern Ther Health Med. 2023;29(6):30–5.
60. Liebell D. Perspectives on the pathophysiology, management, and relevance of olfactory and gustatory dysfunction to COVID-19, part one. Altern Ther Health Med. 2023;29(2):76–81.
61. Wu TJ, Yu AC, Lee JT. Management of post-COVID-19 olfactory dysfunction. Curr Treat Options Allergy. 2022:1–18. https://doi.org/10.1007/s40521-021-00297-9.
62. Fernandez-de-Las-Penas C, Nijs J, Neblett R, et al. Phenotyping post-COVID pain as a nociceptive, neuropathic, or nociplastic pain condition. Biomedicine. 2022;10(10). https://doi.org/10.3390/biomedicines10102562.
63. Limerick G, Christo DK, Tram J, et al. Complex regional pain syndrome: evidence-based advances in concepts and treatments. Curr Pain Headache Rep. 2023;27(9):269–98. https://doi.org/10.1007/s11916-023-01130-5.
64. Suzuki K, Suzuki S, Haruyama Y, et al. Associations between the burdens of comorbid sleep problems, central sensitization, and headache-related disability in patients with migraine. Front Neurol. 2024;15:1373574. https://doi.org/10.3389/fneur.2024.1373574.
65. Srikanth S, Boulos JR, Dover T, Boccuto L, Dean D. Identification and diagnosis of Long COVID-19: a scoping review. Prog Biophys Mol Biol. 2023;182:1–7. https://doi.org/10.1016/j.pbiomolbio.2023.04.008.
66. Chang R, Yen-Ting Chen T, Wang SI, Hung YM, Chen HY, Wei CJ. Risk of autoimmune diseases in patients with COVID-19: a retrospective cohort study. EClinicalMedicine. 2023;56:101783. https://doi.org/10.1016/j.eclinm.2022.101783.
67. Ciaffi J, Vanni E, Mancarella L, et al. Post-acute COVID-19 joint pain and new onset of rheumatic musculoskeletal diseases: a systematic review. Diagnostics (Basel). 2023;13(11). https://doi.org/10.3390/diagnostics13111850.
68. Kioi Y, Yorifuji H, Higami Y, Katada Y. Serositis and lymphopenia are common features of systemic lupus erythematosus following SARS-CoV-2 infection: a case report and literature review. Int J Rheum Dis. 2023;26(11):2267–71. https://doi.org/10.1111/1756-185X.14767.
69. Aggarwal R, Ringold S, Khanna D, et al. Distinctions between diagnostic and classification criteria? Arthritis Care Res (Hoboken). 2015;67(7):891–7. https://doi.org/10.1002/acr.22583.
70. Stewart JM, Pianosi P, Shaban MA, et al. Postural hyperventilation as a cause of postural tachycardia syndrome: increased systemic vascular resistance and decreased cardiac output when upright in all postural tachycardia syndrome variants. J Am Heart Assoc. 2018;7(13). https://doi.org/10.1161/JAHA.118.008854.
71. Boulding R, Stacey R, Niven R, Fowler SJ. Dysfunctional breathing: a review of the literature and proposal for classification. Eur Respir Rev. 2016;25(141):287–94. https://doi.org/10.1183/16000617.0088-2015.
72. Younossi ZM, Bernstein D, Shiffman ML, et al. Diagnosis and management of primary biliary cholangitis. Am J Gastroenterol. 2019;114(1):48–63. https://doi.org/10.1038/s41395-018-0390-3.

73. Ursini F, Ciaffi J, Mancarella L, et al. Fibromyalgia: a new facet of the post-COVID-19 syndrome spectrum? Results from a web-based survey. RMD Open. 2021;7(3). https://doi.org/10.1136/rmdopen-2021-001735.
74. Colatutto D, Sonaglia A, Zabotti A, Cereser L, Girometti R, Quartuccio L. Post-COVID-19 arthritis and sacroiliitis: natural history with longitudinal magnetic resonance imaging study in two cases and review of the literature. Viruses. 2021;13(8). https://doi.org/10.3390/v13081558.
75. El-Rhermoul FZ, Fedorowski A, Eardley P, et al. Autoimmunity in Long COVID and POTS. Oxf Open Immunol. 2023;4(1):iqad002. https://doi.org/10.1093/oxfimm/iqad002.
76. Schou TM, Joca S, Wegener G, Bay-Richter C. Psychiatric and neuropsychiatric sequelae of COVID-19 – a systematic review. Brain Behav Immun. 2021;97:328–48. https://doi.org/10.1016/j.bbi.2021.07.018.
77. Luedke JC, Vargas G, Jashar DT, Malone LA, Morrow A, Ng R. Neuropsychological functioning of pediatric patients with Long COVID. Clin Neuropsychol. 2024:1–18. https://doi.org/10.1080/13854046.2024.2344455.
78. Graham EL, Clark JR, Orban ZS, et al. Persistent neurologic symptoms and cognitive dysfunction in non-hospitalized Covid-19 "long haulers". Ann Clin Transl Neurol. 2021;8(5):1073–85. https://doi.org/10.1002/acn3.51350.
79. Fry L, Logemann A, Waldron E, et al. Emotional functioning in Long COVID: comparison to post-concussion syndrome using the Personality Assessment Inventory. Clin Neuropsychol. 2024;38(4):963–83. https://doi.org/10.1080/13854046.2023.2264546.
80. Merikanto I, Dauvilliers Y, Chung F, et al. Disturbances in sleep, circadian rhythms and daytime functioning in relation to coronavirus infection and Long-COVID – a multinational ICOSS study. J Sleep Res. 2021:e13542. https://doi.org/10.1111/jsr.13542.
81. O'Driscoll DM, Young AC. Contemporary concise review 2022: sleep. Respirology. 2023;28(6):518–24. https://doi.org/10.1111/resp.14500.
82. Rogers JP, Chesney E, Oliver D, et al. Psychiatric and neuropsychiatric presentations associated with severe coronavirus infections: a systematic review and meta-analysis with comparison to the COVID-19 pandemic. Lancet Psychiatry. 2020;7(7):611–27. https://doi.org/10.1016/S2215-0366(20)30203-0.
83. Sumantri S, Rengganis I. Immunological dysfunction and mast cell activation syndrome in Long COVID. Asia Pac Allergy. 2023;13(1):50–3. https://doi.org/10.5415/apallergy.0000000000000022.
84. da Silveira Gorman R, Syed IU. Connecting the dots in emerging mast cell research: do factors affecting mast cell activation provide a missing link between adverse COVID-19 outcomes and the social determinants of health? Med Sci (Basel). 2022;10(2). https://doi.org/10.3390/medsci10020029.
85. Pot M. Epistemic solidarity in medicine and healthcare. Med Health Care Philos. 2022;25(4):681–92. https://doi.org/10.1007/s11019-022-10112-0.
86. Shah R, Clarke R, Ahluwalia S, Launer J. Finding meaning in the consultation: working in the hermeneutic window. Br J Gen Pract. 2021;71(707):282–3. https://doi.org/10.3399/bjgp21X716105.
87. Shah R, Clarke R, Ahluwalia S, Launer J. Finding meaning in the consultation: supporting the hermeneutic window in practice. Br J Gen Pract. 2022;72(715):83–4. https://doi.org/10.3399/bjgp22X718493.
88. Shah R, Clarke R, Ahluwalia S, Launer J. Finding meaning in the consultation: introducing the hermeneutic window. Br J Gen Pract. 2020;70(699):502–3. https://doi.org/10.3399/bjgp20X712865.
89. Stevens S, Snell C, Stevens J, Keller B, VanNess JM. Cardiopulmonary exercise test methodology for assessing exertion intolerance in myalgic encephalomyelitis/chronic fatigue syndrome. Front Pediatr. 2018;6:242. https://doi.org/10.3389/fped.2018.00242.

90. Thaweethai T, Jolley SE, Karlson EW, et al. Development of a definition of postacute sequelae of SARS-CoV-2 infection. JAMA. 2023;329(22):1934–46. https://doi.org/10.1001/jama.2023.8823.
91. Twomey R, DeMars J, Franklin K, Culos-Reed SN, Weatherald J, Wrightson JG. Chronic fatigue and postexertional malaise in people living with Long COVID: an observational study. Phys Ther. 2022;102(4). https://doi.org/10.1093/ptj/pzac005.
92. Vernon SD, Hartle M, Sullivan K, et al. Post-exertional malaise among people with Long COVID compared to myalgic encephalomyelitis/chronic fatigue syndrome (ME/CFS). Work. 2023;74(4):1179–86. https://doi.org/10.3233/WOR-220581.
93. Wernhart S, Weihe E, Totzeck M, Balcer B, Rassaf T, Luedike P. Cardiopulmonary profiling of athletes with post-exertional malaise after COVID-19 infection-a single-center experience. J Clin Med. 2023;12(13). https://doi.org/10.3390/jcm12134348.
94. Balcom EF, Nath A, Power C. Acute and chronic neurological disorders in COVID-19: potential mechanisms of disease. Brain. 2021;144(12):3576–88. https://doi.org/10.1093/brain/awab302.
95. Johnson J, Rodriguez MA, Al Snih S. Life-space mobility in the elderly: current perspectives. Clin Interv Aging. 2020;15:1665–74. https://doi.org/10.2147/CIA.S196944.
96. Chu L, Valencia IJ, Garvert DW, Montoya JG. Deconstructing post-exertional malaise in myalgic encephalomyelitis/chronic fatigue syndrome: a patient-centered, cross-sectional survey. PLoS One. 2018;13(6):e0197811. https://doi.org/10.1371/journal.pone.0197811.
97. Thoma M, Froehlich L, Hattesohl DBR, Quante S, Jason LA, Scheibenbogen C. Why the psychosomatic view on myalgic encephalomyelitis/chronic fatigue syndrome is inconsistent with current evidence and harmful to patients. Medicina (Kaunas). 2023;60(1). https://doi.org/10.3390/medicina60010083.
98. Clutterbuck D, Ramasawmy M, Pantelic M, et al. Barriers to healthcare access and experiences of stigma: findings from a coproduced Long COVID case-finding study. Health Expect. 2024;27(2):e14037. https://doi.org/10.1111/hex.14037.
99. Ireson J, Taylor A, Richardson E, Greenfield B, Jones G. Exploring invisibility and epistemic injustice in Long COVID-a citizen science qualitative analysis of patient stories from an online Covid community. Health Expect. 2022;25(4):1753–65. https://doi.org/10.1111/hex.13518.
100. Au L, Capotescu C, Eyal G, Finestone G. Long COVID and medical gaslighting: dismissal, delayed diagnosis, and deferred treatment. SSM Qual Res Health. 2022;2:100167. https://doi.org/10.1016/j.ssmqr.2022.100167.
101. Soranzo A, Taddio L. Perceptual phenomena cannot be approached from a single perspective. J Intelligence. 2023;11(11). https://doi.org/10.3390/jintelligence11110214.
102. Mehta N. Mind-body dualism: a critique from a health perspective. Mens Sana Monogr. 2011;9(1):202–9. https://doi.org/10.4103/0973-1229.77436.
103. Bonilla H, Quach TC, Tiwari A, et al. Myalgic encephalomyelitis/chronic fatigue syndrome is common in post-acute sequelae of SARS-CoV-2 infection (PASC): results from a post-COVID-19 multidisciplinary clinic. Front Neurol. 2023;14:1090747. https://doi.org/10.3389/fneur.2023.1090747.
104. Jason LA, Dorri JA. ME/CFS and post-exertional malaise among patients with Long COVID. Neurol Int. 2022;15(1):1–11. https://doi.org/10.3390/neurolint15010001.
105. Legler F, Meyer-Arndt L, Modl L, et al. Long-term symptom severity and clinical biomarkers in post-COVID-19/chronic fatigue syndrome: results from a prospective observational cohort. EClinicalMedicine. 2023;63:102146. https://doi.org/10.1016/j.eclinm.2023.102146.
106. Rivera J, Rodriguez T, Pallares M, et al. Prevalence of post-COVID-19 in patients with fibromyalgia: a comparative study with other inflammatory and autoimmune rheumatic diseases. BMC Musculoskelet Disord. 2022;23(1):471. https://doi.org/10.1186/s12891-022-05436-0.
107. Jahng J, Kim YS. Irritable bowel syndrome: is it really a functional disorder? A new perspective on alteration of enteric nervous system. J Neurogastroenterol Motil. 2016;22(2):163–5. https://doi.org/10.5056/jnm16043.

108. Sanal-Hayes NEM, Hayes LD, McLaughlin M, Berry ECJ, Sculthorpe NF. Post-traumatic stress disorder and complex post-traumatic stress disorder in people with Long COVID, ME/CFS, and controls. Am J Med. 2023. https://doi.org/10.1016/j.amjmed.2023.12.006.
109. Wu KK, Lee D, Sze AM, et al. Posttraumatic stress, anxiety, and depression in COVID-19 survivors. East Asian Arch Psychiatr. 2022;32(1):5–10. https://doi.org/10.12809/eaap2176.
110. Agoston DV. Traumatic brain injury in the Long-COVID era. Neurotrauma Rep. 2024;5(1):81–94. https://doi.org/10.1089/neur.2023.0067.
111. Victor MM, Muller Haas L, Grevet EH, Rohde LA. Successful treatment of post-COVID-19 ADHD-like syndrome: a case report. J Atten Disord. 2023;27(10):1092–8. https://doi.org/10.1177/10870547231168338.
112. Koonce RM, Martin BC. The association between suspected long-COVID and stimulant prescribing in the United States. Psychiatry Res. 2024;331:115686. https://doi.org/10.1016/j.psychres.2023.115686.
113. National Academies of Sciences E, Medicine. Long-term health effects of COVID-19: disability and function following SARS-CoV-2 infection. Washington, DC: The National Academies Press; 2024.
114. Espinosa-Gonzalez AB, Master H, Gall N, Halpin S, Rogers N, Greenhalgh T. Orthostatic tachycardia after covid-19. BMJ. 2023;380:e073488. https://doi.org/10.1136/bmj-2022-073488.
115. Tariq SH, Tumosa N, Chibnall JT, Perry MH 3rd, Morley JE. Comparison of the Saint Louis University mental status examination and the mini-mental state examination for detecting dementia and mild neurocognitive disorder—a pilot study. Am J Geriatr Psychiatry. 2006;14(11):900–10. https://doi.org/10.1097/01.JGP.0000221510.33817.86.
116. Wang XJ, Ebbert JO, Loftus CG, Rosedahl JK, Philpot LM. Comorbid extra-intestinal central sensitization conditions worsen irritable bowel syndrome in primary care patients. Neurogastroenterol Motil. 2023;35(4):e14546. https://doi.org/10.1111/nmo.14546.
117. Nijs J, George SZ, Clauw DJ, et al. Central sensitisation in chronic pain conditions: latest discoveries and their potential for precision medicine. Lancet Rheumatol. 2021;3(5):e383–92. https://doi.org/10.1016/S2665-9913(21)00032-1.
118. Zou XY, Liu XH, Lu CL, et al. Traditional Chinese medicine for post-viral olfactory dysfunction: a systematic review. Integr Med Res. 2024;13(2):101045. https://doi.org/10.1016/j.imr.2024.101045.
119. Trager RJ, Brewka EC, Kaiser CM, Patterson AJ, Dusek JA. Acupuncture in multidisciplinary treatment for post-COVID-19 syndrome. Med Acupunct. 2022;34(3):177–83. https://doi.org/10.1089/acu.2021.0086.
120. Lam WC, Wei D, Li H, et al. The use of acupuncture for addressing neurological and neuropsychiatric symptoms in patients with Long COVID: a systematic review and meta-analysis. Front Neurol. 2024;15:1406475. https://doi.org/10.3389/fneur.2024.1406475.
121. Chen XY, Lu CL, Wang QY, et al. Traditional, complementary and integrative medicine for fatigue post COVID-19 infection: a systematic review of randomized controlled trials. Integr Med Res. 2024;13(2):101039. https://doi.org/10.1016/j.imr.2024.101039.
122. Romeyke T. A multimodal approach in the treatment of persistent post-COVID. Diseases. 2022;10(4). https://doi.org/10.3390/diseases10040097.
123. Kleim JA, Jones TA. Principles of experience-dependent neural plasticity: implications for rehabilitation after brain damage. J Speech Lang Hear Res. 2008;51(1):S225–39. https://doi.org/10.1044/1092-4388(2008/018).
124. Zimmermann P, Curtis N. Coronavirus infections in children including COVID-19: an overview of the epidemiology, clinical features, diagnosis, treatment and prevention options in children. Pediatr Infect Dis J. 2020;39(5):355–68. https://doi.org/10.1097/INF.0000000000002660.
125. Zimmermann P, Curtis N. Why is COVID-19 less severe in children? A review of the proposed mechanisms underlying the age-related difference in severity of SARS-CoV-2 infections. Arch Dis Child. 2020. https://doi.org/10.1136/archdischild-2020 320338.

126. Rao S, Gross RS, Mohandas S, et al. Postacute sequelae of SARS-CoV-2 in children. Pediatrics. 2024;153(3). https://doi.org/10.1542/peds.2023-062570.
127. Stephenson T, Allin B, Nugawela MD, et al. Long COVID (post-COVID-19 condition) in children: a modified Delphi process. Arch Dis Child. 2022;107(7):674–80. https://doi.org/10.1136/archdischild-2021-323624.
128. Lopez-Leon S, Wegman-Ostrosky T, Ayuzo Del Valle NC, et al. Long-COVID in children and adolescents: a systematic review and meta-analyses. Sci Rep. 2022;12(1):9950. https://doi.org/10.1038/s41598-022-13495-5.
129. Kompaniyets L, Bull-Otterson L, Boehmer TK, et al. Post-COVID-19 symptoms and conditions among children and adolescents – United States, March 1, 2020-January 31, 2022. MMWR Morb Mortal Wkly Rep. 2022;71(31):993–9. https://doi.org/10.15585/mmwr.mm7131a3.
130. Feldstein LR, Rose EB, Horwitz SM, et al. Multisystem inflammatory syndrome in U.S. children and adolescents. N Engl J Med. 2020;383(4):334–46. https://doi.org/10.1056/NEJMoa2021680.
131. Morris SB, Schwartz NG, Patel P, et al. Case series of multisystem inflammatory syndrome in adults associated with SARS-CoV-2 infection – United Kingdom and United States, March-August 2020. MMWR Morb Mortal Wkly Rep. 2020;69(40):1450–6. https://doi.org/10.15585/mmwr.mm6940e1.
132. Osmanov IM, Spiridonova E, Bobkova P, et al. Risk factors for post-COVID-19 condition in previously hospitalised children using the ISARIC Global follow-up protocol: a prospective cohort study. Eur Respir J. 2022;59(2). https://doi.org/10.1183/13993003.01341-2021.
133. Pellegrino R, Chiappini E, Licari A, Galli L, Marseglia GL. Prevalence and clinical presentation of Long COVID in children: a systematic review. Eur J Pediatr. 2022;181(12):3995–4009. https://doi.org/10.1007/s00431-022-04600-x.
134. Morello R, Mariani F, Mastrantoni L, et al. Risk factors for post-COVID-19 condition (Long COVID) in children: a prospective cohort study. EClinicalMedicine. 2023;59:101961. https://doi.org/10.1016/j.eclinm.2023.101961.
135. Razzaghi H, Forrest CB, Hirabayashi K, et al. Vaccine effectiveness against Long COVID in children. Pediatrics. 2024;153(4). https://doi.org/10.1542/peds.2023-064446.
136. Kharel M, Sakamoto JL, Carandang RR, et al. Impact of COVID-19 pandemic lockdown on movement behaviours of children and adolescents: a systematic review. BMJ Glob Health. 2022;7(1). https://doi.org/10.1136/bmjgh-2021-007190.
137. Malone LA, Morrow A, Chen Y, et al. Multi-disciplinary collaborative consensus guidance statement on the assessment and treatment of postacute sequelae of SARS-CoV-2 infection (PASC) in children and adolescents. PM R. 2022;14(10):1241–69. https://doi.org/10.1002/pmrj.12890.
138. Morrow AK, Malone LA, Kokorelis C, et al. Long-term COVID 19 sequelae in adolescents: the overlap with orthostatic intolerance and ME/CFS. Curr Pediatr Rep. 2022;10(2):31–44. https://doi.org/10.1007/s40124-022-00261-4.
139. Morrow AK, Ng R, Vargas G, et al. Postacute/Long COVID in pediatrics: development of a multidisciplinary rehabilitation clinic and preliminary case series. Am J Phys Med Rehabil. 2021;100(12):1140–7. https://doi.org/10.1097/PHM.0000000000001896.
140. Toepfner N, Brinkmann F, Augustin S, Stojanov S, Behrends U. Long COVID in pediatrics-epidemiology, diagnosis, and management. Eur J Pediatr. 2024;183(4):1543–53. https://doi.org/10.1007/s00431-023-05360-y.
141. Chen EY, Morrow AK, Malone LA. Exploring the influence of pre-existing conditions and infection factors on pediatric Long COVID symptoms and quality of life. Am J Phys Med Rehabil. 2023. https://doi.org/10.1097/PHM.0000000000002363.
142. Jimeno-Almazan A, Franco-Lopez F, Buendia-Romero A, et al. Rehabilitation for post-COVID-19 condition through a supervised exercise intervention: a randomized controlled trial. Scand J Med Sci Sports. 2022;32(12):1791–801. https://doi.org/10.1111/sms.14240.

143. Chen EY, Burton JM, Johnston A, Morrow AK, Yonts AB, Malone LA. Considerations in children and adolescents related to coronavirus disease 2019 (COVID-19). Phys Med Rehabil Clin N Am. 2023;34(3):643–55. https://doi.org/10.1016/j.pmr.2023.03.004.
144. Roge I, Smane L, Kivite-Urtane A, et al. Comparison of persistent symptoms after COVID-19 and other non-SARS-CoV-2 infections in children. Front Pediatr. 2021;9:752385. https://doi.org/10.3389/fped.2021.752385.
145. Mat Hassan N, Salim HS, Amaran S, et al. Prevalence of mental health problems among children with Long COVID: a systematic review and meta-analysis. PLoS One. 2023;18(5):e0282538. https://doi.org/10.1371/journal.pone.0282538.
146. Bergmans RS, Chambers-Peeple K, Aboul-Hassan D, et al. Opportunities to improve Long COVID care: implications from semi-structured interviews with black patients. Patient. 2022;15(6):715–28. https://doi.org/10.1007/s40271-022-00594-8.
147. Maclean A, Hunt K, Brown A, et al. Negotiation of collective and individual candidacy for Long COVID healthcare in the early phases of the Covid-19 pandemic: validated, diverted and rejected candidacy. SSM Qual Res Health. 2023;3:100207. https://doi.org/10.1016/j.ssmqr.2022.100207.
148. Rushforth A, Ladds E, Wieringa S, Taylor S, Husain L, Greenhalgh T. Long COVID – the illness narratives. Soc Sci Med. 2021;286:114326. https://doi.org/10.1016/j.socscimed.2021.114326.
149. Baz SA, Fang C, Carpentieri JD, Sheard L. 'I don't know what to do or where to go'. Experiences of accessing healthcare support from the perspectives of people living with Long COVID and healthcare professionals: a qualitative study in Bradford, UK. Health Expect. 2023;26(1):542–54. https://doi.org/10.1111/hex.13687.
150. Chou R, Herman E, Ahmed A, et al. Long COVID definitions and models of care: a scoping review. Ann Intern Med. 2024. https://doi.org/10.7326/M24-0677.
151. Alliance LC. The Long COVID Alliance. https://longcovidalliance.org.
152. List JM, Long TG. Community-based primary care management of 'Long COVID': a Center of Excellence Model at NYC Health+ hospitals. Am J Med. 2021;134(10):1232–5. https://doi.org/10.1016/j.amjmed.2021.05.029.
153. Buonsenso D, Di Gennaro L, De Rose C, et al. Long-term outcomes of pediatric infections: from traditional infectious diseases to Long COVID. Future Microbiol. 2022;17:551–71. https://doi.org/10.2217/fmb-2022-0031.
154. Global Burden of Disease Long CC, Wulf Hanson S, Abbafati C, et al. Estimated global proportions of individuals with persistent fatigue, cognitive, and respiratory symptom clusters following symptomatic COVID-19 in 2020 and 2021. JAMA. 2022;328(16):1604–15. https://doi.org/10.1001/jama.2022.18931.
155. Nittas V, Gao M, West EA, et al. Long COVID through a public health lens: an umbrella review. Public Health Rev. 2022;43:1604501. https://doi.org/10.3389/phrs.2022.1604501.
156. Gonzalez-Aumatell A, Bovo MV, Carreras-Abad C, et al. Social, academic, and health status impact of Long COVID on children and young people: an observational, descriptive, and longitudinal cohort study. Children (Basel). 2022;9(11). https://doi.org/10.3390/children9111677.

Chapter 13
Policy Changes Before and After the COVID-19 Pandemic and Their Impact on Health Care Coverage and Access

Nathalie Huguet and Jennifer E. DeVoe

Abbreviations

ACA	Patient Protection and Affordable Care Act
ACIP	Advisory Committee on Immunization Practices
BIPOC	Black, indigenous, and people of color
CHC	Community health centers
CHCF	Community Health Center Fund
CHIP	Children's Health Insurance Program
CMS	Centers for Medicare and Medicaid
DC	District of Columbia
FPL	Federal poverty level
FQHCs	Federally qualified health centers
HRSA	US Health Resources and Services Administration
IRA	Inflation Reduction Act
PEUC	Pandemic Emergency Unemployment Compensation
RHC	Rural health clinics
US	United States

> *I worry a lot about our ability to care for and be reimbursed when patients whose insurance was tied to their employment are now unemployed. Opening enrollment in ACA plans is one solution but I fear [it] won't be enough. Expanding Medicaid eligibility would be helpful.*
> —Primary Care Provider

N. Huguet (✉)
Department of Family Medicine, Oregon Health & Science University School of Medicine, Portland, OR, USA
e-mail: huguetn@ohsu.edu

J. E. DeVoe
OHSU Center for Primary Care Research and Innovation and OHSU-PSU School of Public Health, Portland, OR, USA

A. Cheng et al. (eds.), *Primary Care in a Public Health Emergency*,
https://doi.org/10.1007/978-3-032-12487-6_13

Introduction

Health care and public health services have a direct impact on health; however, it is policies that shape the organization and delivery of these services—from payment to workforce training and readiness. Health policies have a profound impact on health care and public health programs [1], especially those programs serving people in the United States (US) who live in poverty and have experienced marginalization and disadvantage. For example, various policies in US history have increased access to health insurance, such as the enactment of Medicare and Medicaid in the 1960s and three decades later, the State Children's Health Insurance Program (CHIP) to expand coverage for low-income children, which led to a reduction in child mortality [2]. Most recently, the Patient Protection and Affordable Care Act (ACA) further expanded coverage to millions more people. Health policies are laws, regulations, procedures, and decisions implemented to promote health within a society [3]. In this chapter, we describe several health policies and their impact on access to care before, during, and after the COVID-19 pandemic and provide recommendations to inform policy makers and advocacy groups.

The health care legal and policy landscape changed drastically in the decade preceding the COVID-19 pandemic prompted by the passage of the ACA in 2010 [4]. State and federal government decisions affected the implementation of the ACA in the years leading up to the pandemic (Jan 2010–Jan 2020), during the early years of the pandemic (Feb 2020–May 10, 2023), and after the federal public health emergency declaration had ended on May 11, 2023.

The ACA has had far-reaching positive impacts on access to care and population health, and it has bolstered support and sustainability for safety net clinics. Prior to the pandemic, legal and political actions strengthened the ACA in some ways and weakened it in other ways. During the early years of the pandemic, temporary policies were put into place to mitigate the impact of the pandemic on access to health insurance coverage and health care. Some of these policies have expired or have been rolled back, predicted to cause a ripple effect on communities hit hardest by the pandemic. Throughout these time periods, important lessons have been learned about how policy changes can positively and negatively impact health.

Part 1—Pre-pandemic (Jan 2010–Jan 2020)

The Affordable Care Act's Impact on Access to Health Insurance

The ACA, the largest health care-related legislation in the US since the 1960s, was enacted with the goal of expanding health insurance coverage to all citizens and legal residents [4]. The ACA's path to expanding Medicaid was one of its most impactful provisions. It laid the legislative groundwork for a uniform, nationwide coverage option for working-age adults with incomes up to 138% of the federal poverty level (FPL), who had not previously been eligible for coverage in most states. Prior to the ACA, Medicaid eligibility widely varied by state and was often based on age (children), pregnancy status, a disability diagnosis, or status as a parent or caretaker of one or more minor children. The ACA also led to the development of a health insurance Marketplace and subsidies for qualified individuals to purchase private coverage. It was envisioned that once an individual's income reached 138% of FPL, they would seamlessly transition from Medicaid to Marketplace plans using an integrated eligibility determination system with coverage accessible through generous premium subsidies [5]. In 2012, the Supreme Court ruled that states were not legally required to implement Medicaid expansions, and those opting out could not be penalized [6]. Twenty-six states and the District of Columbia (DC) expanded Medicaid in 2014. The uninsurance rates dropped more in states that expanded Medicaid (percent uninsured in 2013 = 13%, in 2014 = 9%, 25% drop) than in states that did not expand (percent uninsured in 2013 = 16%, in 2014 = 13%, 13% drop) [7]. Since 2014, the number of states that have expanded Medicaid eligibility has increased to 41 by December 2024 (Fig. 13.1). Eligibility requirements (e.g., work requirements) vary by state. Expansion of Medicaid eligibility has been a successful strategy to not only reduce the number of people without health insurance but also to improve the health and well-being of millions of Americans.

Following the passage of the ACA and implementation of insurance expansion policies, the number of individuals in the U.S. without health insurance significantly

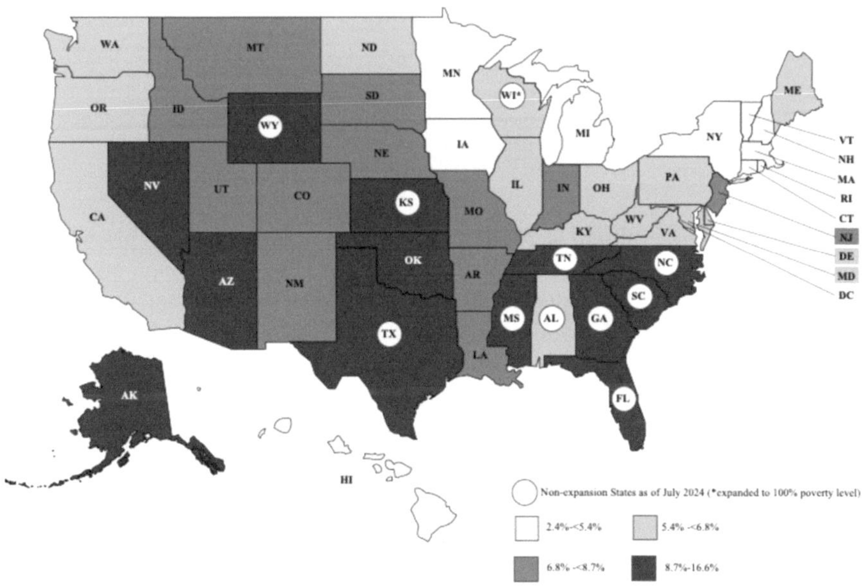

Fig. 13.1 State expansion status as of December 2024 and percent uninsurance (quartile) in 2022. (Source: Health Insurance Historical Tables, US Census Bureau [7])

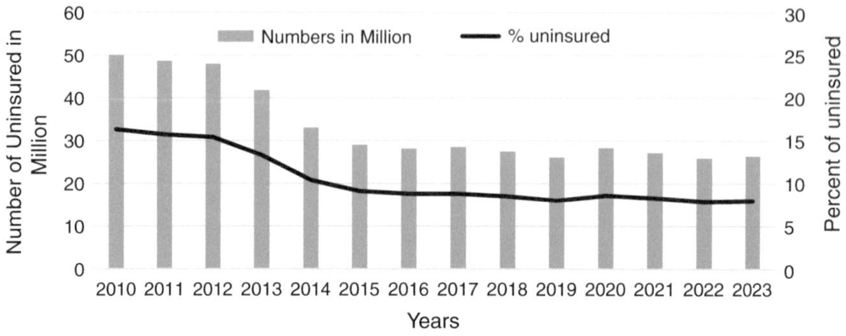

Fig. 13.2 Number and percent of uninsured adults, 2010 to 2023. (Source: Health Insurance Historical Tables, US Census Bureau [8])

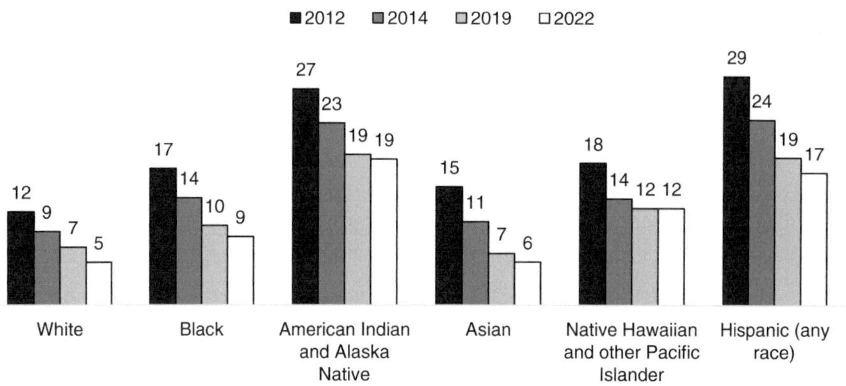

Fig. 13.3 Percent of uninsured by race and ethnicity, 2012–2022. (Source: Health Insurance Historical Tables, US Census Bureau [7])

decreased from 46.5 million in 2010 to 26.7 million in 2016 and then has had relatively small upward or downward fluctuation (Fig. 13.2) [8]. Although all race and ethnic groups experienced a decline in uninsurance rate following the implementation of the ACA, Hispanic and American Indian/Alaska Native have the highest rates of uninsurance relative to the other groups (Fig. 13.3). Notably, these inequities are partially driven by the high number of BIPOC (black, indigenous, and people of color) individuals living in non-expansion states [9]. If all states were to expand Medicaid, racial and ethnic coverage gaps would likely be significantly narrowed.

It is important to note that the ACA created insurance coverage options for millions in the US who had previously been uninsured; however, it did not guarantee continuous coverage or make enrollment processes easy for everyone to navigate successfully. Discontinuous coverage has health impacts [10]. Churn, defined as the "temporary loss of coverage in which enrollees disenroll and then re-enroll within a short period of time," has been shown to impact continuity of care and to have major repercussions on accessing services, needed medication, and treatment; churn also causes delays in diagnoses of chronic health conditions [11–16]. Churn happens not only when people move out of Medicaid to being uninsured and then back into Medicaid again, but for people who, because of slight fluctuations in income, must move between Medicaid and Marketplace plans to find affordable coverage [10]. Policies aimed at reducing churn were implemented during the pandemic and demonstrated significant effectiveness [17], as will be discussed in Part 2.

The ACA's Impact on Access to Care

The ACA's scope extends beyond historically disadvantaged populations who benefit from increased health insurance options because it explicitly requires all health insurance plans to provide essential health benefits covering ambulatory, laboratory, and preventive services; chronic disease management; and mental health and substance use disorder treatment [4]. Since these ACA provisions were put into place, many studies [18–31] have shown increased utilization of ambulatory care, preventive services, medications, behavioral and mental health care, and chronic disease management post-ACA [23, 31]. The ACA has been associated with increases in timely diagnoses of health conditions, improved cardiac surgery outcomes, and reduction in infant mortality rates. Overall, access to health insurance and comprehensiveness of health benefits consistently shows positive impact on health care access and outcomes; however, gaps remain. For example, there is significant variation in medication access across payors and particularly for state Medicaid plans [32]. Payors can determine a list of medications (preferred drug list) covered by the plan without requiring prior authorization. These lists change over time. These variations in access to medications perpetuate disparities [33–35]. More efforts are needed to provide insurance for all and equity in availability of health care services, regardless of payor. In the following section, we will describe the impact of the ACA on preventive care, chronic disease management, and mental health and substance use disorder treatment.

Preventive Care

Of particular importance to all Americans, the ACA mandated that insurers cover preventive services without cost-sharing requirements. Improving access to preventive services and reducing cost barriers is associated with increased life expectancy [36]. Care such as mammography reduces the burden of illness and is now free for beneficiaries, regardless of their deductible or co-payment amounts. A report from the US Assistant Secretary for Planning and Evaluation estimated that in 2020, more than 150 million people with private insurance coverage, 20 million enrollees in Medicaid expansion, and 61 million Medicare beneficiaries had access to preventive services without cost-sharing under the ACA provision [37]. Free access to preventive care services has been associated with increased utilization of these services for people from low socioeconomic groups and those who experience the greatest financial barriers benefiting the most [38]. Studies evaluating the impact of this policy show an increase in preventive services rates overall, with some evidence denoting larger improvement in Medicaid expansion states than non-expansion states [30, 39–41].

Chronic Disease Management

In combination with greater access to preventive services, another important ACA provision was that children <19 years old (enacted in 2010) and adults (enacted in 2014) could no longer be declined health insurance for having a "pre-existing health condition." These provisions allowed for better detection and management of chronic conditions [23, 42]. For example, many people in the US have diabetes mellitus and have benefited greatly from ACA policies. Patients with diabetes showed increased access to preventive care [19, 26, 43] and eye examinations [44], improved diabetes control [45, 46], and a reduction in diabetes expenditures [28, 47]. There has also been a steep decline in uninsurance rates among people with diabetes, and a higher percentage of people with undiagnosed diabetes is getting timely diagnosis and treatment [48]. And although the pre-existing condition protection applied to all adults, evidence shows better outcomes in states that expanded Medicaid. For example, one study found that people with chronic conditions reported better self-assessed health post-ACA than pre-ACA but only in states that had expanded Medicaid [49].

Behavioral and Mental Health

It is estimated that one in four adults in the US live with mental illness [50]. The ACA mandated behavioral health, mental health, and substance abuse services as essential health benefits [51], increasing parity in insurance coverage and prohibiting caps on annual and lifetime benefits, removing cost barriers. Following the ACA, there was an improvement in insurance access [52], diagnosis [23, 53], treatment [54], and reduction in cost barriers for adults with mental illness [52]. Additionally, since the implementation of the ACA, community health centers, who care for all patients regardless of health insurance and ability to pay, have progressively increased the delivery of behavioral and mental health services, with more than 98% offering services [55], facilitating access for socioeconomically disadvantaged adults. A limited number of studies showed greater improvement in insurance coverage among patients with mental illness in Medicaid expansion states than in non-expansion states but did not observe an increase in treatment [56, 57]. One study noted positive changes in Medicaid expansion with regards to mental illness treatment facilities [57]. Despite these improvements, access to mental health care remains limited, especially in states that did not expand Medicaid, by mental health provider shortage and lower reimbursement or restricted access to certain services (i.e., inpatient services) [58, 59].

Substance Use Disorder Treatment

Access to substance use disorder services was also improved as a result of the ACA reforms [60]. Evidence has shown increased rates of opioid treatment [61–63], improvement in access to and admission in treatment facilities [64], an increase in timely diagnosis of substance use disorders [23], and a reduction in cost barriers to treatment [65]. A few studies compared outcomes in Medicaid expansion versus non-expansion states [57, 66, 67]. One study, in particular, found a greater reduction in opioid-related deaths in Medicaid expansion states relative to non-expansion states [66]. Others noted a reduction in racial disparities with regard to access for medication for opioid use disorder in Medicaid expansion states [66].

The ACA's Impact on Supporting and Expanding the Safety Net's Capacity

In addition to improving patients' access to insurance, health care, and health outcomes, the ACA led to an expansion in the number of safety net clinics receiving federal support, especially federally qualified health centers (FQHCs) and other community health centers (CHCs) such as rural health clinics (RHCs) and other types of safety net clinics—collectively referred to as CHCs thereafter. These CHCs serve over 30 million people, including 10% of the nation's children and adolescents, 14% of the US population who identify as racial and ethnic minorities, 16% of all Medicaid beneficiaries, 20% of uninsured individuals, and 33% of people living in poverty in the US [55]. Moreover, they serve nearly 400,000 veterans, 1.3 million people experiencing homelessness, 1 million agricultural workers, and 7.4 million people preferring a language other than English. In some regions, CHCs are the only providers of primary and preventive care services for underserved rural and urban populations. The disappearance of CHCs from any region of the country would eliminate services and/or worsen access for many people.

CHCs have been in place since 1965 when the US Office of Economic Opportunity created the Neighborhood Health Center Program from which CHCs are descendants [68, 69]. Today's health centers include CHCs funded in part by the US Health Resources and Services Administration (HRSA), health center look-alikes not receiving HRSA funding, and rural health clinics [70]. All health centers provide primary care services to improve the health of underserved populations [71]. They are differentiated based on their designations and certifications (i.e., HRSA Section

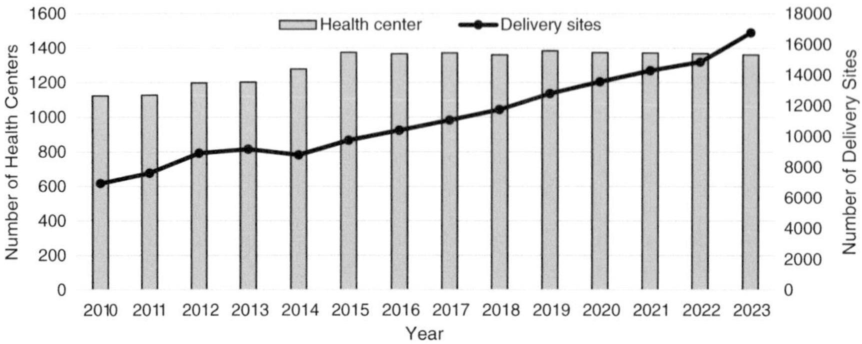

Fig. 13.4 Number of health centers and delivery sites in the United States, 2010–2023. (Source: National health center program Uniform Data System awardee data [74])

330 authorization or Centers for Medicare and Medicaid certification). CHCs are required to provide services to everyone, regardless of insurance status or ability to pay out of pocket [72]. The number of CHCs increased significantly over time (Fig. 13.4) from more than 100 health centers supported by the Neighborhood Health Center Program in 1972 [73], to over 1300 CHCs across the US, operating more than 16,000 delivery sites in 2024 [74]. CHC delivery sites are in a variety of settings including on urban and rural tribal lands and in other urban and rural sites.

The ACA provisions to support the operations of CHCs were important because these centers do not operate in highly profitable health care segments and their revenue is directly affected by government policies that increase or decrease insurance coverage (or lack of), care utilization, and reimbursement rates. To cover the cost of care, clinics who deliver care to uninsured patients receive limited reimbursements dependent on awarded block grants. Recognizing that insurance payments do not cover the operating costs of CHCs, additional funding was needed for these clinics to be able to continue to serve uninsured patients and expand their health care services (e.g., mental health services) to align with the ACA reforms. As a result, the ACA provided $9.5 billion as part of the Community Health Center Fund (CHCF) to increase support for operating costs between 2011 and 2015, accounting for 70% of CHCs' total funding [75].

Overall, sources of revenue for these CHCs include payments from payors (Medicaid, Medicare, private insurance), federal funds, and out-of-pocket payments. Over half (Fig. 13.5) of patients served by CHCs have Medicaid insurance, as such Medicaid funding plays an important role in CHCs' ability to continue to serve their patients and to expand their services. Medicaid expansion under the ACA led to increased revenue for CHCs in states that expanded their Medicaid programs, as patients who had previously been uninsured now had insurance coverage that provided more robust funding and payment for CHC services. The increased revenue and financial security [76–78] from the ACA led to CHCs being able to expand their reach in medically underserved areas [79], (especially in urban areas), add services (e.g., treatment for opioid use disorder, dental care) [80], increase

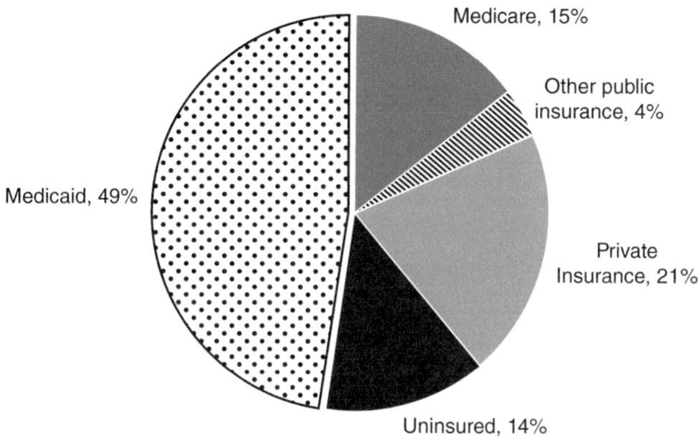

Fig. 13.5 Community health centers payor mix, 2023. (Source: National health center program Uniform Data System awardee data [74])

capacity (e.g., more staff, mental health providers), add capacity for social services, and improve quality of care [81]. Thus, the support from the ACA, especially Medicaid expansion, had a significantly positive impact on these safety net clinics.

Efforts to Strengthen or Weaken the ACA's Impact

Since the passage of the ACA, subsequent litigation and policymaking decisions have affected the impact of the legislation. In this section, we will outline some areas of discourse.

Pregnancy Care and Vaccinations

Since the implementation of the ACA, related policies have been implemented to improve maternal care and vaccinations. Pregnant individuals are typically eligible for Medicaid while pregnant and 60 days postpartum. In states that did not expand Medicaid eligibility following the ACA, pregnancy is often a qualifying condition for coverage; however, many individuals lose coverage 60 days postpartum, which disproportionally impacts BIPOC communities [82, 83]. Congress allowed states to increase this coverage to 12 months postpartum in April 2022, regardless of expansion status [84]. As of January 17, 2025, 49 states had or were in the process of expanding postpartum coverage to 12 months to eligible beneficiaries [85]. This extended coverage period is critical to ensure continuous coverage at a time when new mothers are at increased risk for cardiovascular mortality [86]. Effective October 1, 2023, as part of the Inflation Reduction Act (IRA, Section 11405) [87], all ACIP (Advisory Committee on Immunization Practices) [88] recommended vaccines must be covered at no cost to the beneficiaries by all Medicaid programs [89].

Although all states are mandated to provide no-cost vaccines, states can choose who can offer these vaccines (e.g., pharmacists) and the reimbursement level for the services, opening the door for state variations and health disparities [90].

Demonstration Waivers

Various state-based innovation and demonstration waivers (Section 1332, Section 1115) have been granted by the US Centers for Medicare and Medicaid Services (CMS) and implemented in specific states. These programs or projects are approved (or denied) through a process by which individual states apply and are granted waivers from certain federal insurance requirements. These are approved by CMS if they provide coverage and cost-sharing that is equivalent or better than the coverage that would be provided without the waiver.

Section 1332 waivers allow states to implement innovative strategies aimed at controlling insurance premium costs [91]. Similarly, Section 1115 demonstration projects waive specific rules about Medicaid provision to benefit beneficiaries' health services and access [92]. These demonstration projects can target specific populations (e.g., elderly, people with disabilities, children), cost reduction, services, technology, and more. For example, an approved demonstration project in Nevada will provide limited dental benefits to non-pregnant adults with diabetes [93]. This project will increase access to dental care to this specific subgroup of Medicaid recipients.

Executive Orders and Litigation

In 2024, the administration updated a 2022 executive order [84] to improve continuous coverage [94], remove enrollment barriers for children, and mitigate state operating and processing variations [94]. A few examples of other, smaller in scope, litigations to strengthen the ACA included extending the time of open enrollment for Marketplace insurance (American Rescue Plan Act of 2021; Public Law 117-2) or simplifying the enrollment application processes. There was also legislation specific to the COVID-19 pandemic (discussed in Part 2) [95, 96].

Additionally, there have been thousands [97] of legal challenges to the ACA at all levels of government, and each state has created policies to implement ACA-supported policies and programs differently. Some judicial decisions and other policies have weakened the ACA. One such decision impacted Medicaid eligibility expansion to adults with lower income. The original ACA legislation included a provision that states choosing not to expand Medicaid would lose their Medicaid funding. This portion of the law was contested as unconstitutional, and the US Supreme Court (June 28, 2012) voted to make Medicaid expansion optional for states. This Supreme Court decision also specified that if a state decided to expand, they must follow all the rules regarding expansion.

Another major effort to weaken the ACA focused on removal of the individual mandate. The individual mandate required all eligible individuals to have health insurance or incur a tax penalty unless eligible for an exemption. The main objectives of this mandate were to (1) ensure access to health insurance and (2) control the cost of insurance premiums by including healthy individuals. This mandate was challenged as unconstitutional early on, but the Supreme Court ruled it constitutional. As part of the Tax Cuts and Jobs Act (2017), the tax penalty related to the individual mandate was eliminated in 2019, essentially repealing the mandate. Studies have shown that "repealing" the mandate did not impact enrollment but was predicted to increase premium costs for some plans [98].

Additional policies implemented between 2017 and 2020 weakened the ACA, such as cessation of subsidies (2017) to insurers to encourage them to remain in the insurance exchange and control premium costs; allowing less comprehensive short-term plans (2019); reduced funding for health insurance navigators (2018) and shortening enrollment periods; and allowing states to implement work requirements for Medicaid [99]. Work requirements were approved in 13 states during the Trump Administration under Section 1115 waivers [100]. Strict work requirements coupled with complicated and burdensome reporting requirements led to loss of coverage for many beneficiaries in these states [101]. The Biden Administration withdrew Section 1115 work requirement waivers in February 2021.

Legal challenges to the ACA continue, such as the effort to remove the no-cost coverage for preventive services [102]. *Braidwood Management v Becerra* is a legal challenge to the ACA's requirement that insurers cover preventive benefits without cost sharing [102]. If this challenge is successful, all insured individuals will lose free preventive benefits as a basic coverage guarantee, including over 231 million children and adults (150 million with private insurance, 20 million with Medicaid, and 61 million with Medicare) [37]. If cost sharing is required for preventive care, it is likely that fewer people will seek evidence-based preventive care resulting in increased rates of morbidity and mortality from preventable conditions [103], and patients in low-income areas will be most affected [104]. Removing this access to free preventive services and the resulting drop in screenings could be devastating, as evidenced by what happened after the decline in receipt of preventive services in early 2020. Specifically, the temporary decline in receipt of preventive services (such as cancer screening) early in the COVID-19 pandemic has led to an estimated 10,000 excess deaths [105] from breast and colorectal cancers; removing access to free preventive services could similarly lead to higher rates of preventable morbidity and mortality.

Policymaking in Health Care Has Been Unstable and Unpredictable

Unfortunately, policymaking in health care has been tumultuous due to the contentious backdrop of American democracy. Section 1115 waivers have been used to strengthen and weaken the ACA and to reflect divergent beliefs about the role of government in creating a social safety net. For example, Section 1115 waivers allowing Medicaid work requirements were put in place during President Trump's first term and later rescinded under President Biden.

Congressional leadership changes also impact the availability of funding for programs that support socioeconomically disadvantaged individuals, such as safety net clinics. The ACA implemented the CHCF that needs regular re-appropriation (initial 5 years and then varying). Congress has delayed these funds several times (2015, 2018) causing financial difficulties for safety net clinics, resulting in layoffs, location closures, and limiting access to and delivery of services [106]. Fortunately, these funds were reauthorized in December 2019 until 2023, as delays in funding prior to the pandemic could have weakened these vital services just prior to the massive needs of patients during the pandemic. The funds were reauthorized in 2024 up to 2025; however, availability of the funds is dependent on the government operating and would be unavailable in a shutdown. Fluctuation and uncertainty in the renewal of CHC funds over time has been and will continue to be challenging and can lead to clinics closing, reduction in or limited staff capacity, and loss of access for patients [107].

The ongoing policy changes and unpredictable funding appropriations can be challenging for primary care clinics to deliver care and for patients to continue receiving reliable and timely care. During the early years of the pandemic, these processes became even more chaotic as many decisions needed to be made and hastily implemented to respond to the national public health emergency and how it impacted local communities across the country.

Part 2—The COVID-19 Pandemic (Feb 2020–May 10, 2023)

The COVID-19 pandemic tested American democratic institutions—broad policies were developed to mitigate the impacts of unemployment and uninsurance, increase telehealth use, and increase access to medications. In this section, we will discuss some of these policies. Specific policies related to COVID-19 surveillance and treatment are out of the scope of this chapter but are covered in more details throughout the book.

The Need for Unemployment Payments Drastically Increased

To reduce the spread of the COVID-19 virus, state and local governments took many actions (e.g., closing schools, mandating social distancing, issuing stay-at-home orders), which contributed to many people losing their jobs and an abrupt rise in unemployment rates. The number of unemployment claims in the US surged early in the pandemic to levels not seen in 80 years (Fig. 13.6) [108]. Most of these claims were from temporary layoffs. Unemployment rates increased in nearly all sectors and for almost all occupations but were more significant in food preparation, personal care, and transportation services. In nearly all US states, unemployment rates doubled between 2019 and 2020. In 2019, unemployment rates varied from

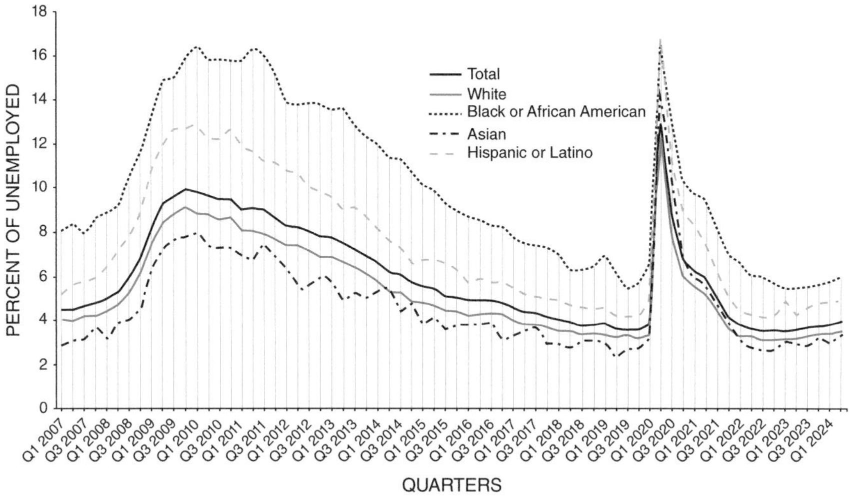

Fig. 13.6 US unemployment rate by race and ethnicity, 2007–2014. (Source: US Bureau of Labor Statistics [111])

≤2.5% (VT, HI, UT, ND) to ≥5% (WV, NM, MS, DC, AK). In 2020, unemployment rates varied from 4.2% (SD) to ≥10% (MI, CA, HI, NV) [109]. Women were more impacted by unemployment than men during the pandemic, and this was particularly true for single mothers as most schools transitioned to online learning in a virtual environment and childcare was extremely limited. Job loss was also more frequent among racial and ethnic minorities, those with less education, and younger adults [110].

To reduce economic hardship, federal and state policy makers expanded unemployment insurance via the Pandemic Unemployment Assistance (PUA) and the Pandemic Emergency Unemployment Compensation (PEUC) [112]. Unemployment insurance was created in 1935 and temporarily (usually for a maximum of 26 weeks) provides a portion of laid-off workers' wages while they are looking for work [113]. During the pandemic, PUA provided temporary benefits to workers who lost work due to COVID-19 related disruptions [114, 115]. These disruptions could include care giving, childcare due to school closure, and temporary or permanent job loss due to COVID-19 state/federal restrictions. The PEUC extended the benefit length of unemployment insurance to 53 weeks. Unemployment insurance was not equally distributed [116, 117]. Although workers in low-wage jobs were more likely to become unemployed and are disproportionately women, Black, and Hispanic workers, the demographics of those who received unemployment benefits did not reflect those who were most likely to be unemployed [118]. In fact, Black and Hispanic workers were less likely to have received unemployment insurance following job loss compared to White workers [115]. One study found that 34% of Black and 33% of Hispanic workers received unemployment insurance and pandemic-related supplements (e.g., Federal Pandemic Unemployment Compensation) compared to 53% of White workers [115]. Similarly, women were less likely to receive unemployment insurance than men [119].

People Needed Access to Health Insurance Coverage, Expanded Coverage Options, and Consistent Coverage.

For many people, loss of employment meant loss of health insurance coverage that was tied to that employment. Over half of laid-off workers lost health insurance [120]. One source reported that between 23% and 50% of employers continued to provide employer-sponsored insurance to laid-off employees (at least temporarily) [120]. Another source estimated that at least 7 million workers and their dependents lost coverage abruptly in the early months of the pandemic. It is important to note that collecting data during this time was challenging. For example, the 2020 American Community Survey, which reports yearly national uninsured rates, was not released due to data collection interruption. However, there are enough data available from this time to demonstrate that major shifts in employment and health insurance coverage took place over a very short timeframe.

During the pandemic, following the Coronavirus Preparedness and Response Supplemental Appropriations Act [121] and the Coronavirus Aid, Relief, and Economic Security Act (2020) [96], CMS and private insurers implemented various waivers and amendments to facilitate continuous enrollment (1135 waiver), the capacity of health care facilities (1135 waiver), reimbursement for telehealth and virtual visits, and prescription early refill and waiver of fill limits. These actions also removed barriers to COVID-19 testing and treatment. The goal of these waivers was to improve patients' health outcomes while also reducing virus exposure and supporting strained health care facilities.

Health Insurance Coverage Options

People who abruptly lost employer-sponsored health insurance coverage could enroll in Medicaid or Marketplace insurance programs. Those in Medicaid expansion states were less likely to remain uninsured and more likely to gain Medicaid (Fig. 13.7), as compared to those who lost employer-sponsored coverage in non-expansion states [122]. Between December 2019 and December 2022, Medicaid saw an increase of 23 million enrollees (a 30% increase). Similarly, people not eligible for Medicaid could enroll in Marketplace insurance [123]. Early in the pandemic, most of the state-based Marketplace programs expanded enrollment periods to facilitate access to people who lost health insurance. In 2021, Federally-facilitated Marketplaces also extended their enrollment periods [124]. The American Rescue Plan Act of March 2021 raised the premium subsidies for Marketplace enrollees for

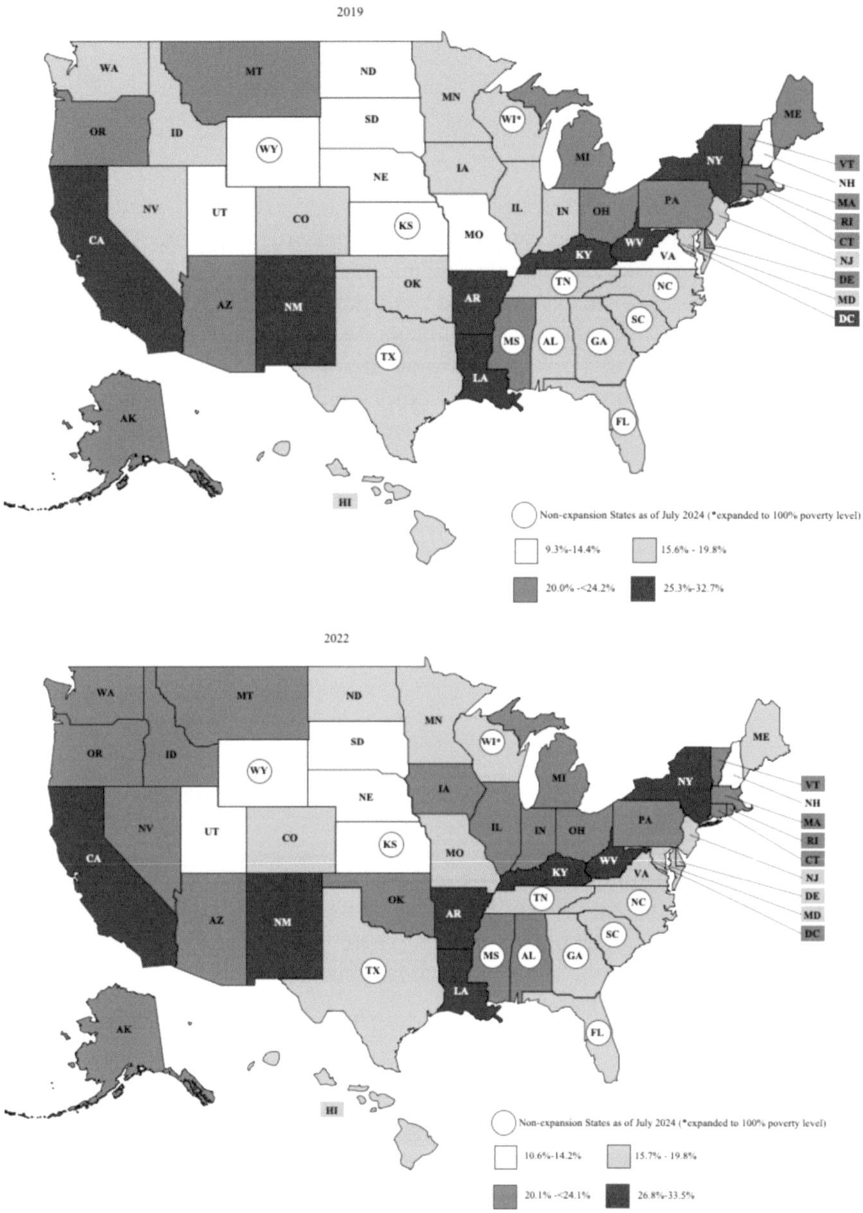

Fig. 13.7 Percent of population with Medicaid insurance in 2019 and 2022 by state. (Source: Health Insurance Coverage of the Total Population, KFF. https://www.kff.org/other/state-indicator/totalpopulation/?activeTab=map&currentTimeframe=1&selectedDistributions=employer&sortModel=%7B"colId":"Location","sort":"asc"%7D-notes. Reprinted with permission [127].)

2 years and for those receiving unemployment insurance for 1 year [125], Between December 2019 and 2022, Marketplace enrollment increased by 3 million (30%) [126].

Continuous Coverage

In March 2020, as part of the Families First Coronavirus Response Act (FFCRA) [95], states were provided additional funding for their Medicaid programs if they allowed beneficiaries to remain enrolled until the end of the public health emergency—referred to as continuous enrollment. Medicaid enrollment rates significantly increased during this period due to new eligibility for millions of unemployed individuals and continuous enrollment from 71 million to 84 million in January 2024 (Fig. 13.8). Evidence shows greater increase in states that expanded Medicaid (Fig. 13.7) [128]. Moreover, Hispanic, Asian, Native Hawaiian and Pacific Islander groups showed greater increases in enrollment between 2019 and 2022 (Fig. 13.9) compared to other race and ethnic groups. Similarly, the percentage of Medicaid enrollment by males increased more than by females (Fig. 13.9).

In addition to policies that expanded unemployment payments and facilitated health insurance coverage access, state and federal policies were implemented to ensure continuous access to health care, including access to remote care, and medications.

Consistent Access to Care

Accessing care in traditional ways was not possible for many people and not safe due to the need to maintain social distancing. Thus, care was interrupted for many people who receive it on a consistent basis. There was a need to create innovative modes of virtual care delivery and adequate reimbursement for that care.

Telehealth Flexibilities

At the onset of the pandemic, stay-at-home, social distancing orders, and recommendations to keep patients out of health care facilities to reduce viral spread led to rapid adoption and widespread use of telehealth [131, 132]. The use of video and phone visits rapidly grew by >600% over a 6-week period, as shown in Fig. 13.10. Pre-COVID reimbursement policies and payment rates for services provided via telehealth were inconsistent and insufficient to support the professionals providing the services [133]. Further, some of the technologies and associated privacy regulations were still in development, which limited the use of telehealth. The public health emergency prompted several federal and state-based actions to quickly put into place telehealth use, privacy, and reimbursement rules and regulations to allow

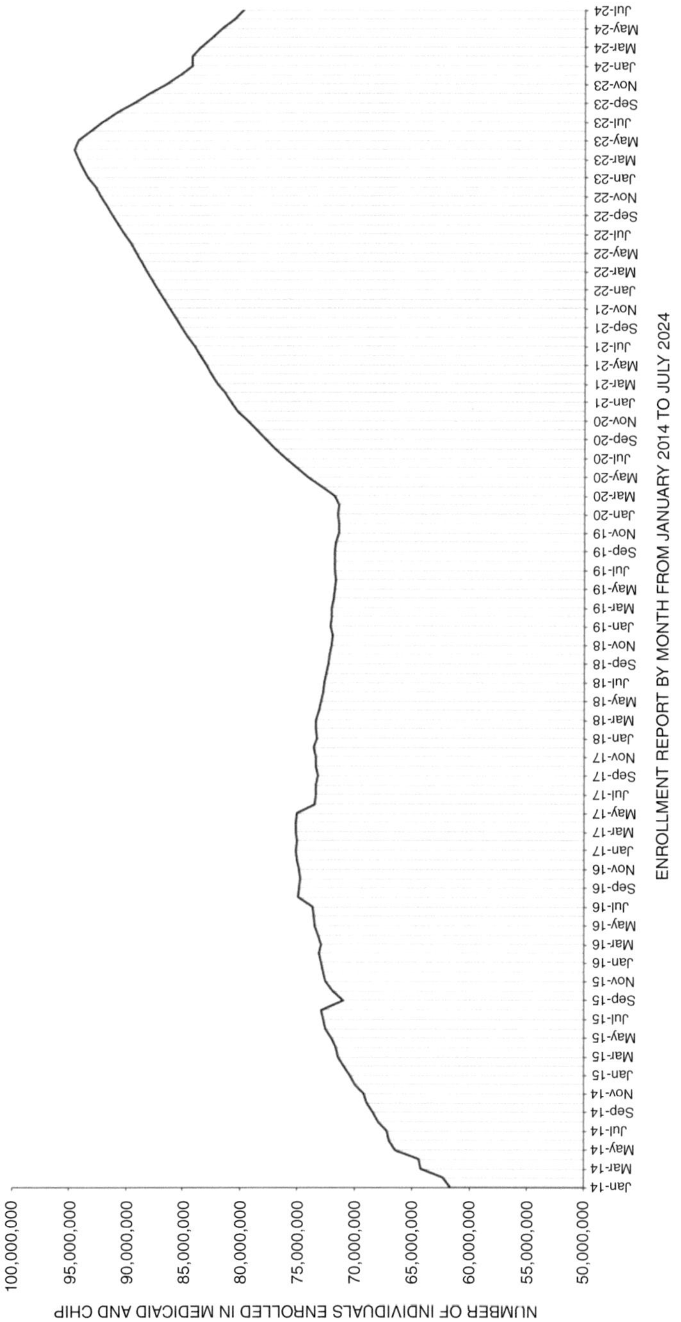

Fig. 13.8 Medicaid and CHIP enrollment, January 2014-January 2024. (Source: Centers for Medicare and Medicaid enrollment [129])

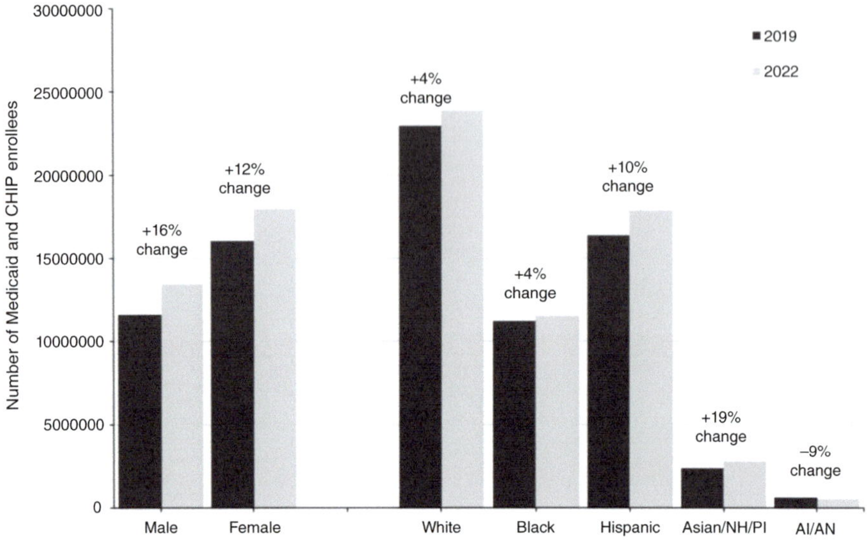

Fig. 13.9 Medicaid enrollment by race and ethnicity and by sex in 2019 and 2022. (Note: NH/PI: Native Hawaiian and Pacific Islander; AI/AN: American Indian/Alaska Natives. Source: Health Coverage & Uninsured Indicators, KFF https://www.kff.org/state-category/health-coverage-uninsured/nonelderly-with-medicaid/. Reprinted with permission [130].)

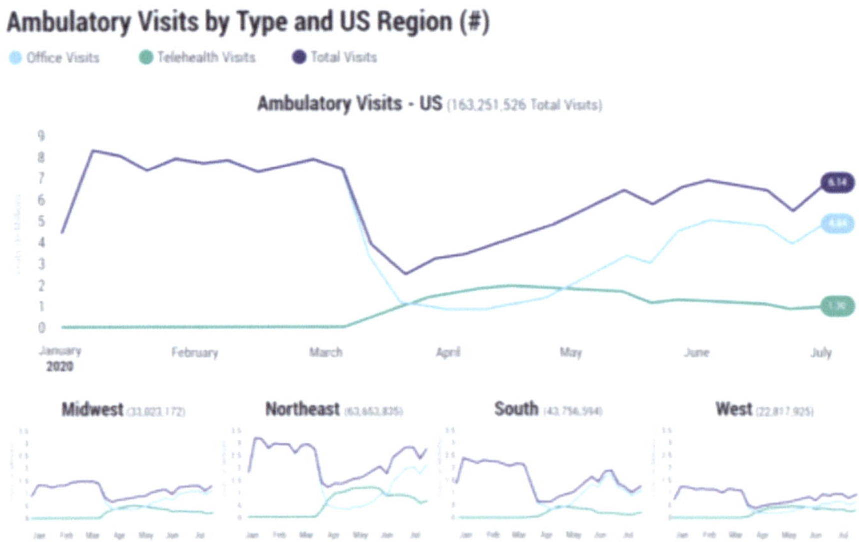

Fig. 13.10 Ambulatory Visits by Type and US Region (%). (Source: Fox B and Sizemore JO, "Telehealth: Fad or the Future," Epic Research, 2020 (available at https://www.epicresearch.org/articles/telehealth-fad-or-the-future). Reprinted with permission.)

for and facilitate the rapid increase in telehealth that was needed. Some of the specific changes were essential to promote equitable care, including parity in reimbursement between telehealth and in-person visits, allowance of and equal reimbursement for telephone visits and, permitting telehealth for a wide range of services (e.g., mental and behavioral health). The rapid uptick in telehealth care enabled researchers to better understand its advantages and disadvantages. Telehealth is discussed in greater detail in Chapter 9.

Advantages Studies have noted that telehealth reduced some health care access disparities by mitigating barriers to care such as transportation, childcare, or sick leave access [134–137]. Many patients appreciated the convenience of telehealth [136, 138–140] and reported being satisfied with this medium of care [141]. Studies also found that telehealth likely opened up new avenues for patients without a primary care physician [135] and those without health insurance [136] as both underserved subgroups were more likely to choose telehealth than their counterparts. For some, telehealth also facilitated medication management and reduced referral wait times [142]. Enhancements made to enable telehealth visits also bolstered many health care systems' patient portals, and communication with clinicians via patient portals also increased substantially [143].

Disadvantages Access to the internet, especially high-speed internet, is critical to use telehealth and patient portal platforms to access care [144]. Access to the technology required to successfully participate in telehealth visits is not universal and limited or no access to these technological capabilities was more likely to negatively impact use and the quality of telehealth care received by low-income people [145, 146]. Use of the phone for health care, though better than no care, is limited by audio interaction [144] and reimbursed at a lower rate than video visits. Patients in rural areas, older adults, racial and ethnic minority populations, and those with low socioeconomic status experienced greater barriers (e.g., poor quality or no broadband) to telehealth use than their counterparts [147, 148]. Nonetheless, regulatory changes during the pandemic, especially to state-based Medicaid telehealth policy, were essential to allow audio-only (telephone) visits and reimbursement at equal rates and to facilitate access to those with limited broadband or technology access.

Medication access

The need for social distancing also impacted access to prescription refills, particularly for patients with Medicaid coverage. Policy changes related to the public health emergency allowed patients to more easily receive their medications. For example, prior to these changes, Medicaid prescription dispensing and refills were limited to 1-month supply for most medications with some exceptions that allowed for a 90-day supply for a few medication types [149]. In contrast, many commercial insurers authorize 90-day supplies for nearly all regular medication prescriptions. During the pandemic, some states opted to amend their Medicaid programs and

Table 13.1 State-based policy changes that were made to increase medication access during the COVID-19 pandemic [150]

Actions taken	Action taken under Approved Disaster-Relief State Plan Amendments to Address COVID-19 and/or Other State-Reported Actions
Waive or extend prior authorization requirements	AK, AR, AZ, CA, CO, DC, DE, GA, IL, IN, KS, KY, LA, MA, ME, MI, MO, MT, NC, ND, NH, NJ, NY, OH, OK, OR, RI, SD, TN, TX,WI
Exceptions and changes to preferred drug list	AK, AR, AZ, CO, DC, DE, FL, GA, IL, IN, KS, KY, LA, MA, ME, MO, MT, NC, ND, OR, PA, TX, RI, VA, VT, WA, WI, WV
Allow early refills for most medications	AK, AL, AR, AZ, CA, CO, CT, DC, DE, FL, GA, IA, IL, IN, KS, KY, LA, MA, MD, ME, MI, MN, MT, NC, ND, NJ, OH, OK, OR, PA, RI, SD, TN, TX, UT, VA, VT, WI, WV
Increase maximum supply or quantity limit of certain medications	AK, AL, AR, AZ, CA, CO, CT, DC, DE, FL, GA, IA, IL, IN, KS, KY, LA, MA, MD, ME, MI, MN, MT, NC, ND, NJ, NM, NY, OH, OK, OR, PA, RI, SD, TN, TX, VA, VT, WI, WV
Eliminate cost-sharing for medications	IA, IN, LA, MA, ME, MO, NE, OH
Add temporary supplemental payment to the professional dispensing fee for costs of delivery of medication	AK, KS, MA, NC, NM

This table reflects actions up to 7/1/2021
Medicaid Emergency Authority Tracker: Approved State Actions to Address COVID-19
KFF, 2021. https://www.kff.org/medicaid/issue-brief/medicaid-emergency-authority-tracker-approved-state-actions-to-address-covid-19/. Reprinted with permission

facilitate enhanced access to prescription medications. Another example of a beneficial change was a pause placed on requiring prior authorization to fill certain medications. Table 13.1 summarizes many of the state-based changes made to increase access to medications.

Workforce Scope

To enable the delivery of critical services to people in need, several policies were amended to expand the scope of many health care professionals. For example, pharmacists were granted expanded licenses to give immunizations in states that had previously not allowed them to do so [151]. This expanded scope was critical to enable COVID-19 vaccinations to reach millions of people as retail pharmacies are more accessible to some people, especially in rural areas, and some of them have longer hours of operation. Moreover, in response to the need for broadening access to COVID-19 vaccines, the federal government partnered with 21 large retail pharmacies (e.g., Walgreens, CVS) representing more than 41,000 locations nationwide, under the Federal Retail Pharmacy Program to provide access to the COVID-19 vaccine in the community. By August 2023, over 300 million doses of COVID-19 vaccines were administered by community pharmacists [152, 153]. In addition, prior to the pandemic, scope of practice for nurse practitioners varied by state, with some allowing full practice ($n = 23$) and others imposing restrictions such as physician supervision [154]. The scope of practice for nurse practitioners was temporarily broadened in all states which expanded access to care in medically underserved and health professional shortage areas. Expanding the scope of practice for pharmacists and nurse practitioners was beneficial to serving the needs of communities and did not have an adverse impact on patient safety [155, 156].

With the end of the public health emergency, some of these pandemic-related policy changes are being de-implemented, while others are being scaled down, impacting clinics' ability to care for their patients and patients' ability to get continuous care.

Part 3—After the Federal Public Health Emergency Ended (Post-MAY 11, 2023)

Although there is no clear "end date" to mark the end of the COVID-19 pandemic, for the purposes of this chapter, we describe the beginning of the "post pandemic" period as the date the federal public health emergency was lifted. The end of the public health emergency, on May 11, 2023, marked the expiration date of many temporary policies implemented in the early months of the pandemic. Even prior to this official end date, federal legislation enacted late in 2022 ordered an unwinding of policies, such as those in the Families First Coronavirus Response Act. The repeal of several policies has led to increased uninsurance rates and churn, reductions in telehealth utilization, and return to restrictions on health care professional scope of practice.

Higher Rates of Insurance Coverage Instability

A major protection of Families First Coronavirus Response Act ensured that Medicaid beneficiaries who experienced changes in family income or life circumstances could remain continuously enrolled without risk of coverage loss and not churn off coverage [157]. Without this protection, large-scale coverage losses began in April 2023 with over 25 million children and adults losing insurance coverage by September 2024 [158]. Data suggest that one in five Medicaid beneficiaries (1 in 10 children) were disenrolled and that 23% remain uninsured [159]. Fortunately, nearly half of those disenrolled (47%) were able to re-enroll in Medicaid and 16% enrolled in employer-sponsored insurance. However, less than 10% enrolled in a Marketplace plan [159]. Despite having these other insurance types, most (>60%) of those disenrolled beneficiaries report financial difficulties associated with monthly premiums and out-of-pocket costs [159]. The impact was especially severe in the Medicaid non-expansion states, as people who lost coverage, such as young adults and postpartum women, had no affordable coverage options [159]. Patients impacted by the disenrollment face loss of continuity of care, which has been associated with increased utilization of preventive care, fewer ED or hospitalizations, and lower health care expenditures [160]. Medicaid disenrollment is particularly challenging for CHCs caring for a large proportion of Medicaid beneficiaries [161, 162]. These clinics are losing significant revenue while expanding staff resources to assist patients with re-enrollment and in securing other insurance coverage [55]. Moreover, 23% of these CHCs report reducing staff, services, and appointments to account for the losses.

Limited or no Access to Telehealth Care Options

Although many of the pandemic-driven changes (e.g., reimbursement parity, remote patient monitoring, online prescribing) remain available, the federal government and many state governments have repealed or altered these policy changes which had facilitated enhanced access to telehealth care [163]. As a result, millions of people in the US lost access to comprehensive telehealth care.

Telephone visits, for example, are regulated by a patchwork of policies that vary across the country. This is important because evidence shows that socioeconomically disadvantaged patients, racial and ethnic minorities, older adults, those living in rural areas, and those with Medicaid coverage used telephone visits more frequently than video visits [164–166]. Unfortunately, concerns about quality of care, fraud, and misuse have led to telephone visits being regulated differently than other types of telehealth. For example, although video visits are available in all states, reimbursements vary by state based on services provided, health care provider eligibility to provide the service, and location of the patients [167]. Telephone visits are reimbursed in varying capacity in 43 Medicaid state programs and in DC, with some states only reimbursing telephone visits occurring in underserved or rural areas. In addition, many states (43+DC) have some regulations or laws governing private insurance related to telehealth reimbursement.

The patchwork of regulations also creates complexity for billing entities such as CHCs, who may not be eligible to bill for some services. CMS does not allow FQHCs or RHCs (who seek reimbursement as organizations, not individual providers) to bill as distant site providers (delivering services from a remote location), while 39 state Medicaid programs do. The variability, complexity, and changing nature of state regulations specific to telehealth reimbursement may perpetuate racial, ethnic, geographic, and socioeconomic disparities in access to care.

Workforce Scope Reduction and Shortages

As noted above, expanding the scope of practice for pharmacists and nurse practitioners was beneficial to serve communities, especially in medically underserved areas. Repeal of these expanded authorities upends gains in health care system capacity, which has been accelerated by higher rates of health professionals leaving the workforce prior to retirement age due to burnout and turnover [168–171]. Notably, although expanding the scope of practice was beneficial to improve access in underserved areas, it also led to increased workload and burnout [172, 173], which is compounding workforce shortages. Job vacancies in the health care workforce have increased substantially since the start of the pandemic; for example, vacancies for nurses have increased by 18% to 30% [174]. Workforce shortages in rural areas can have dramatic effects on the community leading to hospital closure, limited availability of services (e.g., obstetrical care), and delayed care [175]. These workforce shortages have been associated with poor patient health outcomes, such as pregnancy and childbirth adverse outcomes and mortality [176, 177]. Compounding this crisis is the fact that communities of color are more likely to live in rural areas, exacerbating health inequities [178]. It is estimated that by 2026, the health care system will face a shortage of 3.2 million health care workers.

In summary, post-pandemic changes to policies and waivers target access to health insurance, health services, and health care workforce scope and capacity. Regulations are continuing to change and vary widely across US states. These changes will contribute to inequities in access to care and health outcomes among underserved populations and perpetuate health inequities.

Part 4—Lessons Learned—Benefits, Harms, Recommendations

Promoting Continuous Access to Health Insurance

Facilitating access to health insurance via Medicaid or the Marketplace was critical for people with lower income who lost their jobs during the pandemic. As of summer 2024, no studies have evaluated whether the protections to ensure continuous Medicaid coverage enabled timely access to health care, especially primary care and preventive care, and/or limited ED use and preventable hospitalizations, reduced disparities, and reduced insurance gaps. However, we can suspect that continuous enrollment facilitated access to care, promoted positive health outcomes, and reduced health disparities based on the evidence from the ACA implementation described in Part 1.

These policies allowed for the uninsured rate to drop by 18% during the pandemic [179]. Importantly, there is evidence that expanding Medicaid benefits helped strengthen state economies via enhanced federal funding, offsetting costs in other areas (e.g., mental health care), and reducing mortality [180]. Thus, avoiding insurance gaps and facilitating Medicaid eligibility expansion is beneficial to state economies.

Undeniably, the rise in insurance enrollment during the pandemic was associated with increased federal spending by $137 billion for new Medicaid enrollees and further increases due to premium tax credits (estimated at $35.5 billion). However, to put this in perspective, the estimated federal cost of other pandemic-era assistance such as the recovery rebates was $413.6 billion [181]. Importantly, the cost to states for new Medicaid enrollees was absorbed by the federal government [182]. Also notable is that the percent change in total Medicaid expenditures during 2020–2023 was lower or equal to the percent change in enrollees; suggesting that new enrollees did not overuse or incur large expenditures. Previous studies assessing changes in Medicaid expenditures following the ACA expansion, found similar results [28, 29, 183]. It is unknown what cost is or has been associated with the post-pandemic disenrollment. *We recommend* that federal and state policies facilitate continuous enrollment such as developing systems to streamline enrollment and eligibility determination. Moreover, ACA-related Medicaid expansion is shown to be a success without overexpanding state financial resources. *We recommend* that all states expand Medicaid coverage to support low-income adults, without imposing burdensome provisions such as work requirement reporting. Further, several states have expanded eligibility regardless of citizenship status to promote health care for all. Lessons from the ACA Medicaid expansion suggest that such eligibility expansion will benefit the overall population health of the state. *We recommend* that states broaden their eligibility criteria to encompass all individuals and reduce disparities in access.

Facilitate Adoption of Telehealth

In addition to ensuring continuous access to health insurance, pandemic-era policies facilitated access to care via telehealth and augmented the scope of practice for various health care providers. Telehealth has become a standard of care. Emerging evidence shows that the quality of care received during a telehealth visit is equivalent to that of an in-person visit [184–187]. Notably, telehealth has been found to be cost saving for health care system expenditures and patient-related expenditures. Health care system savings included preventing costly care (e.g., ED visits) by facilitating access to needed care and reducing no-show rates [188–190]. Estimates suggest that CMS could save more than $1 billion per year in expenditures from telehealth services [191]. Telehealth also reduced health systems' carbon footprint, which could assist health systems that pledged to reduce their greenhouse gas emissions 50% by 2030 [192, 193]. Most importantly, telehealth reduces patient costs associated with receiving care such as travel expenses, missing work, and family expenses (e.g., childcare) [190, 194, 195]. These savings are particularly important for socioeconomically disadvantaged patients, women, and patients in rural areas [194]. Learnings from the pandemic suggest that telehealth is an effective modality to deliver care and reduce access disparities and health care expenditures. *We recommend* that federal policies be established to (1) standardize telehealth regulations across states; (2) include a comprehensive set of services; and (3) ensure parity of reimbursement for all services to all providers or organizations, including audio-only services.

Promote Efforts to Ensure an Adequate Health Care Workforce

The pandemic opened the door to expanding the scope of practice for certain providers without impeding the quality of care received but also led to a tsunami of health care workforce turnover and burnout leading to an unprecedented shortage. Shortages will have a compounding impact in rural areas who were already experiencing health care workforce shortages prior to the pandemic [196]. Strategies to address workforce shortages have been put forth [175, 196]. For instance, there have been calls to increase funding to support pipeline programs for rural care, relocation and retention of providers, provider incentives (e.g., student debt relief), and rural residency programs. Another example is to facilitate pathways to training (such as virtual programs) for underrepresented minorities and people with low incomes to advance their health care certifications (e.g., registered nurses becoming nurse practitioners). Learnings from the pandemic were two-fold. On the one hand, it showed that relaxing regulations limiting who can deliver what services improved access to needed care and could help address workforce shortages (e.g., pharmacists delivering vaccinations). On the other hand, it showed the toll of a system failing their workforce. The demand on underpaid health care workers, such as nurses and medical assistants, and the undervaluing of primary care clinicians led to alarming rates of burnout and turnover [197, 198]. *We recommend* the following: (1) a comprehensive review of the scope of practice be completed to expand service delivery, which could assist with workforce shortages; (2) efforts be accelerated to promote and facilitate an expansion of the health care workforce in specialties and areas of greatest need by providing financial incentives and increased availability of community-based residencies and curriculum; (3) alignment of federal and state funding (and ongoing accountability) with training benchmarks targeting the nation's needs (e.g., primary care, mental health care) and (4) narrow the salary gaps between providers in different specialties to not dissuade future graduates from entering specialties with the greatest needs (e.g., primary care, mental health care).

Conclusion

Even with all the emergency policy interventions, the COVID-19 public health crisis shortened life expectancy for people living in the US and occurred alongside other growing population health threats such as alarming rates of maternal mortality, a worsening opioid crisis, and increasing rates of mental health diagnoses [199]. This demonstrates the inadequacy of the US health care system prior to the pandemic and suggests the ongoing fragility of the safety net considering efforts to roll back many of the policy interventions that had positive impacts of reducing inequities and improving access to health insurance coverage and health care services for millions of people.

The removal of evidence-based policies that have been shown to improve health is analogous to removing a new life-saving medication from a person who needs it to survive. We cannot ignore lessons learned. Discoveries made during the pandemic cannot be undiscovered and should guide policies and regulation promoting continuous access to high-quality primary care for all.

Acknowledgment The authors would like to thank Ms. Kathryn Bonuck and Mr. Jeremy Erroba for their assistance with gathering public data and permission for reproduction of material.

Competing Interest The authors have no conflicts of interest to declare that are relevant to the content of this chapter.

References

1. Smith K. A (brief) history of health policy in the United States. Dela J Public Health. 2023;9(5):6–10. https://doi.org/10.32481/djph.2023.12.003.
2. Currie J, Chorniy A. Medicaid and child health insurance program improve child health and reduce poverty but face threats. Acad Pediatr. 2021;21(8S):S146–53. https://doi.org/10.1016/j.acap.2021.01.009.
3. Pollack Porter KM, Rutkow L, McGinty EE. The importance of policy change for addressing public health problems. Public Health Rep. 2018;133(1_suppl):9S–14S. https://doi.org/10.1177/0033354918788880.
4. US Congress. Patient Protection and Affordable Care Act. In: US Congress, editor. Public Law 111-1482010.
5. Keith K. Congress extends enhanced ACA subsidies. Health Aff (Millwood). 2022;41(11):1542–3. https://doi.org/10.1377/hlthaff.2022.01293.
6. Supreme Court of the United States. National Federation of Independent Business v Sebelius. 2012.
7. United States Census Bureau. Health Insurance Historical Tables – HHI Series. https://www.census.gov/data/tables/time-series/demo/health-insurance/historical-series/hic.html. Accessed 7 Aug 2024.
8. KFF. Key Facts about the Uninsured Population. https://www.kff.org/uninsured/issue-brief/key-facts-about-the-uninsured-population/. Accessed 12 Apr 2024.
9. Tolbert J, Rudowitz R, Damico A. How many uninsured are in the coverage gap and how many could be eligible if all states adopted the medicaid expansion? https://www.kff.org/

medicaid/issue-brief/how-many-uninsured-are-in-the-coverage-gap-and-how-many-could-be-eligible-if-all-states-adopted-the-medicaid-expansion/. Accessed 11 Nov 2024.

10. Sommers BD, Rosenbaum S. Issues in health reform: how changes in eligibility may move millions back and forth between medicaid and insurance exchanges. Health Aff (Millwood). 2011;30(2):228–36. https://doi.org/10.1377/hlthaff.2010.1000.
11. Ela EJ, Vizcarra E, Thaxton L, White K. Insurance churn and postpartum health among texas women with births covered by medicaid/CHIP. Womens Health Issues. 2022;32(2):95–102. https://doi.org/10.1016/j.whi.2021.11.002.
12. Kressin NR, Terrin N, Hanchate AD, et al. Is insurance instability associated with hypertension outcomes and does this vary by race/ethnicity? BMC Health Serv Res. 2020;20(1):216. https://doi.org/10.1186/s12913-020-05095-8.
13. Brown AGM, Kressin N, Terrin N, et al. The influence of health insurance stability on racial/ethnic differences in diabetes control and management. Ethn Dis Winter. 2021;31(1):149–58. https://doi.org/10.18865/ed.31.1.149.
14. Banerjee R, Ziegenfuss JY, Shah ND. Impact of discontinuity in health insurance on resource utilization. BMC Health Serv Res. 2010;10:195. https://doi.org/10.1186/1472-6963-10-195.
15. Albright BB, Chino F, Chino JP, Havrilesky LJ, Aviki EM, Moss HA. Associations of insurance churn and catastrophic health expenditures with implementation of the affordable care act among nonelderly patients with cancer in the United States. JAMA Netw Open. 2021;4(9):e2124280. https://doi.org/10.1001/jamanetworkopen.2021.24280.
16. Corallo BSM. Analysis of national trends in medicaid and CHIP enrollment during the COVID-19 pandemic. https://www.kff.org/coronavirus-covid-19/issue-brief/analysis-of-recent-national-trends-in-medicaid-and-chip-enrollment/. Accessed 12 Apr 2024.
17. Nelson DB, Goldman AL, Zhang F, Yu H. Continuous medicaid coverage during the COVID-19 public health emergency reduced churning, but did not eliminate it. Health Aff Sch. 2023;1(5) https://doi.org/10.1093/haschl/qxad055.
18. Angier H, Ezekiel-Herrera D, Marino M, et al. Racial/ethnic disparities in health insurance and differences in visit type for a population of patients with diabetes after medicaid expansion. J Health Care Poor Underserved. 2019;30(1):116–30. https://doi.org/10.1353/hpu.2019.0011.
19. Angier H, Hoopes M, Marino M, et al. Uninsured primary care visit disparities under the affordable care act. Ann Fam Med. 2017;15(5):434–42. https://doi.org/10.1370/afm.2125.
20. Bailey SR, Marino M, Ezekiel-Herrera D, et al. Tobacco cessation in affordable care act medicaid expansion states versus non-expansion states. Nicotine Tob Res. 2019; https://doi.org/10.1093/ntr/ntz087.
21. Holderness H, Angier H, Huguet N, et al. Where do oregon medicaid enrollees seek outpatient care post-affordable care act medicaid expansion? Med Care. 2019;57(10):788–94. https://doi.org/10.1097/MLR.0000000000001189.
22. Hoopes MJ, Angier H, Gold R, et al. Utilization of community health centers in medicaid expansion and nonexpansion states, 2013–2014. J Ambul Care Manage. 2016;39(4):290–8. https://doi.org/10.1097/JAC.0000000000000123.
23. Huguet N, Angier H, Hoopes MJ, et al. Prevalence of pre-existing conditions among community health center patients before and after the affordable care act. J Am Board Fam Med. 2019;32(6):883–9. https://doi.org/10.3122/jabfm.2019.06.190087.
24. Huguet N, Angier H, Rdesinski R, et al. Cervical and colorectal cancer screening prevalence before and after Affordable Care Act Medicaid expansion. Prev Med. 2019;124:91–7. https://doi.org/10.1016/j.ypmed.2019.05.003.
25. Huguet N, Hoopes MJ, Angier H, Marino M, Holderness H, DeVoe JE. Medicaid expansion produces long-term impact on insurance coverage rates in community health centers. J Prim Care Community Health. 2017;8(4):206–12. https://doi.org/10.1177/2150131917709403.
26. Huguet N, Springer R, Marino M, et al. The Impact of the Affordable Care Act (ACA) medicaid expansion on Visit Rates for Diabetes in Safety Net Health Centers. J Am Board Fam Med. 2018;31(6):905–16. https://doi.org/10.3122/jabfm.2018.06.180075.

27. Huguet N, Valenzuela S, Marino M, et al. Following uninsured patients through medicaid expansion: ambulatory care use and diagnosed conditions. Ann Fam Med. 2019;17(4):336–44. https://doi.org/10.1370/afm.2385.
28. Lindner SR, Marino M, O'Malley J, et al. Health care expenditures among adults with diabetes after Oregon's Medicaid Expansion. Diabetes Care. 2019; https://doi.org/10.2337/dc19-1343.
29. Springer R, Marino M, O'Malley JP, Lindner S, Huguet N, DeVoe JE. Oregon Medicaid Expenditures after the 2014 affordable care act medicaid expansion: over-time differences among new, returning, and continuously insured enrollees. Med Care. 2018;56(5):394–402. https://doi.org/10.1097/mlr.0000000000000907.
30. Tilhou AS, Huguet N, DeVoe J, Angier H. The affordable care act medicaid expansion positively impacted community health centers and their patients. J Gen Intern Med. 2020; https://doi.org/10.1007/s11606-019-05571-w.
31. Rudowitz RLL. Implications of the ACA medicaid expansion: a look at the data and evidence. The Henry Kaiser Family Foundation. https://www.kff.org/medicaid/issue-brief/implications-of-the-aca-medicaid-expansion-a-look-at-the-data-and-evidence/. Accessed 10 Jan 2020.
32. Ovsag K, Hydery S, Mousa SA. Preferred drug lists: potential impact on healthcare economics. Vasc Health Risk Manag. 2008;4(2):403–13. https://doi.org/10.2147/vhrm.s926.
33. Werble C. Health policy brief: formularie. Health Affairs. 2017; https://doi.org/10.1377/hpb20170914.000177.
34. Ross-Degnan D, Wallace J, Zhang F, Soumerai SB, Garabedian L, Wharam JF. Reduced cost-sharing for preventive drugs preferentially benefits low-income patients with diabetes in high deductible health plans with health savings accounts. Med Care. 2020;58(Suppl 6 1):S4–S13. https://doi.org/10.1097/MLR.0000000000001295.
35. Sinaiko AD, Ross-Degnan D, Wharam JF, et al. Utilization and spending with preventive drug lists for asthma medications in high-deductible health plans. JAMA Netw Open. 2023;6(8):e2331259. https://doi.org/10.1001/jamanetworkopen.2023.31259.
36. Maciosek MV, Coffield AB, Flottemesch TJ, Edwards NM, Solberg LI. Greater use of preventive services in U.S. health care could save lives at little or no cost. Health Aff (Millwood). 2010;29(9):1656–60. https://doi.org/10.1377/hlthaff.2008.0701.
37. Office of the Assistant Secretary for Planning and Evaluation. Access to Preventive Services without Cost-sharing: evidence from the Affordable Care Act 2022. https://aspe.hhs.gov/sites/default/files/documents/786fa55a84e7e3833961933124d70dd2/preventive-services-ib-2022.pdf
38. Norris HC, Richardson HM, Benoit MC, Shrosbree B, Smith JE, Fendrick AM. Utilization impact of cost-sharing elimination for preventive care services: a rapid review. Med Care Res Rev. 2022;79(2):175–97. https://doi.org/10.1177/10775587211027372.
39. Bloodworth R, Chen J, Mortensen K. Variation of preventive service utilization by state Medicaid coverage, cost-sharing, and Medicaid expansion status. Prev Med. 2018;115:97–103. https://doi.org/10.1016/j.ypmed.2018.08.020.
40. Reynolds GL, Fisher DG. The role of the medicaid expansion in the use of preventive health care services in California Men. Am J Mens Health. 2020;14(1):1557988320903193. https://doi.org/10.1177/1557988320903193.
41. Hatch B, Hoopes M, Darney BG, et al. Impacts of the affordable care act on receipt of women's preventive services in community health centers in medicaid expansion and nonexpansion states. Womens Health Issues. 2021;31(1):9–16. https://doi.org/10.1016/j.whi.2020.08.011.
42. Rosland AM, Kieffer EC, Tipirneni R, et al. Diagnosis and care of chronic health conditions among medicaid expansion enrollees: a mixed-methods observational study. J Gen Intern Med. 2019;34(11):2549–58. https://doi.org/10.1007/s11606-019-05323-w.
43. Ladapo JA, Chokshi DA. Changes in cardiovascular care provision after the Affordable Care Act. Am J Manag Care. 2017;23(11):e366–73.

44. Chen EM, Armstrong GW, Cox JT, et al. Association of the affordable care act medicaid expansion with dilated eye examinations among the United States population with diabetes. Ophthalmology. 2019; https://doi.org/10.1016/j.ophtha.2019.09.010.
45. Marino M, Angier H, Springer R, et al. The affordable care act – effects of insurance on diabetes biomarkers. Diabetes care – under review following invitation to revise and resubmit. 2020;
46. Marino M, Angier H, Fankhauser K, et al. Disparities in biomarkers for patients with diabetes after the affordable care act. Medical Care. (in press)
47. Casagrande SS, McEwen LN, Herman WH. Changes in health insurance coverage under the affordable care act: a national sample of U.S. Adults with diabetes, 2009 and 2016. Diabetes Care. 2018;41(5):956–62. https://doi.org/10.2337/dc17-2524.
48. Myerson R, Romley J, Chiou T, Peters AL, Goldman D. The affordable care act and health insurance coverage among people with diagnosed and undiagnosed diabetes: data from the national health and nutrition examination survey. Diabetes Care. 2019;42(11):e179–80. https://doi.org/10.2337/dc19-0081.
49. Winkelman TNA, Chang VW. Medicaid expansion, mental health, and access to care among childless adults with and without chronic conditions. J Gen Intern Med. 2018;33(3):376–83. https://doi.org/10.1007/s11606-017-4217-5.
50. Substance Abuse and Mental Health Services Administration (SAMHSA). SAMHSA Announces National Survey on Drug Use and Health (NSDUH) Results Detailing Mental Illness and Substance Use Levels in 2021. https://www.samhsa.gov/newsroom/press-announcements/20230104/samhsa-announces-nsduh-results-detailing-mental-illness-substance-use-levels-2021. Accessed 7 Aug 2024.
51. Cowell AJ, Prakash S, Jones E, Barnosky A, Wedehase B. Behavioral health coverage in the individual market increased After ACA parity requirements. Health Aff (Millwood). 2018;37(7):1153–9. https://doi.org/10.1377/hlthaff.2017.1517.
52. Thomas KC, Shartzer A, Kurth NK, Hall JP. Impact of ACA health reforms for people with mental health conditions. Psychiatr Serv. 2018;69(2):231–4. https://doi.org/10.1176/appi.ps.201700044.
53. Angier H, Huguet N, Ezekiel-Herrera D, et al. New hypertension and diabetes diagnoses following the affordable care act medicaid expansion. Fam Med Commun Health. 2020;8(4) https://doi.org/10.1136/fmch-2020-000607.
54. Howell BA, Wang EA, Winkelman TNA. Mental health treatment among individuals involved in the criminal justice system after implementation of the affordable care act. Psychiatr Serv. 2019;70(9):765–71. https://doi.org/10.1176/appi.ps.201800559.
55. National Association of Community Health Centers. Community Health Center Chartbook 2024. https://www.nachc.org/wp-content/uploads/2024/07/2024-2022-UDS-DATA-Community-Health-Center-Chartbook.pdf. Accessed 7 Aug 2024.
56. Zuvekas SH, McClellan CB, Ali MM, Mutter R. Medicaid expansion and health insurance coverage and treatment utilization among individuals with a mental health condition. J Ment Health Policy Econ. 2020;23(3):151–82.
57. Olfson M, Wall M, Barry CL, Mauro C, Feng T, Mojtabai R. Medicaid expansion and low-income adults with substance use disorders. J Behav Health Serv Res. 2021;48(3):477–86. https://doi.org/10.1007/s11414-020-09738-w.
58. Saunders H, Guth MGE. A look at strategies to address behavioral health workforce shortages: findings from a survey of state medicaid programs. 2023. https://www.kff.org/medicaid/issue-brief/a-look-at-strategies-to-address-behavioral-health-workforce-shortages-findings-from-a-survey-of-state-medicaid-programs/?utm_campaign=KFF-2023-Medicaid&utm_source=hs_email&utm_medium=email&utm_content=241088401&_hsenc=p2ANqtz-9C3OXFb9do6iUSNn8DgzRQAHffc8GZmdLgWLJvQrn2ogX89PruDfKoraOXDS_cR8xpD-MDAC8YDBuczpLsvZao1Ucb3wQ. Accessed 7 Aug 2024.

59. Williams MO, Gilroy JR, Chang TY, Seymour DJ. Challenges for insured patients in accessing behavioral health care. Ann Fam Med. 2017;15(4):363–5. https://doi.org/10.1370/afm.2092.
60. Kravitz-Wirtz N, Davis CS, Ponicki WR, et al. Association of medicaid expansion with opioid overdose mortality in the United States. JAMA Netw Open. 2020;3(1):e1919066. https://doi.org/10.1001/jamanetworkopen.2019.19066.
61. McKenna RM. Treatment use, sources of payment, and financial barriers to treatment among individuals with opioid use disorder following the national implementation of the ACA. Drug Alcohol Depend. 2017;179:87–92. https://doi.org/10.1016/j.drugalcdep.2017.06.028.
62. Mojtabai R, Mauro C, Wall MM, Barry CL, Olfson M. The affordable care act and opioid agonist therapy for opioid use disorder. Psychiatr Serv. 2019;70(7):617–20. https://doi.org/10.1176/appi.ps.201900025.
63. Pro G, Montgomery BEE, Zaller N. Tailoring services in opioid treatment programs for patients involved in America's criminal justice system: national associations and variation by state and Medicaid expansion status. Subst Abuse Treat Prev Policy. 2021;16(1):50. https://doi.org/10.1186/s13011-021-00388-5.
64. Mulia N, Lui CK, Bensley KMK, Subbaraman MS. Effects of medicaid expansion on alcohol and opioid treatment admissions in U.S. racial/ethnic groups. Drug Alcohol Depend. 2022;231:109242. https://doi.org/10.1016/j.drugalcdep.2021.109242.
65. Feder KA, Mojtabai R, Krawczyk N, et al. Trends in insurance coverage and treatment among persons with opioid use disorders following the Affordable Care Act. Drug Alcohol Depend. 2017;179:271–4. https://doi.org/10.1016/j.drugalcdep.2017.07.015.
66. Johnson NL, Choi S, Herrera CN. Black clients in expansion states who used opioids were more likely to access medication for opioid use disorder after ACA implementation. J Subst Abuse Treat. 2022;133:108533. https://doi.org/10.1016/j.jsat.2021.108533.
67. Olfson M, Wall M, Barry CL, Mauro C, Mojtabai R. Impact of medicaid expansion on coverage and treatment of low-income adults with substance use disorders. Health Aff (Millwood). 2018;37(8):1208–15. https://doi.org/10.1377/hlthaff.2018.0124.
68. Levitan S. Healing the poor in their backyard. In: Hollister R, Kramer B, Bellin S, editors. Neighborhood health centers. Lexington Books; 1974.
69. ChroniCles. Community health centers: Chronicling their history and broader meaning. https://www.chcchronicles.org/stories/community-health-centers-chronicling-their-history-and-broader-meaning. Accessed 12 Apr 2024.
70. Rural Health Information Hub. Federally Qualified Health Centers (FQHCs) and the Health Center Program. https://www.ruralhealthinfo.org/topics/federally-qualified-health-centers#different-from-rhc. Accessed 12 Apr 2024.
71. Health Resources and Services Administration. About the Health Center Program. https://bphc.hrsa.gov/about-health-center-program. Accessed 12 Apr 2024.
72. CMS (Centers for Medicare & Medicaid Services). Chapter 13 – rural health clinic (RHC) and federally qualified health center (FQHC) services. Medicare Benefit Policy Manual. Centers for Medicare & Medicaid Services, 2019.
73. Zwick DI. Some accomplishments and findings of neighborhood health centers. Milbank Mem Fund Q. 1972;50(4):387–420.
74. Health Resources and Services Administration. National Health Center Program Uniform Data System (UDS) Awardee Data. https://data.hrsa.gov/tools/data-reporting/program-data/national. Accessed 12 Apr 2024.
75. National Association of Community Health Centers. An Overview of Federal Health Center Funding. https://www.nachc.org/policy-advocacy/health-center-funding/federal-grant-funding/. Accessed 12 Apr 2024.
76. Saloner B, Wilk AS, Levin J. Community health centers and access to care among underserved populations: a synthesis review. Med Care Res Rev. 2020;77(1):3–18. https://doi.org/10.1177/1077558719848283.

77. Han X, Luo Q, Ku L. Medicaid expansion and grant funding increases helped improve community health center capacity. Health Aff (Millwood). 2017;36(1):49–56. https://doi.org/10.1377/hlthaff.2016.0929.
78. Lewis C, Coleman A, Abrams MKMMD. The Role of Medicaid Expansion in Care Delivery at Community Health Centers. https://www.commonwealthfund.org/publications/issue-briefs/2019/apr/role-medicaid-expansion-care-delivery-FQHCs. Accessed 12 Apr 2024.
79. Behr CL, Hull P, Hsu J, Newhouse JP, Fung V. Geographic access to federally qualified health centers before and after the affordable care act. BMC Health Serv Res. 2022;22(1):385. https://doi.org/10.1186/s12913-022-07685-0.
80. Lyu W, Wehby GL. The effects of medicaid expansions on dental services at federally qualified health centers. J Am Dent Assoc. 2023;154(3):215–224 e10. https://doi.org/10.1016/j.adaj.2022.11.005.
81. Cole MB, Galarraga O, Wilson IB, Wright B, Trivedi AN. At federally funded health centers, medicaid expansion was associated with improved quality of care. Health Aff (Millwood). 2017;36(1):40–8. https://doi.org/10.1377/hlthaff.2016.0804.
82. Daw JR, Kozhimannil KB, Admon LK. Factors associated with postpartum uninsurance among medicaid-paid births. JAMA Health Forum. 2021;2(6):e211054. https://doi.org/10.1001/jamahealthforum.2021.1054.
83. Kozhimannil KB, Interrante JD, Basile Ibrahim B, et al. Racial/ethnic disparities in postpartum health insurance coverage among rural and urban U.S. residents. J Womens Health (Larchmt). 2022;31(10):1397–402. https://doi.org/10.1089/jwh.2022.0169.
84. Executive Office of the President [Joseph Biden]. Continuing To Strengthen Americans' Access to Affordable, Quality Health Coverage. 5 April 2022. Exec Order No 104070. https://www.whitehouse.gov/briefing-room/presidential-actions/2022/04/05/executive-order-on-continuing-to-strengthen-americans-access-to-affordable-quality-health-coverage/2022.
85. KFF. Medicaid Postpartum Coverage Extension Tracker. https://www.kff.org/medicaid/issue-brief/medicaid-postpartum-coverage-extension-tracker/. Accessed 21 Apr 2025.
86. Luther JP, Johnson DY, Joynt Maddox KE, Lindley KJ. Reducing cardiovascular maternal mortality by extending medicaid for postpartum women. J Am Heart Assoc. 2021;10(15):e022040. https://doi.org/10.1161/JAHA.121.022040.
87. US Congress. Inflation Reduction Act of 2022. Public Law No 117-1692022.
88. Centers for Disease Control and Prevention. Vaccine-specific recommendations. https://www.cdc.gov/acip-recs/hcp/vaccine-specific/index.html. Accessed 22 Aug 2024.
89. Mandatory Medicaid and Children's Health Insurance Program Coverage of Adult Vaccinations under the Inflation Reduction Act. 2023.
90. Polaris JJZ, Eiden AL, DiFranzo AP, Pfister HR, Itzkowitz MC, Bhatti AA. State medicaid coverage and reimbursement of adult vaccines administered by physicians and pharmacists. AJPM Focus. 2024;3(4):100252. https://doi.org/10.1016/j.focus.2024.100252.
91. CMS (Centers for Medicare & Medicaid Services). Data Brief on State Innovation Waivers: State-based Reinsurance Programs. 2022. CCIIO Data Brief Series. https://www.cms.gov/cciio/programs-and-initiatives/state-innovation-waivers/downloads/1332-data-brief-dec2022.pdf
92. Medicaid.gov. State Waivers List. https://www.medicaid.gov/medicaid/section-1115-demo/demonstration-and-waiver-list/index.html. Accessed 29 Mar 2024.
93. Whole Mouth Whole Body Connection for Adults with Diabetes (Centers for Medicare and Medicaid Services). 2024.
94. Biden-Harris Administration Builds on the Success of the Affordable Care Act by Streamlining Enrollment in Medicaid and CHIP Coverage. 2024. https://www.cms.gov/newsroom/press-releases/biden-harris-administration-builds-success-affordable-care-act-streamlining-enrollment-medicaid-and
95. US Congress. Families First Coronavirus Response Act (FFCRA). In: US Congress, editor. Public Law 116-1272020.

96. US Congress. Coronavirus Aid, Relief, and Economic Security Act. In: US Congress, editor. Public Law 116-1362020.
97. Gluck AR, Regan M, Turret E. The affordable care act's litigation decade. Georgetown Law J. 2020;108(6):1471–534.
98. Kamal R, Cox C, Fehr R, Ramirez M, Hortsman K, Levitt L. How repeal of the individual mandate and expansion of loosely regulated plans are affecting 2019 premiums. KFF Henry J Kaiser Family Foundation. 2018. https://www.kff.org/health-costs/issue-brief/how-repeal-of-the-individual-mandate-and-expansion-of-loosely-regulated-plans-are-affecting-2019-premiums/. Accessed 29 Mar 2024.
99. Aron-Dine A. Impact of the Administration's Policies Affecting the Affordable Care Act: Testimony of Aviva Aron-Dine, Vice President for Health Policy, Before the House Appropriations Subcommittee on Labor, Health and Human Services, Education, and Related Agencies. Center on Budget and Policy Priorities. 2019. https://www.cbpp.org/research/health/impact-of-the-administrations-policies-affecting-the-affordable-care-act
100. Guth M, Musumeci M. An overview of medicaid work requirements: what happened under the Trump and Biden Administrations? KFF. 2022; https://www.kff.org/medicaid/issue-brief/an-overview-of-medicaid-work-requirements-what-happened-under-the-trump-and-biden-administrations/
101. Musumeci M, Rudowitz R, Hall C. An early look at implementation of medicaid work requirements in Arkansas. KFF. 2018; https://www.kff.org/medicaid/issue-brief/an-early-look-at-implementation-of-medicaid-work-requirements-in-arkansas/
102. Sobel L, Ranji U, Pestaina K, Dawson C. Explaining litigation challenging the ACA's preventive services requirements: Braidwood Management Inc. v. Becerra. 2023. https://www.kff.org/womens-health-policy/issue-brief/explaining-litigation-challenging-the-acas-preventive-services-requirements-braidwood-management-inc-v-becerra/
103. Artiga S, Ubri PJZ. The effects of premiums and cost sharing on low-income populations: updated review of research findings. 2017. https://www.kff.org/medicaid/issue-brief/the-effects-of-premiums-and-cost-sharing-on-low-income-populations-updated-review-of-research-findings/
104. Chernew M, Gibson TB, Yu-Isenberg K, Sokol MC, Rosen AB, Fendrick AM. Effects of increased patient cost sharing on socioeconomic disparities in health care. J Gen Intern Med. 2008;23(8):1131–6. https://doi.org/10.1007/s11606-008-0614-0.
105. Sharpless NE. COVID-19 and cancer. Science. 2020;368(6497):1290. https://doi.org/10.1126/science.abd3377.
106. KFF. Community Health Centers Prepare for Funding Uncertainty. 2019. https://www.kff.org/medicaid/issue-brief/community-health-centers-prepare-for-funding-uncertainty/. Accessed 29 Mar 2024.
107. Proser M, Bysshe T, Weaver D, Yee R. Community health centers at the crossroads: growth and staffing needs. JAAPA. 2015;28(4):49–53. https://doi.org/10.1097/01.JAA.0000460929.99918.e6.
108. Duggan M, Guo A, Johnston A. Unemployment during the pandemic: how to avoid going for broke. Policy Brief. 2020. https://siepr.stanford.edu/publications/policy-brief/unemployment-during-pandemic-how-avoid-going-broke
109. United States Department of Labor. Unemployment Rates for States. https://www.bls.gov/lau/lastrk20.htm. Accessed 22 Aug 2024.
110. Smith SM, Edwards R, Duong HC. Unemployment rises in 2020, as the country battles the COVID-19 pandemic. US Bureau of Labor Statistics. Monthly Labor Review. 2021. https://doi.org/10.21916/mlr.2021.12
111. United States Department of Labor. Civilian unemployment rate. https://www.bls.gov/charts/employment-situation/civilian-unemployment-rate.htm#. Accessed 12 Nov 2024.
112. Pandemic Emergency Unemployment Compensation (PEUC) Questions and Answers. 2020.

113. United States Department of Labor Employment & Training Administration. Unemployment Insurance Program Fact Sheet. 2024. https://oui.doleta.gov/unemploy/docs/factsheet/UI_Program_FactSheet.pdf. Accessed 12 Apr 2024.
114. United States Department of Labor Employment & Training Administration. Pandemic Unemployment Assistance. 2024. https://oui.doleta.gov/unemploy/docs/factsheet/UI_Program_FactSheet.pdf. Accessed 3 May 2024.
115. Ananat EO, Daniels B, Fitz-Henley Ii J 2nd, Gassman-Pines A. Racial and ethnic disparities in pandemic-era unemployment insurance access: implications for health and well-being. Health Aff (Millwood). 2022;41(11):1598–606. https://doi.org/10.1377/hlthaff.2022.00741.
116. Mar D, Ong P, Larson T, Peoples J. Racial and ethnic disparities in who receives unemployment benefits during COVID-19. SN Bus Econ. 2022;2(8):102. https://doi.org/10.1007/s43546-022-00283-6.
117. Park J, Park D. Racial disparities in unemployment benefits among U.S. mortgage borrowers during COVID-19. J Hous Built Environ. 2023:1–31. https://doi.org/10.1007/s10901-022-10006-w.
118. Kochhar R, Bennett J. U.S. labor market inches back from the COVID-19 shock, but recovery is far from complete. Pew Research Center. Short Reads. 2021. https://www.pewresearch.org/short-read/2021/04/14/u-s-labor-market-inches-back-from-the-covid-19-shock-but-recovery-is-far-from-complete/. Accessed 6 Mar 2024.
119. Spadafora F. U.S. Unemployment insurance through the Covid-19 crisis. J Govern Econ. 2023;9(100069) https://doi.org/10.1016/j.jge.2023.100069.
120. Fronstin P, Woodbury SA. Update: how many Americans have lost jobs with employer health coverage during the pandemic? To the Point. Blog. Common Wealth Fund. 2021. https://www.commonwealthfund.org/blog/2021/update-how-many-americans-have-lost-jobs-employer-health-coverage-during-pandemic. Accessed 8 Mar 2024.
121. US Congress. Coronavirus Preparedness and REsponse Supplemental Appropriations Act. In: US Congress, editor. Public Law 116-1232020.
122. Benitez J. Comparison of unemployment-related health insurance coverage changes in medicaid expansion vs nonexpansion states during the COVID-19 pandemic. JAMA Health Forum. 2022;3(6):e221632. https://doi.org/10.1001/jamahealthforum.2022.1632.
123. Hsu J, Chin CY, Weiss M, et al. Growth in ACA-compliant marketplace enrollment and spending risk changes during the COVID-19 pandemic. Health Affairs. 2021;40(11):1722–30. https://doi.org/10.1377/hlthaff.2021.00501.
124. Swartz K, Graves J. Shifting the open enrollment period For ACA marketplaces could increase enrollment and improve plan choices. Health Affairs. 2014;33(7):1286–93. https://doi.org/10.1377/hlthaff.2014.0007.
125. Pollitz K. How the American Rescue Plan Will Improve Affordability of Private Health Coverage. https://www.kff.org/affordable-care-act/issue-brief/how-the-american-rescue-plan-will-improve-affordability-of-private-health-coverage/. Accessed 3 May 2024.
126. Ortaliza J, Amin K, Cox C. As ACA Marketplace Enrollment Reaches Record High, Fewer Are Buying Individual Market Coverage Elsewhere. https://www.kff.org/private-insurance/issue-brief/as-aca-marketplace-enrollment-reaches-record-high-fewer-are-buying-individual-market-coverage-elsewhere/. Accessed 3 May 2024.
127. KFF. Health Insurance Coverage of the Total Population. https://www.kff.org/other/state-indicator/total-population/?currentTimeframe=1&sortModel=%7B%22colId%22:%22Location%22,%22sort%22:%22asc%22%7D. Accessed 12 Nov 2024.
128. Jacobs PD, Moriya AS. Changes in health coverage during the COVID-19 pandemic. Health Aff (Millwood). 2023;42(5):721–6. https://doi.org/10.1377/hlthaff.2022.01469.
129. CMS (Centers for Medicare & Medicaid Services). Medicaid and CHIP enrollment snapshot. https://www.medicaid.gov/medicaid/program-information/medicaid-chip-enrollment-data/medicaid and-chip-enrollment-trend-snapshot/index.html. Accessed 22 Aug 2024.

130. KFF. Health Coverage & Uninsured Indicators. https://www.kff.org/state-category/health-coverage-uninsured/nonelderly-with-medicaid/. Accessed 22 Aug 2024.
131. Lipton BJ, Pesko MF. State medicaid and private telemedicine coverage requirements and telemedicine use, 2013–2019. Health Serv Res. 2023;58(5):988–98. https://doi.org/10.1111/1475-6773.14173.
132. Shaver J. The state of telehealth before and after the COVID-19 pandemic. Prim Care. 2022;49(4):517–30. https://doi.org/10.1016/j.pop.2022.04.002.
133. Mann DM, Chen J, Chunara R, Testa PA, Nov O. COVID-19 transforms health care through telemedicine: evidence from the field. J Am Med Inform Assoc. 2020;27(7):1132–5. https://doi.org/10.1093/jamia/ocaa072.
134. Chang JE, Lindenfeld Z, Albert SL, et al. Telephone vs. video visits during COVID-19: safety-net provider perspectives. J Am Board Fam Med. 2021;34(6):1103–14. https://doi.org/10.3122/jabfm.2021.06.210186.
135. Liaw WR, Jetty A, Coffman M, et al. Disconnected: a survey of users and nonusers of telehealth and their use of primary care. J Am Med Inform Assoc. 2019;26(5):420–8. https://doi.org/10.1093/jamia/ocy182.
136. Polinski JM, Barker T, Gagliano N, Sussman A, Brennan TA, Shrank WH. Patients' satisfaction with and preference for telehealth visits. J Gen Intern Med. 2016;31(3):269–75. https://doi.org/10.1007/s11606-015-3489-x.
137. Khairat S, Haithcoat T, Liu S, et al. Advancing health equity and access using telemedicine: a geospatial assessment. J Am Med Inform Assoc. 2019;26(8-9):796–805. https://doi.org/10.1093/jamia/ocz108.
138. Robinson MD, Branham AR, Locklear A, Robertson S, Gridley T. Measuring satisfaction and usability of facetime for virtual visits in patients with uncontrolled diabetes. Telemed J E Health. 2016;22(2):138–43. https://doi.org/10.1089/tmj.2014.0238.
139. Peden CJ, Mohan S, Pagán V. Telemedicine and COVID-19: an observational study of rapid scale up in a US academic medical system. J Gener Intern Med. 2020;35(9):2823–5. https://doi.org/10.1007/s11606-020-05917-9.
140. Odeh B, Kayyali R, Nabhani-Gebara S, Philip N, Robinson P, Wallace CR. Evaluation of a telehealth service for COPD and HF patients: clinical outcome and patients' perceptions. J Telemed Telecare. 2015;21(5):292–7. https://doi.org/10.1177/1357633X15574807.
141. Fisher L, Polonsky W, Asuni A, Jolly Y, Hessler D. The early impact of the COVID-19 pandemic on adults with type 1 or type 2 diabetes: a national cohort study. J Diabetes Complicat. 2020;34(12):107748. https://doi.org/10.1016/j.jdiacomp.2020.107748.
142. Khairat S, Pillai M, Edson B, Gianforcaro R. Evaluating the telehealth experience of patients with COVID-19 symptoms: recommendations on best practices. J Patient Exp. 2020;7(5):665–72. https://doi.org/10.1177/2374373520952975.
143. Nath B, Williams B, Jeffery MM, et al. Trends in electronic health record inbox messaging during the COVID-19 pandemic in an ambulatory practice network in New England. JAMA Netw Open. 2021;4(10):e2131490. https://doi.org/10.1001/jamanetworkopen.2021.31490.
144. Benda NC, Veinot TC, Sieck CJ, Ancker JS. Broadband internet access is a social determinant of health! Am J Public Health. 2020;110(8):1123–5. https://doi.org/10.2105/AJPH.2020.305784.
145. Ahn DT. The COVID-19 pandemic: a "Tech"-tonic shift toward virtual diabetes care. J Diabetes Sci Technol. 2020;14(4):708–9. https://doi.org/10.1177/1932296820929719.
146. Kerr D, Warshaw H. Clouds and silver linings: COVID-19 pandemic is an opportune moment to democratize diabetes care through telehealth. J Diabetes Sci Technol. 2020;14(6):1107–10. https://doi.org/10.1177/1932296820963630.
147. Nouri S, Khoon EC, Lyles CRLK. Addressing equity in telemedicine for chronic disease management during the Covid-19 pandemic. NEJM Catalyst. 2020; https://doi.org/10.1056/CAT.20.0123.

148. Drake C, Lian T, Cameron B, Medynskaya K, Bosworth HB, Shah K. Understanding telemedicine's "new normal": variations in telemedicine use by specialty line and patient demographics. Telemed J E Health. 2021; https://doi.org/10.1089/tmj.2021.0041.
149. Alpern JD, Chomilo N, DeSilva M. Drug-dispensing limits within Medicaid during the COVID-19 pandemic. J Manag Care Spec Pharm. 2021;27(10):1489–93. https://doi.org/10.18553/jmcp.2021.27.10.1489.
150. KFF. Medicaid Emergency Authority Tracker: Approved State Actions to Address COVID-19. https://www.kff.org/medicaid/issue-brief/medicaid-emergency-authority-tracker-approved-state-actions-to-address-covid-19/. Accessed 21 May 2024.
151. Schmit CD, Penn MS. Expanding state laws and a growing role for pharmacists in vaccination services. J Am Pharm Assoc (2003). 2017;57(6):661–9. https://doi.org/10.1016/j.japh.2017.07.001.
152. El Kalach R, Jones-Jack N, Elam MA, et al. Federal retail pharmacy program contributions to bivalent mRNA COVID-19 vaccinations across sociodemographic characteristics – United States, September 1, 2022–September 30, 2023. MMWR Morb Mortal Wkly Rep. 2024;73(13):286–90. https://doi.org/10.15585/mmwr.mm7313a2.
153. Centers for Disease Control and Prevention. The Federal Retail Pharmacy Program for COVID-19 Vaccination. https://archive.cdc.gov/www_cdc_gov/vaccines/covid-19/retail-pharmacy-program/index.html. Accessed 3 May 2024.
154. Poghosyan L, Pulcini J, Chan GK, et al. State responses to COVID-19: potential benefits of continuing full practice authority for primary care nurse practitioners. Nurs Outlook. 2022;70(1):28–35. https://doi.org/10.1016/j.outlook.2021.07.012.
155. Le LM, Veettil SK, Donaldson D, et al. The impact of pharmacist involvement on immunization uptake and other outcomes: an updated systematic review and meta-analysis. J Am Pharm Assoc (2003). 2022;62(5):1499–1513 e16. https://doi.org/10.1016/j.japh.2022.06.008.
156. Martin B, Buck M, Zhong E. Evaluating the impact of executive orders lifting restrictions on advanced practice registered nurses during the COVID-19 pandemic. J Nurs Regul. 2023;14(1):50–8.
157. Tolbert J., Ammula M. 10 things to know about the unwinding of the medicaid continuous enrollment provision. 2023. https://www.kff.org/medicaid/issue-brief/10-things-to-know-about-the-unwinding-of-the-medicaid-continuous-enrollment-provision/
158. KFF. Medicaid Enrollment and Unwinding Tracker. https://www.kff.org/report-section/medicaid-enrollment-and-unwinding-tracker-overview/. Accessed 3 May 2024.
159. Lopes L, Sparks G, Presiado M, et al. KFF Survey of Medicaid Unwinding. https://www.kff.org/medicaid/poll-finding/kff-survey-of-medicaid-unwinding/?utm_campaign=KFF-Medicaid&utm_medium=email&_hsenc=p2ANqtz-8eGkR25FgEGNBUid9uPrRNDFoMD0l_wj-M5KO0NQsR-q5GS-VD49WDbYzwFqdCOX_M53AN2efm_Rlf4EFe4Erohcuz_w&_hsmi=302308689&utm_content=302308689&utm_source=hs_email. Accessed 3 May 2024.
160. Bazemore A, Merenstein Z, Handler L, Saultz JW. The impact of interpersonal continuity of primary care on health care costs and use: a critical review. Ann Fam Med. 2023;21(3):274–9. https://doi.org/10.1370/afm.2961.
161. Lester L, Dinh D, Larson A, et al. Insurance instability among community-based health center patients with diabetes post-affordable care act medicaid expansion. JABFM. 2025;
162. Bensken WP, Koroukian SM, McGrath BM, Alberti PM, Cottrell EK, Sills MR. Unwinding of continuous medicaid coverage among patients at community health centers. JAMA Health Forum. 2024;5(1):e234622. https://doi.org/10.1001/jamahealthforum.2023.4622.
163. Koma W, Cubanski J, Neuman T. FAQs on medicare coverage of telehealth. https://www.kff.org/medicare/issue-brief/faqs-on-medicare-coverage-of-telehealth/. Accessed 3 May 2024.

164. Weber E, Miller SJ, Shroff N, Beyrouty M, Calman N. Recent telehealth utilization at a large federally qualified health center system: evidence of disparities even within telehealth modalities. Telemed J E Health. 2023;29(11):1601–12. https://doi.org/10.1089/tmj.2022.0511.
165. Chang JE, Lindenfeld Z, Thomas T, Waldman J, Griffin J. Patient characteristics associated with phone versus video telemedicine visits for substance use treatment during COVID-19. J Addict Med. 2022;16(6):659–65. https://doi.org/10.1097/adm.0000000000000985.
166. Rodriguez JA, Betancourt JR, Sequist TD, Ganguli I. Differences in the use of telephone and video telemedicine visits during the COVID-19 pandemic. Am J Manag Care. 2021;27(1):21–6. https://doi.org/10.37765/ajmc.2021.88573.
167. Center for Connected Health Policy. State Telehealth Laws and Medicaid Program Policies. 2023. https://www.cchpca.org/2023/10/Fall2023_ExecutiveSummaryfinal.pdf
168. Sinsky CA, Brown RL, Stillman MJ, Linzer M. COVID-related stress and work intentions in a sample of US health care workers. Mayo Clin Proc Innov Qual Outcomes. 2021;5(6):1165–73. https://doi.org/10.1016/j.mayocpiqo.2021.08.007.
169. Shanafelt TD, West CP, Dyrbye LN, et al. Changes in burnout and satisfaction with work-life integration in physicians during the first 2 years of the COVID-19 pandemic. Mayo Clin Proc. 2022;97(12):2248–58. https://doi.org/10.1016/j.mayocp.2022.09.002.
170. McNeill M. Extraordinary impacts on the healthcare workforce:: COVID-19 and aging. Dela J Public Health. 2022;8(5):164–7. https://doi.org/10.32481/djph.2022.12.038.
171. Shen K, Eddelbuettel JCP, Eisenberg MD. Job flows into and out of health care before and after the COVID-19 pandemic. JAMA Health Forum. 2024;5(1):e234964. https://doi.org/10.1001/jamahealthforum.2023.4964.
172. Abdelsadig Mohammed H, Elamin SA, El-Awaisi A, El Hajj MS. Use of the job demands-resource model to understand community pharmacists' burnout during the COVID-19 pandemic. Res Social Adm Pharm. 2022;18(9):3568–79. https://doi.org/10.1016/j.sapharm.2022.03.011.
173. McQuade BM, Keller E, Elmes A, DiDomenico RJ, Jarrett JB. Stratification of burnout in health-system pharmacists during the COVID-19 pandemic: a focus on the ambulatory care pharmacist. J Am Coll Clin Pharm. 2022;5(9):942–9. https://doi.org/10.1002/jac5.1672.
174. American Hospital Association. Data Brief: Health Care Workforce Challenges Threaten Hospitals' Ability to Care for Patients. https://www.aha.org/system/files/media/file/2021/11/data-brief-health-care-workforce-challenges-threaten-hospitals-ability-to-care-for-patients.pdf. Accessed 3 May 2024.
175. Joint Economic Committee. Addressing rural health worker shortages will improve population health and create job opportunities. 2024. https://www.jec.senate.gov/public/index.cfm/democrats/2024/1/addressing-rural-health-worker-shortages-will-improve-population-health-and-create-job-opportunities
176. Snyder JE, Stahl AL, Streeter RA, Washko MM. Regional variations in maternal mortality and health workforce availability in the United States. Ann Intern Med. 2020;173(11 Suppl):S45–s54. https://doi.org/10.7326/m19-3254.
177. Needleman J, Buerhaus P, Pankratz VS, Leibson CL, Stevens SR, Harris M. Nurse staffing and inpatient hospital mortality. N Engl J Med. 2011;364(11):1037–45. https://doi.org/10.1056/NEJMsa1001025.
178. RowlandsDW,LoveH.MappingruralAmerica'sdiversityanddemographicchange.2021.https://www.brookings.edu/articles/mapping-rural-americas-diversity-and-demographic-change/
179. Centers for Disease Control and Prevention. U.S. Uninsured Rate Dropped 18% During Pandemic. https://www.cdc.gov/nchs/pressroom/nchs_press_releases/2023/202305.htm. Accessed 3 May 2024.
180. Guth M, Ammula M. Building on the evidence base: studies on the effects of medicaid expansion, February 2020 to March 2021. 2021. https://www.kff.org/report-section/building-on-the-evidence-base-studies-on-the-effects-of-medicaid-expansion-february-2020-to-march-2021-report/

181. Congressional Budget Office. Cost estimate. 2021. https://www.cbo.gov/system/files/2021-02/hwaysandmeansreconciliation.pdf
182. Willaims E, Burns ARR. Fiscal Implications for Medicaid of Enhanced Federal Funding and Continuous Enrollment. 2023. https://www.kff.org/medicaid/issue-brief/fiscal-implications-for-medicaid-of-enhanced-federal-funding-and-continuous-enrollment/. Accessed 3 May 2024.
183. Springer R, Marino M, Bailey SR, et al. Prescription opioid use patterns, use disorder diagnoses and addiction treatment receipt after the 2014 Medicaid expansion in Oregon. Addiction. 2019;114(10):1775–84. https://doi.org/10.1111/add.14667.
184. Quinton JK, Ong MK, Sarkisian C, et al. The impact of telemedicine on quality of care for patients with diabetes after March 2020. J Gen Intern Med. 2022;37(5):1198–203. https://doi.org/10.1007/s11606-021-07367-3.
185. Baughman DJ, Jabbarpour Y, Westfall JM, et al. Comparison of quality performance measures for patients receiving in-person vs telemedicine primary care in a large integrated health system. JAMA Netw Open. 2022;5(9):e2233267. https://doi.org/10.1001/jamanetworkopen.2022.33267.
186. Hailu R, Mehrotra A, Huskamp HA, Busch AB, Barnett ML. Telemedicine use and quality of opioid use disorder treatment in the US during the COVID-19 pandemic. JAMA Netw Open. 2023;6(1):e2252381. https://doi.org/10.1001/jamanetworkopen.2022.52381.
187. Wilcock AD, Huskamp HA, Busch AB, et al. Use of telemedicine and quality of care among medicare enrollees with serious mental illness. JAMA Health Forum. 2023;4(10):e233648. https://doi.org/10.1001/jamahealthforum.2023.3648.
188. NCQA. Findings and Recommendations: Telehealth Effect on Total Cost of Care. https://www.ncqa.org/programs/data-and-information-technology/telehealth/taskforce-on-telehealth-policy/taskforce-on-telehealth-policy-findings-and-recommendations-telehealth-effect-on-total-cost-of-care/. Accessed 3 May 2024.
189. Buysse H, De Moor G, Van Maele G, Baert E, Thienpont G, Temmerman M. Cost-effectiveness of telemonitoring for high-risk pregnant women. Int J Med Inform. 2008;77(7):470–6. https://doi.org/10.1016/j.ijmedinf.2007.08.009.
190. Snoswell CL, Taylor ML, Comans TA, Smith AC, Gray LC, Caffery LJ. Determining if telehealth can reduce health system costs: scoping review. J Med Internet Res. 2020;22(10):e17298. https://doi.org/10.2196/17298.
191. Bipartisan Policy Center. Medicare Telehealth Spending Estimator. https://bipartisanpolicy.org/blog/medicare-telehealth-spending-estimator/. Accessed 3 May 2024.
192. Sharma S, Yellowlees PM, Gotthardt CJ, Luce MS, Avdalovic MV, Marcin JP. Environmental impact of ambulatory telehealth use by a statewide university health system during COVID-19. Telemed J E Health. 2023;29(8):1134–42. https://doi.org/10.1089/tmj.2022.0396.
193. US Department of Health and Human Services. Health Sector Commitments to Emissions Reduction and Resilience. https://www.hhs.gov/climate-change-health-equity-environmental-justice/climate-change-health-equity/actions/health-sector-pledge/index.html. Accessed 3 May 2024.
194. Bynum AB, Irwin CA, Cranford CO, Denny GS. The impact of telemedicine on patients' cost savings: some preliminary findings. Telemed J E Health Winter. 2003;9(4):361–7. https://doi.org/10.1089/153056203772744680.
195. Patel KB, Turner K, Alishahi Tabriz A, et al. Estimated indirect cost savings of using telehealth among nonelderly patients with cancer. JAMA Netw Open. 2023;6(1):e2250211. https://doi.org/10.1001/jamanetworkopen.2022.50211.
196. Council on Graduate Medical Education. Strengthening the Rural Health Workforce to Improve Health Outcomes in Rural Communities. Vol. 24. 2022. https://www.hrsa.gov/sites/default/files/hrsa/advisory-committees/graduate-medical-edu/reports/cogme-april-2022-report.pdf

197. Gumas ED, Gunja MS, Shah A, WIlliams II RD. Overworked and undervalued: unmasking primary care physicians' dissatisfaction in 10 high-income countries. 2023. https://www.commonwealthfund.org/publications/issue-briefs/2023/aug/overworked-undervalued-primary-care-physicians-10-countries
198. Sirkin JT, Flanagan E, Tong ST, et al. Primary care's challenges and responses in the face of the COVID-19 pandemic: insights from AHRQ's learning community. Ann Fam Med. 2023;21(1):76–82. https://doi.org/10.1370/afm.2904.
199. Shmerling RH. Why life expectancy in the US is falling. Havard Health Publishing; 2022. https://www.health.harvard.edu/blog/why-life-expectancy-in-the-us-is-falling-202210202835

Chapter 14
Conclusion: Together, Our Lights Shine Brighter

Anthony Cheng, Jennifer E. DeVoe, and Lauren S. Hughes

If we are lucky, life is punctuated by deeply meaningful experiences that shape our understanding of ourselves and the world. It's much easier to reminisce on joyful memories, but it is just as useful to remember and make meaning of painful times. We were honored to serve as the editors of this book and recognize that it dives deep into many painful and sad memories from the COVID-19 pandemic. We hope the book and the experiences it documents also serve as a backstop for healing, growth, and preparedness.

The early years of the COVID-19 pandemic were marked by death, isolation, and upheaval. We will never forget the images of refrigerated trailers that served as makeshift New York City hospital morgues: in one day on April 7, 2020, 598 people died in New York City—an early warning to the rest of our country that the worst was still to come. Alongside health care workers everywhere, primary care teams scrambled to serve their communities while worrying about what would happen to their families if they brought home the virus. So, even though this book focuses on an incredibly difficult time in our lives, we hope it reminds readers about how primary care teams showed up with purpose, compassion, and love, working together to re-discover shared goals and a common purpose. As one primary care clinician remarked during the early months of the pandemic:

> I have had to share my frailties and limitations as a primary care clinician as we struggle to patch together calls, messages, and visits to try to meet needs. It reminded me (and my

A. Cheng (✉)
Department of Family Medicine, Oregon Health & Science University, Portland, OR, USA
e-mail: chengan@ohsu.edu

J. E. DeVoe
OHSU Center for Primary Care Research and Innovation and OHSU-PSU School of Public Health, Portland, OR, USA

L. S. Hughes
Farley Health Policy Center, University of Colorado, Aurora, CO, USA

A. Cheng et al. (eds.), *Primary Care in a Public Health Emergency*,
https://doi.org/10.1007/978-3-032-12487-6_14

> patients) that we are humans, working together imperfectly, to make life better and more meaningful. This has helped me cope with burnout and restored a sense of purpose to this helping profession.

Health care workers were initially seen as heroes, greeted by cheers and ringing bells from neighbors participating in a global nightly tradition that celebrated their service and signaled: *We were in this together!* As days turned into months, and months turned into years, primary care teams faced frequent changes and impossible choices while continuing to fear for their patients, families, and themselves. One primary care clinician recalls:

> …there was this kind of fear and anxiety about the unknown, and many changing circumstances, along with this very deep sense of purpose that 'This is the work that we are called to do, and we are prepared to do it.'

Another clinician remarked:

> For both testing and later for vaccinations, we just jumped in and did it, built the plane as we flew it, because we knew our patients needed it. Because we were guided by what our patients needed and what was right, we were successful and had that inspiration to keep our momentum.

As the pandemic dragged on, divergent opinions emerged about how to navigate through uncertainty and conflicting evidence. Trust fractured. In some cases, medical and public health professionals were targeted with ridicule and death threats. For many, the power of community and collective action remained a source of motivation and strength during the seemingly impossible moments, drawing some teams closer together.

> …we came together to problem solve and strategize every day during the pandemic (in a morning all-clinic huddle), which allowed us to maintain relationships, laugh, cry, and troubleshoot the challenges of the day.

In many places, teams grew bigger and stronger as everyone stepped up to help, bravely learning new skills and taking on new roles. Researchers, students, residents, administrators, public health officials, and clinicians all worked together.

> …Our residents are routinely stepping up to support one another when burn-out risk rises or when one of us is out for illness or quarantine. Primary care is a team sport, and keeping your team safe and healthy (physically and mentally) is part of winning!

While writing and editing this book over the last two years, we were reminded again about how being "in the trenches" was intense and exhausting, but it was also exhilarating because primary care teams are strong, resilient, and capable. We were inspired by hope and the realization that primary care teams would not hesitate to serve again. In the darkness, our collective lights shine brighter. What we accomplished was the result of a massive joint effort—a crucible which showed us how strong we really are, when we are bound together with trusting relationships. Our multiple overlapping communities—our neighborhoods, our clinics, our cities and our states—all interlocked and strengthened to care for the most vulnerable.

> The experiences of the pandemic …reinforced what I already knew, that the basic unit of health care is not the test or medication or intervention – it's the trusting relationship.

> Walking patients and families through the trials and tribulations of this pandemic has been a blessing. Whether due to medical concerns, financial concerns, or mental health, our community needs this resource. Primary care is uniquely positioned for this task. We remain here for our patients and our community. Thank you, fellow family docs, for placing yourself potentially in harm's way to protect your community.

There is not enough gratitude to go around, but let us simply say, thank you, to everyone who strengthened our communities. From enduring isolation, to sharing small acts of kindness, to team leadership, to crisis communication, every act contributed to our survival. And today, we are present and ready for the next big challenge.

> The courage, resilience, inventiveness, and dedication of my primary care colleagues is a huge inspiration. The nation owes them all an enormous debt of gratitude.

Index

A. Cheng et al. (eds.), *Primary Care in a Public Health Emergency*,
https://doi.org/10.1007/978-3-032-12487-6

MIX
Papier aus verantwortungsvollen Quellen
Paper from responsible sources
FSC® C105338

If you have any concerns about our products,
you can contact us on
ProductSafety@springernature.com

In case Publisher is established outside the EU,
the EU authorized representative is:
Springer Nature Customer Service Center GmbH
Europaplatz 3, 69115 Heidelberg, Germany

Printed by Libri Plureos GmbH
in Hamburg, Germany